ETHICAL AND LEGAL ISSUES FOR DOCTORAL NURSING STUDENTS

HOW TO ORDER THIS BOOK

BY PHONE: 877-500-4337 or 717-290-1660, 9AM–5PM Eastern Time

BY FAX: 717-509-6100

BY MAIL: Order Department
DEStech Publications, Inc.
439 North Duke Street
Lancaster, PA 17602, U.S.A.

BY CREDIT CARD: American Express, VISA, MasterCard, Discover

BY WWW SITE: http://www.destechpub.com

Ethical *and* Legal Issues *for* Doctoral Nursing Students

A Textbook for Students and Reference for Nurse Leaders

Edited by

Anne G. Peirce, RN, PhD
Associate Dean for Academic Affairs
Adelphi University School of Nursing

Jennifer A. Smith, RN, MBA, MPH, DNP
Senior Associate Dean
Columbia University School of Nursing

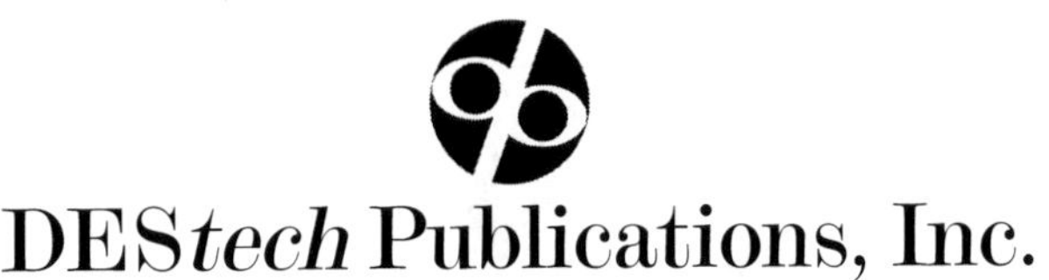

Ethical and Legal Issues for Doctoral Nursing Students

DEStech Publications, Inc.
439 North Duke Street
Lancaster, Pennsylvania 17602 U.S.A.

Printed in the United States of America
10 9 8 7 6 5 4 3 2 1

Main entry under title:
Ethical and Legal Issues for Doctoral Nursing Students: A Textbook for Students and Reference for Nurse Leaders

A DEStech Publications book
Bibliography: p.
Includes index p. 325

Library of Congress Catalog Card No. 2013940138
ISBN No. 978-1-60595-058-7

To our husbands,
Nathaniel W. Peirce, EdD
and
Daniel H. Smith, MD
for their constant support and encouragement.

Contents

Preface

Advanced practice nurses and researchers prepared at the doctoral level must be equipped with specialized knowledge and skills in all aspects of medical, research, legal and business ethics relevant to evidence-based practice and research in underserved and other populations. The editors of this text realized the need for such content after completing an article together in 2008 for the *Journal of Professional Nursing,* "The ethics curriculum for doctor of nursing practice programs" (24(5): September–October, 270–274).

Traditional bioethics content often does not address these issues and therefore there is need for an expanded view of required ethics content in the curriculum of Doctor of Nursing Practice (DNP) and PhD programs nationwide. Thus, we have edited this new textbook, *Ethical and Legal Issues for Doctoral Nursing Students: A Textbook for Students and Reference for Nurse Leaders.* In today's healthcare workplace, whether in practice, academia or in research settings, doctoral nursing students and faculty may face the following ethical dilemmas:

- Determining that a bodega (Spanish market) owner was selling unprescribed antibiotics over the counter
- Voting, as part of a committee, on whether a noncompliant patient deserved a second liver transplant
- Being asked by a collaborating physician to collect clinical information before IRB and HIPAA forms were completed
- Having to care for a child who was declared dead but whose parents refused to allow the ventilator to be shut down
- Deciding how to handle a suspected case of billing irregularity

These examples demonstrate that the rapidly expanding scope of advanced practice requires doctorally prepared-advanced practice nurses and nurse researchers to make more complex ethical decisions, often without the necessary background to do so competently and comfortably. This curricular gap can have serious consequences in access, quality and patient safety and can also mean that nurses may not be able to fully contribute to the ethical decision-making process. DNP and PhD graduates must understand how the legal definition of death, assisted suicide and euthanasia may affect medication prescription and decisions about site of care. DNPs and PhDs must fully comply with HIPAA regulations and understand how the Stark Acts and the False Claims Act affect their practices. Medicare, Medicaid and private insurer reimbursement also requires a deep understanding of how coding irregularities might be considered fraud. As is true with clinical knowledge, traditional APN or undergraduate nursing ethics curricula do not reflect the expanded vision needed to practice in the twenty-first century. Nursing education at the doctoral level necessitates stronger ethical knowledge and application in clinical practice.

By the year 2015, nurse practitioner education will transition from the master's level to the doctorate. This represents a fundamental change that will require a curriculum that reflects the advanced level of a doctoral degree program. PhD nursing programs also require an advanced level of ethical education. This text will utilize a definition of nursing ethics which includes elements of medical, legal, research and business ethics. The expanded content is taught within one major core course and provides a foundation for all major courses.

The rationale for expanded expertise is based on five premises that directly influence health care quality:

- As the scope and independence of practice of DNPs have expanded, so too have ethical dilemmas that directly influence such practice. There are major, unaddressed ethical dilemmas that influence DNPs' ability to provide quality care to all. Consider that as part of a transplant team, DNP-prepared nurses may directly influence who is placed on organ transplant lists.
- Knowledge of bioethics, with its focus on patient care and research, is important but not sufficient for DNP practice. Nurses who practice at an advanced level must also understand other ethical frameworks, including legal and business arenas. Coding practices may influence reimbursement as well as patient costs. A nurse prepared at the DNP level must understand the ramifications of under- and over-coding.
- As health care becomes more interdisciplinary, DNPs must understand how different ethical frameworks impact the workplace. Having an expanded foundational base for ethical decision-making

will increase the DNP's ability to participate at the highest level with multiple professions.
- There are tremendous issues of access and disparity in care provided to the underserved. These problems are directly influenced by ethical reasoning and in turn lead to further ethical discourse. Knowledge of funding mechanisms and cultural differences are necessary but not sufficient to solve these problems. These issues will not be solved by health professionals who do not have a firm grounding in ethics.

We believe that *Ethical and Legal Issues for Doctoral Nursing Students: A Textbook for Students and Reference for Nurse Leaders* will help guide faculty and students in the complex healthcare arena faced by both.

Throughout this text, the LACE (Licensure, Accreditation, Certification and Education) 2008 APRN Consensus Model definition of advanced practice nursing is used. The model was developed by the APRN Consensus Work Group and the National Council of State Boards of Nursing APRN Advisory Committee with input from the stakeholder communities. There are four roles defined in this model: certified registered nurse anesthetist (CRNA), certified nurse-midwife (CNM), clinical nurse specialist (CNS) and certified nurse practitioner. When the title APRN is used in the text, it represents all four of these roles.

The contents of the book reflect current knowledge and legislation. We would like to thank all the authors for their thoughtful and wise contributions to this volume.

ANNE G. PEIRCE, RN, PhD
Associate Dean for Academic Affairs
Adelphi University School of Nursing

JENNIFER A. SMITH, ANP, DNP
Senior Associate Dean
Columbia University School of Nursing

Contributors

PAMELA BJORKLUND, PhD, RN, CNS, PMHNP-BC
Associate Professor, Department of Graduate Nursing
The College of St. Scholastica

ELIZABETH W. COCHRANE, Esq.

CAROLINE M. HEWITT, DNS, RN, WHNP-BC, ANP-BC
Assistant Professor
School of Nursing
Fairfield University

RITA MARIE JOHN, EdD, DNP, CPNP, PMHS
Associate Professor of Clinical Nursing
PNP/NNP Program Director
School of Nursing
Columbia University

NANCY KING REAME, MSN, PhD, FAAN
Mary Dickey Lindsay Professor of Nursing
Director, Pilot Studies Resource of the Irving Institute for
Clinical & Translational Research
School of Nursing
Columbia University

COURTNEY REINISCH, DNP, FNP-BC, DCC
Clinical Assistant Professor
Specialty Director – Family Nurse Practitioner Program
College of Nursing
Rutgers, The State University of New Jersey

JOAN VALAS, PhD, RN, ACNP-BC
Associate Professor of Nursing
Chair, Department of Graduate Studies
School of Nursing
Adelphi University

CHAPTER 1

Ethics: What it is, What it is Not and What the Future May Bring

ANNE G. PEIRCE

1.1. OVERVIEW

> *It must be asked who in the health care system will protect the vulnerable and what knowledge and resources are needed for that protection. If not nurses, than whom?*

The ethics of care has been a strong thread in the fabric of nursing. We have advised patients, negotiated with families, and argued for and against treatment, all in the name of nursing care. These singular efforts have not been in vain, but are not enough for the changing role of advanced practice nurses. Nurses at the forefront of advanced practice (APRNs) must have an in-depth knowledge of the foundations of ethics in order to understand the future of ethics and how to best apply current ethics knowledge in the health care arena. With in-depth knowledge of ethics comes the voice to assist patients when needed and to speak for them when they cannot, as well as to ensure fiduciary and legal compliance (Peirce and Smith, 2008). APRNs today cannot, and should not, only be employees who carry out bioethical decisions made by others. Doctorally prepared nurses, either in practice or research, must be the leaders to their colleagues, students, and other members of the healthcare team. This chapter will discuss the earliest writings on ethics as well as the newest work on neuroethics. This background can then be used as foundation for the chapters to come, where specific patient populations and situations are explored by experts in those areas.

Ethics, bioethics, morals, morality and even the law have overlapping definitions and in fact may sometimes be used interchangeably. The following are brief definitions of some of the major terms used in this chapter:

ETHICS: A theory or system surrounding moral practices and beliefs. Ethics is also called the philosophy of morality or moral philosophy.

MORALITY: A specific judgment about actions or character. It is sometimes used to define right and wrong actions.

MORALS: A standard of behavior used to define a good act or action.

BIOETHICS: Applied ethical inquiry and moral responses specific to health care.

NORMATIVE ETHICS: The study of the norms that make an act right or wrong.

VIRTUE ETHICS: The aspects of the human character that makes actions right or wrong.

UTILITARIANISM: The doctrine that an act is right if it produces happiness or benefits. It describes ethical acts that produce the greatest good for the greatest number of people.

DEONTOLOGY: The ethical approach regarding adherence to rules and obligations regardless of consequences.

PRAGMATIC ETHICS: This approach is situation dependent. In pragmatic ethics, all ethical dilemmas and their solutions are modifiable if the situation warrants.

NEUROETHICS: The view that some ethical decisions are intuitive and may be automatic, deriving in part from our genetic backgrounds and neural processing.

1.2. HISTORICAL VIEW

1.2.1. Greeks

The earliest Greek philosophers, including Plato, Socrates and Aristotle, explored the questions that we ask today: what is a good life and what is needed to live such a life? A significant part of that early discussion focused on virtue. Aristotle (384–322 BC), in the Nicomachean Ethics, wrote that a good life is living a life of virtue (Aristotle, 1980). To Aristotle, the virtues of a life well lived were somewhat dependent upon role. Whereas a soldier might need the virtue of courage, a nurse might need the virtue of compassion. He did, however, acknowledge the importance of core virtues needed by all, such as justice and wisdom (Pellegrino and Thomasma, 1993). Today, nurses continue to be influenced by Aristotle; just consider that undergraduate fundamentals and professionalism books often contain a list or description of the implied virtues of nursing, including but not limited to caring, honesty, and integrity (Chitty and Black, 2011).

Aristotle distinguished between moral and intellectual virtues (Aristotle, 1980). The former is knowledge based and the latter is character or habit based. To have a good life, it was important to both know what was good and act in ways that affirmed that good. But this thought of goodness, or what Aristotle called eudaimonia, is a term that is not fully captured in translation. In part, Artistotle referred to the need for balance, or the Doctrine of the Mean (Armstrong, 2007; Kuczewski and Polansky, 2000). The Doctrine of the Mean is evocative of the Eastern philosophies in which balance, evidenced by the concepts of yin and yang, underlie health and wellness. Aristotle considered that there is a necessary balance, and someone who is too virtuous can be as problematic as someone who is not at all.

Aristotle believed that there is a difference between being virtuous and acting virtuously. If one's character is virtuous, then one's action will be the same—it is part of the whole. However, a non-virtuous person can be taught to act in a virtuous way through education, and in time achieve the habits of virtue. To do what is right for the right reasons, to the right extent, to the right person and at the right time is goodness (Armstrong, 2007).

1.2.2. Romans

Similar to the Greeks, Roman Stoics considered virtues critical to a well-lived life. They perceived these virtues as so embedded in human life that they became a form of natural law. The notion that there are laws of nature that provide a guiding force is something we consider today as well (Baltzly, 2010). The human abhorrence of murder could be considered a reflection of natural law, as could the instinctive reaction to incest. These forms of natural law virtues are seen by biologists, most notably Wilson (2007), as critical to genetic survival. Sociobiologists see the value of cooperation and altruism in increasing fitness for survival. They point to the presence of cooperation and altruism in both animal and human behavior as evidence of its deep-rooted presence in nature (Houchmandzadeh and Vallade, 2012; Roughgarden, 2012).

Natural law has at least two important ethical doctrines that were defined by later thinkers. One is the Doctrine of Double Effect, which is credited to Thomas Aquinas (Moore, 2011). This doctrine proposes that if an act has two expected results, then both should be considered in making the decision (McIntyre, 2011). The use of morphine to reduce pain (primary effect), with its known effect of respiratory suppression (secondary effect), is a classic example.

The second doctrine of natural law is the Principle of Totality (Moore, 2011). Stoics, and later religious philosophers, believed that when we are whole, we are perfect. Cicero wrote that "The primary duty is that the creature should maintain itself in its natural constitution; next, that it should cleave to all that is in harmony with nature and spurn all that is not . . ." (Cicero, 1914).

This principle of totality would indicate that health care should only occur in instances when that wholeness is threatened. For example, surgery for illness or trauma would be considered permissible under the Principle of Totality. Surgery to alter the body for cosmetic reasons would not meet the strictest standard of natural law. The Principle of Totality may become even more important in the future as medical research allows us to consider the possibility of genetic enhancement. The debate as to whether it is good for humankind is bound to echo the early work of the Stoics.

1.2.3. Hippocrates, Galen and Maimonides: Physicians as Philosophers

"As to diseases, make a habit of two things—to help, or at least to do no harm. The art (sic) of medicine has three factors: the disease, the patient, and the physician. The physician is the servant of the art. The patient must co-operate with the physician in combating the disease." (Hippocrates quoted in Bartz, 2000, p. 14).

The time of Hippocrates (460–370 BC) was one of magic as well as medicine. Hippocrates sought to codify the acts of medicine in order to prevent harm by charlatans. Early physicians were compelled to write about basic behaviors of physicians in order to create a moral or ethical bottom line. Many of these writings are attributed to Hippocrates, a contemporary of Socrates, who lived around 460 BC. His approach to medicine was one of vigilant watchfulness, allowing healing to occur naturally, but if it did not, to wait to intervene until it was clear that healing would not occur without intervention (Bartz, 2000).

Galen (131–200 AD) is considered one of the greatest physicians of all time. His influence on medicine remained strong up to the time of the Enlightenment. Of all his contributions, his work on the circulatory system was the most important. In addition to his work as an anatomist, Galen was also a philosopher. In fact, he wrote a treatise entitled *The Best Physician is also a Philosopher* (Drizis, 2008). His ethical focus, derived from the works of Hippocrates, was on the duties of the physician and not the patient-physician relationship.

At a later time, Maimonides (1138–1204) wrote similarly about the virtues of medicine (Nuland, 2006). A disciple of Galen and Hippocrates, he sought to solidify his religious life with his practice of medicine (Collins, 2007). The duty of medicine was important to Maimonides because a healthy body was important to God. He did not think that prayer alone was enough to restore health. He also wrote of the importance of knowledge to the patient. While knowledge is important to autonomy, Maimonides did not see patients as fully autonomous but rather as somewhat dependent upon the knowledge of the physician and the will of God (Collins, 2007; Gesundheit, 2011).

1.2.4. Western Philosophy and Ethics

To the early European philosophers, moral goodness was less about education and character and more about faith. Important contributions to the thinking about ethics reemerged in medieval times with the writings of St. Thomas Aquinas and St. Augustine. Aquinas sought to reconcile the virtue ethics of Aristotle with the theological virtues of the Christian church. To Augustine and Aquinas, the duty to God as manifested in faith, hope, charity and obedience, were more important than the reasoned life advocated by Aristotle (Pellegrino and Thomasma, 1993).

The 17th century was a time of great philosophical debate. Labeled the Enlightenment or the Age of Reason, it was dominated by European philosophers, many of whom were also scientists. This group, including Spinoza, Locke, Newton, Rousseau and Voltaire, advocated the primacy of science in explaining the world around us. With this new world view, the notion of unreasoned action was questioned. If murder was a sin, why was the taking of life in war not the same? The dialogue between the obedience to God and the reasoned action according to conscience continues today as evidenced by the early discussions surrounding AIDS when it was seen by some as a punishment for sinful behavior.

1.2.5. The Reformation, Kant and Deontology

Immanuel Kant (1724–1804) is credited with the development of one of the major ethical schools of thought that of deontology or what is sometimes called rule-utilitarianism (Kant, 1998). Writing after the time of the Reformation, he conceptualized *Moral Law* as not so much a replacement of Divine Law, but as an outgrowth. Kant was raised as a deeply religious conservative Protestant but began his career as a mathematical physicist. He later turned to the broader questions of philosophy. He strove to identify those actions or virtues that can be universally accepted. Kant wrote of the Moral Imperative, saying that there are certain acts that all agree are right. According to Kant, if one knows of these acts, then one should follow them. Kant's basic premise was that "A person ought to act in accordance with the rule that, if generally followed, would produce the greatest balance of good over evil, everyone considered." (Mappes and DeGrazia, 2001, p.13). He focused on adherence to the rules but not the consequences of such adherence. Kant argued instead for the respect of rules as guiding forces as long as they are universal in acceptance or can be universally accepted. In other words, one's actions should be such that they could serve as a model for universal law if everyone were to adopt them. A high standard indeed!

Kant's influence on ethics can be summarized as follows (Blackburn, 2001; Johnson, 2008; Kant, 1998; Rohlf, 2010):

1. Ethics should not be concerned with consequences of the act but with duty to the act (rule adherence).
2. The right act can be universalized. Others can and should act in the same way.
3. The right act treats humans as ends in themselves, not as a means to an end.
4. The right act is a rational act, not a habit but rather one of free will.

1.2.6. Mill, Bentham and Utilitarianism

While Kant wrote that duty to laws and rules was more important than the outcome of that duty, not all philosophers concurred. There were many who felt that the consequences of actions do matter. To ignore the consequences seemed wrong-sighted when such acts could result in harm. As a result, the consequentialist or utilitarian view evolved. The consequentialists said that the outcome was what was important; therefore the right actions that lead to the wrong outcome was the wrong thing to do. The two main proponents of this thinking were Jeremy Bentham (1748–1832) and John Stuart Mill (1806–1873).

Bentham's Utilitarianism was based on the notion of pleasure, or 'happiness', as the ultimate good (Bentham, 1861). To Bentham, acts that bring happiness are morally better than those that do not. In general, we now understand the Utilitarian view, not as Bentham did in terms of the individual but rather as the collective decisions whose actions bring the greatest good to the greatest number of people. The utility of the act is the happiness, pleasure, or goodness that it produces.

John Stuart Mill expanded upon the work of Bentham, considering not only the amount of pleasure but the quality of the pleasure (Mill,

1971). To Mill, some pleasures were worth more than others. The more a pleasure contributes to a human's growth—whether it be intellectually, spiritually or aesthetically—the better the quality of that pleasure. For example, the pleasure obtained from a successful work day as a nurse may be of better quality than a night spent in a bar, even though both could bring pleasure. Mill argued that it is also the long-term outcomes of such acts that are important. Thus moral guidelines that are developed should be devoted to maximization of pleasure and minimization of pain.

While Bentham and Mill focused on pleasure, in health care we use the notion of health utility to examine what health care actions produce the greatest good for the greatest number of people (Ahronheim, Moreno, and Zuckerman, 2000; Faden and Shebaya, 2010). Is it better to provide free immunizations for those who can't afford them or to rely on the herd response from those who can afford to be immunized? In the utilitarian view, costs (financial and otherwise) would be considered in relation to the benefits derived.

Utilitarianism can be summarized as follows (Beauchamp and Childress, 2008; Bentham, 1961; Blackburn, 2001; Driver, 2009; Mill, 1871):

1. Consequences are of ultimate concern. Intentions are only as important as the consequences they produce.
2. The more people who benefit from the consequences the better.
3. The best consequences produce pleasure or what the person desires.
4. Each person's consequence is important but no more important than another's.

1.3. ETHICS IN HEALTHCARE

Ethical dilemmas in the health care system are different from those in other professions, such as education and business. This has to do, in part, with the life and death results that may flow directly from any given decision and also from the sense that health care decisions should be made in such a way that reflects care for the group as well as the individual.

Many of the codes of ethics that guide health care share a history with research codes of ethics. The first general code of ethics grew out of the Nuremberg trials following World War II, when the world was first alerted to the human devastation wrought by Nazi doctors and nurses (Benedict and Kuhla, 1999; Mappes and DeGrazia, 2001). The trials uncovered evidence of the horrible experiments done on humans in the name of science. As a result, the following code, still used today, was developed. Its ten tenets (ORI, 2012) are:

1. The voluntary consent of the human subject is absolutely essential.
2. The experiment should be such as to yield fruitful results for the good of society.
3. The experiment should be so designed and based on the results of animal experimentation and a knowledge of the natural history of the disease.
4. The experiment should be so conducted as to avoid all unnecessary physical and mental suffering and injury.
5. No experiment should be conducted where there is an a priori reason to believe that death or disabling injury will occur.
6. The degree of risk to be taken should never exceed that determined by the humanitarian importance of the problem to be solved by the experiment.
7. Proper preparations should be made and adequate facilities provided to protect the experimental subject against even remote possibilities of injury, disability, or death.
8. The experiment should be conducted only by scientifically qualified persons.
9. During the course of the experiment the human subject should be at liberty to bring the experiment to an end.
10. During the course of the experiment the scientist in charge must be prepared to terminate the experiment at any stage if he has probable cause to believe, in the exercise of the good faith, superior skill and careful judgment required of him, that a continuation of the experiment is likely to result in injury, disability, or death to the experimental subject.

Following the Nuremberg Code, the Declaration of Helsinki sought to clarify and strengthen protection of humans. This document underscores the fundamental importance of human self-determination in participation in research. It also emphasizes the role the researcher has in protecting the individual in the process, as well as the care that must be given to vulnerable populations under study (Bulger, Heitman and Reiser, 2002). The Belmont Report, put forth by the National Commission for the Protection of Human Subjects of Biomedical and Behavioral

Research in 1979, first identified three principles important with human research as being respect for persons, beneficence and justice (Bulger, Heitman and Reiser, 2002).

In addition to concerns with human research, the development of bioethics was driven by the technological advances of the 20th century. Antibiotics, the heart-lung machine, organ transplants, in vitro fertilization and other discoveries changed the health care landscape from one where nature had the last word to one where life could be prolonged and altered. It wasn't until 1968 that the Harvard Medical School first defined brain death in conjunction with transplants. At that time brain death, labelled irreversible coma, had three major criteria: unresponsiveness to painful stimuli, no movement and no reflexes (Ad Hoc Committee, Harvard, 1968).

1.3.1. Ethical Principles

Four major ethical principles have been identified as critical in health care by Beauchamp and Childress (2008). These so-called major bioethical principles are autonomy, beneficence, nonmaleficence and justice. While these four principles are considered foundational, there are others that are also important. Ross (1930) speaks to prima facie duties that include fidelity, reparation, gratitude, and self-improvement. Other writers have added veracity and even care (Held, 2005; Thomasa, 2008).

1.3.2. Autonomy

Provision One of the ANA Code of Ethics for Nurses (Fowler, 2010) states that:

> *"The nurse, in all professional relationships, practices with compassion and respect for the inherent dignity, worth, and uniqueness of every individual, unrestricted by considerations of social or economic status, personal attributes, or the nature of health problems." (p. 1)*

Autonomy is the notion that competent adults have the right of self-determination and this right should be respected by health care providers. Many ethicists consider autonomy to be the major overriding bioethical principle (Fry and Veatch, 2006). That is, adults have the right to decide what health care they want, as well as when, how and who will be involved in that care. It is taken for granted by most that no competent adult can be forced to have surgery or to undergo treatment if they do not want to do so. In fact, the ideal of autonomy posits that adults do not even have to seek care. In reality, the concept of autonomy is not so absolute. Tuberculosis patients can be forced into care if they are contagious, and soldiers can be forced to be immunized.

In another deviation, children are not generally considered fully autonomous agents until they reach the age of 18. But even legal age is fungible and has changed over time. For example, an emancipated minor is in a different legal class than one who is not. A child undergoing surgery may not give consent but rather assent. The nuances of ethics and children's health care are more fully explored in Chapter 6.

Although autonomy is defined as self-determination or self-governance, there are qualifiers even for competent adults. To be autonomous and be able to self-govern health care decisions, an individual must have the will to do so and also the intention, understanding or knowledge, and freedom from extensive internal and external constraints. In other words, to qualify as an autonomous act it must be an intentional act, a knowledgeable act and the person must want to act in the way he or she did (Beauchamp and Childress, 2008). An accident is not an autonomous act. Nor is a person who agrees to experimental treatment without fully understanding the side effects acting autonomously, or thoughtfully. In the rush and confusion of hospitalization it is not unusual for accidental or non-autonomous decisions to be made. Decisions may be made without complete information or real understanding of what the information means. Research subjects may not truly understand what random assignment implies; that they may not receive the experimental treatment. Surgical patients may not comprehend the unintended consequences of surgery. Understanding may be best thought of as a continuum, in which the goal is to achieve as complete an understanding as possible.

There are other barriers to autonomous actions. In fact, it may not always be a singular decision made by an individual; sometimes autonomous-type decisions are shared by family and patient or by patient and provider. Other external barriers may include judicial laws and physical restraints. Internal constraints may result from substance abuse, psychological disease or pain. Thus autonomy becomes the desired ideal, but not always the realized ideal.

Informed consent is an everyday occurrence representative of the principle of autonomy. When patients sign an informed consent document, it is assumed that they do so of their own free will, with an understanding of what is involved, and free from any constraints in coming to their decision. In reality, an individual may not fully understand what is involved and it also may not be possible to explain every possible outcome. Patients may feel obligated to consent because of pressure from their physicians or family or they may be signing in times of pain or other physical constraints to autonomy.

1.3.3. Beneficence

According to Beauchamp (2008), the word 'beneficence' implies mercy, kindness and charity. While beneficence is the act, the moral virtue is benevolence. Many philosophers have explored what beneficence means in life. The philosopher David Hume (Morris, 2009) thought that beneficence was a central principle of human goodness, while Kant saw it as a duty (Kant, 1998). More recently, Beauchamp and Childress (2008) wrote of two aspects of this principle—positive beneficence and utility beneficence—both of which are important to bioethics.

Positive beneficence refers to the principle that individuals have positive obligations to others (Beauchamp and Childress, 2008). Beauchamp and Childress give examples of positive beneficence, including rescuing people in danger, helping people with disabilities and so forth. They refer to these as moral rules of obligation.

There has been much recent discussion about moral obligations and how far they extend (Scheffler, 1997). In general terms, it appears that individuals feel more obligated to those with whom they are close in terms of friendship, kinship or proximity and less obligation is felt to those further away (Murphy, 1993). Some modern philosophers see this as wrong and write that our concern should be for every human soul, not just the ones we may know (Singer, 1972; 1999). Singer is a strong advocate for the general obligation of beneficence—to do what is good no matter our relationship. Other writers speak of situational or specific beneficence where one's obligation is only to those known (Murphy, 1993). There may be limits to our obligation to be beneficent. No one has the perfect gift of time, money, strength, and compassion to meet all needs, yet that is what beneficence would ideally have us do.

We all want health care providers to do good and contribute to the overall welfare of patients. Within the professional nursing role there is an obligation, a duty to provide care. This also implies there is a duty to beneficence, although this is not directly stated in the ANA Code of Ethics. In part, the duty of beneficence is a reflection of reciprocity (Rawls, 1971). Nurses are paid to care, or at least to provide care, thus illustrating reciprocity. Within that arrangement, care is the unspoken obligation to work towards the welfare of the patient. The social contract between patient and nurse is one that is focused on what is best for the patient, both because it is a paid obligation but also because it is a professional and societal expectation.

The utility of beneficence is that the resultant good should outweigh the bad in all ethically-based decisions (Beauchamp and Childress, 2008). Many decisions in health care are firmly situated within utilitarianism, especially those of public health. For example, immunizations greatly benefit the whole population but still may entail harm to individuals. Every year a handful of people have bad outcomes (including death) from basic immunizations. These results are accepted, in the utilitarian sense, because the good so strongly outweighs the few bad outcomes. The utility approach is sometimes difficult, as the individual is not considered except as part of the whole.

Peirce and Ekhardt write of their ethical concerns (unpublished manuscript) with the wholesale acceptance of evidence-based practice. Evidence-based practice is predicated on the view that one treatment, one medication and so forth is good for all, yet it may not be. Rather, evidence-based practice is good for the average and not for the outlier. Thus utilitarianism principles may override the rights of the individual in order to care for the whole. Because nursing's mandate has always been the care of the individual, there may be ethical issues for some compulsory aspects of evidence-based practice.

Paternalism may come into play with beneficence. Beneficence carries the "odor" of paternalism, in that health care providers sometimes use their own judgment to do what they believe is best for those who are ill or infirm, perhaps overriding the patients' preferences or failing to ascertain the preferences. There are no set rules for who decides what is good and what benchmarks are used for these decisions. There have been instances in the not too distant past in which women were sterilized without consent because the physician thought it wise (ACOG, 2007; Zumpano-Canto, 1996).

However, paternalism is not always problematic. Sometimes input cannot be obtained and then paternalism can make the difference between a good outcome and a bad one. Paternalistic decisions are made frequently in emergency rooms and surgical suites as well as in times of natural and man-made disasters. At those times, it is desirable for a knowledgeable person to take charge and make decisions. While someone has to make decisions in times of crisis, it is hoped that the decision is in the best interest of those affected.

Beauchamp and Childress (2008) propose that while beneficence may be the goal, paternalism is sometimes needed. Paternalism is used to justify both beneficence and nonmaleficence. They list the four criteria that must be met before paternalism can be justified as follows:

1. The patient is at risk for significant preventable harm.

2. The paternalistic act will probably prevent the harm.
3. The benefits of the act outweigh the risk to the patient.
4. The least restrictive act is followed.

1.3.4. Nonmaleficence

Nonmaleficence is distinguished by active, intentional actions that prevent the infliction of harm. To "not do harm" is viewed as separate from preventing harm or promoting good, both of which are generally labeled beneficence (Armstrong, 2007). Many ethicists write that the obligation to not cause or prevent harm is more important, "more stringent", to quote Beauchamp and Childress (2001) than the obligation to do good.

The distinction between these clearly overlapping concepts of preventing harm and promoting good are difficult for many to distinguish. Similar to Frankana's arguments (1988), it can be posited that there is a continuum over which these acts occur. At one end is the obvious intention to do harm solely for the sake of harm and on the other, the obvious intention to do good solely for the sake of good. In between there are acts—intentional or not—which promote the motion towards one end or another. Immunizing a child is done for good, both for the child and for the herd immunity it promotes. Yet this act also carries within it harm; at minimum it hurts and upsets the child, at maximum it leads to death. At the adult level, nurses who work in hospitals may be required to receive booster immunizations. This is done not on the volition of the individual, but as a mandate from the system. Is this a matter of nonmaleficence, of doing no harm, or of beneficence, the promotion of good and how does it relate to autonomy and justice? The answer varies as the viewpoint changes from person to system.

Nursing has always taken the threat of harm seriously. The Nightingale Pledge and the Hippocratic Oath both echo one of the most common statements in medicine, *above all do no harm* or in Latin: *primum non nocere*. In practice, nurses expend energy in preventing problems, whether it be falls, decubitus ulcers, or nosocomial infections. In fact, the prevention of harm often serves as a nursing marker of quality. Organizations concerned with health care quality, including QSEN, IOM and JCAH, have all converged on preventable events as those that indicate quality, but is this correct? Is the absence of harm or reduction in harm the same as quality? Is quality goodness, or is it the promotion of goodness? If so, shouldn't it be measured by activities that reflect beneficence?

1.3.5. Justice

Justice has many definitions, but at its simplest, it is the act of being fair. Hume pointed out that it is only when there is a scarcity of resources, is justice questioned (Cohen, 2010). We all want what is fair, or our fair share of limited resources, whether it is food, fuel or health care. Justice is also the punishment that is meted out when fairness is breached.

Fair allocation of scarce resources seems to be a Natural Law as it seems instinctive in humans and even some animals (Murphy, 2011). We instinctively respond to the idea that all are accorded what is due to them. There are no simple answers to questions of justice and it is difficult to fairly allocate resources (distributive justice) and yet reconcile the common and individual good (commutative justice).

The principle (and the virtue) of justice requires health care decisions to be fair and equal (Fry and Veatch, 2006). Americans have come to expect that all have the same rights when it comes to access to care, the provision of care and that health care be fairly distributed. All of this, of course, may not be true but rather it is the ideal. Allocation of limited resources poses many real as well as potential dilemmas in health care. Recently there have been debates as to how scarce influenza vaccine reserves might be allocated in a pandemic influenza outbreak. Various solutions have been discussed including vaccination of all first line providers, distribution based upon age, or even random distribution through a lottery. In each case, the choice to make the vaccine available to one group would mean that others would not have access to the resource. A system based upon immunizing the caregivers first might ensure better health care for the sick; a system based upon a national lottery would ensure fair distribution across all constituencies. Immunizing caregivers suggests utilitarianism as regulators look at the consequences of an act designed to care for as many of the sick as possible. The lottery system involves distributive justice, or the equitable allocation of resources among people. In either case, there will be devastating consequences for some but not for all.

Philosophers have begun to develop the concept of capability as a way of exploring social justice as well as beneficence. Capability theory proposes that the achievement of well-being is the primary moral driver, and that to achieve well-being it is necessary to foster an individual's capabilities (Nussbaum, 2003; Sen, 2005). Nussbaum delineated ten capabilities that are important to consider when there are questions of social justice. They include:

1. Having a normal, expected life span.

2. Being able to have good health and the elements that contribute to it, such as food and shelter.
3. To be secure in movement and other abilities, such as reproductive choice.
4. To be able to think, reason and imagine.
5. To be emotionally connected.
6. To have practical reason in order to critically evaluate one's life.
7. To have the ability to affiliate with others.
8. To live with and have concern for the earth, its animals and plants.
9. To be able to play and enjoy life.
10. To be able to control one's environment through political participation and property rights.

To achieve justice within this framework, it is necessary to promote acts that help achieve these ten capabilities. Many of the capabilities proposed by Nussbaum echo the nursing literature's emphasis of the bio-psycho-social care of the individual (Smeltzer, Bare, Hinkle and Cheever, 2010). As a result, nurses make justice-based decisions daily, from triage in the emergency room to who receives the first or most care during a shift or in a clinic.

1.3.6. Veracity

Another guiding ethical principle is that of veracity, or truth-telling. Truth is a difficult concept because there is little that is known to be absolutely true. Truth telling and its opposite, lying, are the center of a long history of debate. Many, but not all of the early philosophers, including Augustine and Aquinas, saw lying as a moral wrong and truth telling as the moral right (Bok, 1978). Later, Kant would say that there are no circumstances under which lying was acceptable (Kant, 1993). This would seem to be a statement with which many would initially agree. Yet there may be times when individuals lie and see it to be a moral good. In a famous example it is posed to the reader that if you were hiding an innocent person in your house and a murderer came to the door, would you be justified in lying to the murderer? Many would argue that in this case, the lie was justified. Yet Kant would have disagreed. While extreme, this example demonstrates that an absolute statement against lying, or for truth telling, is not always desirable. It appears that not all lies are created equal, for as Grotius described it, an unacceptable lie is only the one that causes harm or violation of rights (Bok, 1978).

Sissela Bok, in her book *Lying*, describes four conditions in which lying could be justified, if justification is warranted (1978). These four conditions reflect the ethical principles of preventing harm, doing good, justice and veracity. First, Bok writes that it is acceptablc to tell a lie if it will prevent harm, as in the example of the murderer seeking the innocent person. Second, it may be acceptable to lie if it promotes good. Not telling a dying patient the futility of treatment in order to maintain hope could be considered acceptable. Third, lies may be justified if it is known that the other party has already lied and it is seen as equalizing the situation. Fourth, one could justify a lie in order to protect a previous lie and so uphold the virtue of veracity. Yet even as these justifications are discussed, the possibility of abuse is real. It would be difficult to discern a clear line between a justified lie and one which was not. What if the person at the door was a policeman or a trusted friend, would you be justified in protecting the person who asked for refuge? As with all the principles, there is a continual struggle with what it means to hold veracity as an ideal.

1.3.7. Fidelity

Another important principle in bioethics is fidelity, or responsibility. Fidelity is more closely associated with the provider of care than with the recipient of care. Nurses have a responsibility to their patients and to their employers as outlined in the ANA Code of Ethics (Fowler, 2010). Nurses rarely speak of patients in terms of fidelity unless it is in terms of fidelity to another principle, such as fidelity to truth-telling.

Ross (1930) refers to fidelity as promise-keeping. Patients inherently want a professional relationship with providers. Lying, failing to deliver and other acts break the promise and threatens the relationship. It is promise-keeping in its broadest sense that ensures the relationship necessary for patient care. Nurses make a commitment to provide the care necessary because they are being paid to do so and because they see it as a societal/professional obligation.

As with veracity, there are situations in which the keeping of a promise is questioned. There are some who, like Kant and Aquinas, may feel that a promise must be kept no matter what the consequences; there are other more moderate advocates, like Grotius, who write that breaking a promise is acceptable if harm will result if the promise is not broken.

1.4. NEUROETHICS

Ethics discussions in health care are generally based upon the ideal of rational thought; that there will be one best solution to a dilemma if enough information, time and resources are expended in its pursuit. Neuroethicists are challenging the importance, as well as the ability, to logically think through all decisions. As Greene *et al.* (2009) note, "There is a growing consensus that moral judgments are based largely on intuition—'gut feelings' about what is right or wrong in particular cases."

Kahneman (2011) writes that there are two primary decision making processes. One is the instinctive, and/ or intuitive; the second is the logical rational process. He refers to these two processes as system 1 and system 2. According to Kahneman, system 1 is fast, instinctive and tied to emotions while system 2 is slower, deliberate and logical. Some of the decisions within system 1 are based upon instinctive evolutionary development, such as the reaction to sudden loud noises, while other more intuitive decisions develop as a result of deep experience.

Harris (2012) and others (Gazzaniga, 2005, Eagleman, 2012, Greene, 2007) propose that genetic makeup, neurological systems and perhaps the effects of environment have a profound influence on ethical choices, making individuals more dependent on intuition and physics than rational thought and philosophy. These neuroethicists base their reasoning on recent studies which appear to show that some actions start to occur before the person is conscious of the need to make a decision. Soon and colleagues (2008), using a functional MRI, had participants make a choice about an ethical decision. They found that the unconscious brain was activated in advance of the conscious brain by up to ten seconds, indicating a bias against free will. In another study, Greene and Paxton (2008) examined patterns of brain activity in moral decisions related to honest and dishonest actions. They found that, with subjects who faced a decision related to dishonest gain, the MRI revealed neural activity more closely related to unconscious control than conscious control.

While the debate rages over neuroethics, free will, biochemical responses and genetics in the moral landscape, nurses should consider that some, but not all ethical decisions may have an unconscious or automatic nature. If this is true, then the mediating effect of the environment should be strengthened, thus strengthening collective support for individual decisions.

1.5. ETHICAL REASONING

The history of ethical thinking and some of the many principles that go into discussions surrounding ethics and specifically bioethics has been discussed. With this background, how does one make ethical decisions, if in fact one does? Some have asked why does one even need to make these decisions; don't people know instinctively what is right and what is wrong? (Richardson, 2007) None of the overarching ethical principles are absolutely adhered to without debate. Researchers believe that two main ethical decision making approaches exist: the automatic—including instinct and intuition—and the reasoned (Hauser, 2008; Kahneman, 2011; Levy, 2011). Even if the neuroethics theory is accepted with its reliance on instinct and intuition, there will still be a need to review dilemmas, or to debrief about those decisions where instinct ruled.

Also, there are many questions that are not even asked because of prevailing world view. Just a few years ago, the mentally ill were institutionalized. This world view was not questioned; it was accepted. Now forced institutionalization is thought to be wrong and the mentally ill are housed in the community to the extent possible. Similarly, women and children have often been the recipients of decisions that may not have been in their best interest, because they were deemed incapable of self-determination. This world view has now been shown to have ethical implications in many parts of the world.

1.5.1. Instinct, Intuition and Ethical Decision Making

The instinctive response is helpful in times when reasoned judgment cannot occur, for example in times of a natural disaster. The instinct to help can override a more logical decision. These thoughts come to mind quickly, without much reflection (Kehneman, 2002). There are many examples in the popular press of instances when someone has risked their own life to save another—not a logical decision or even an intuitive act, but one that feels right to most people nonetheless.

The other variant of automatic decision making is the intuitive. Klein (2004) writes that intuition is the way we translate experience into decisions using pattern recognition. Klein is not referring to uninformed decisions, but experience informed intuition or what he refers to as "recognition-primed decisions" (2004, p. 27). Experts, who have more experience, also have more recognizable patterns of cues and what Klein calls 'action scripts' (2004). He cites his own research and that of others showing that expert decision makers, whether they be military, police, firemen or nurses, rely on intuition 80–90% of the time in their decisions. Recent work is indicating that such adaptive decision making may be even more beneficial than previously thought (Klein, 2009; Kahneman, 2011). In fact, Klein (2009) has shown that many of our preconceived notions about good decision-making, such as checklist and rules, are not always accurate or helpful. He advocates listening to gut feelings, positing that they are often more right than a logically reasoned decision. Intuitive decision making reflecting the "gut feeling" about what is right and what is wrong in an ethical dilemma (Greene, 2003) may also be what Klein (2004) calls recognition-primed decision making.

1.5.2. Logical Reasoning

Does someone with a criminal history deserve the same consideration when it comes to a kidney transplant? What arguments could and should be used to determine this? Arguments for and against a transplant could be made on the basis of finance, justice, policy, adherence or a myriad of other factors. Health care professionals who use logical reasoning to solve health care dilemmas will consider each of these aspects and more in trying to come to the right decision.

Logical reasoning is the basis for the nursing process and therefore a very familiar and comfortable approach for nurses when considering ethical issues. In the logical approach, there is first the thoughtful identification of a problem, followed by the collection of relevant information, the development and implementation of a solution, and the evaluation of the outcome. For example, in a kidney transplant case a tremendous amount of information—from pre-existing health to psychosocial status—will be collected to reach a logically derived decision. Information that may be collected includes social support, work history, age, co-morbidities, disease state, and ability to comply with medical regime. All these pieces of information and more will go into the decision about transplant status providing a reasoned, justifiable decision. In many cases it also provides the correct decision, but not always. The rational decision based upon logical reasoning assumes that all the factors that go into a decision are quantifiable. They may not be. Indeed, there is a subjective nature to at least some of the decisions made through logical reasoning.

Klein's work (2009) has identified ten factors where myths and misconceptions may lead us to either put more faith in the rational process than should be or to dismiss decisions made outside of the rubrics. For example, his research has shown that more information may not lead to a better decision or less uncertainty. Instead the additional information may serve to obscure a judicious decision. He also warns about the limitations that occur when roles are assigned, goals are set as the first step and ground rules are generated. All these seemingly rational steps in a thorough and thoughtful process can have the undesirable effect of shutting down creative problem solving by focusing on the process and not the outcome.

1.5.3. Religious Arguments

There are many cases in bioethics where there are profound moral disagreements which have a religious basis:

- The right of Jehovah Witnesses to refuse blood products for themselves or their children.
- The right of Christian Scientists to use prayer for healing.
- The use of the "morning after" pill to prevent pregnancy.

A competent adult has the right to self-determination in any of these decisions as long as the decision is not illegal. The practitioner may disagree but it is the patient's right to do as he/she sees fit. Children fall into a different category and will be discussed in Chapter 6.

It should always be kept in mind that the patient's wishes—not what the family says the wishes are—are paramount. This may be particularly important in fundamentalist/patriarchal religions and cultures where the husband may see it as his right to make the health care decisions for both his wife and children. In these cases, a private conversation with the patient may ensure the patient's voice is heard.

An important cornerstone of theology is the concept of choice, or free will. Free will is defined as the ability to choose among alternatives. Until recently, free will was considered essential for human morality (O'Connor, 2010). Anyone could choose to make the right decision, and if they did not, their moral thinking was flawed. Sam Harris, in his book *Free Will* (2012), concludes that human biochemistry may have more influence over many of our actions than does conscience thought. The automatic nature of decision making is profoundly disturbing to many. But as Owen Jones (2012) has pointed out, one cannot will oneself out of many mental states, such as love and anger, so why would free will be seen as an absolute?

Sometimes the patient is unable to make the decision and the providers are left in the uncomfortable position of trying to interpret religious beliefs that may be at odds with the preferred course of medical care. Pence (2004) notes that when there is a religious nature to an ethical disagreement among professionals, it is sometimes helpful to try to steer it away from religion and into a more philosophical approach. He asks how do we know it is the deity's will? If the answer depends on interpretation of religious writings, then many different interpretations are possible. Murder is considered morally wrong and there are many religious treatises that say just that. But if murder is wrong, what of war? What of cultures where it is permitted to murder a woman who marries against her parent's wishes? Most religions do not condemn war specifically. How is killing justified? If war is justified, what of civilians' deaths? Are the accidental killings of children during times of war morally defensible?

1.5.4. Philosophical Talking Points and the Ethical Discussion

There will always be discussion surrounding health care decisions. Sometimes the discussions seem minor in nature, and at other times, they have a feeling of critical significance. Regardless, all ethical decisions, large and small, are important. There are several philosophical talking points and argument strategies that all nurses should have in their ethical tool kits. They are discussed in the following paragraphs.

1.5.5. Reductio ad Absurdum

Reductio ad absurdum is an attempt to reduce the premise of an argument to the absurd (Rescher, 2005). Nurses may recognize this as a common approach used in health care. Consider the following example:

The town is proposing to close the local hospital. One of the doctors argues if the hospital is closed no one in that town will receive the health care that they deserve.

That is an example of an argument to the absurd. If a hospital closes, people will find other ways to receive care. It may not be as convenient but it would be extremely unlikely that all people in a town would never have health care again. That would be absurd! When faced with this form of argument the best strategy is to point out its absurdity—not to treat the argument as rational.

1.5.6. Ad Hominem

Ad hominem, also known as argumentum ad hominem, is the attempt to undermine an argument by pointing out a negative characteristic or belief of the person supporting it (Goarke, 2011). Ad hominem decisions are made based upon the characteristics of the person involved. For example, the patient does not deserve a transplant because his family is a well-known crime family. Or a woman is homeless and therefore she should not be given certain medications that have to be taken at specific times. In both cases, a negative thought about crime families or homelessness carries over to the individual without any proof that it would impact the decision. An ad hominem argument generally implies a negative halo effect that covers both the information and the person involved. A positive halo effect is also possible, although less common, in ethical arguments. This may be seen when a celebrity or politician is used to present an ethical argument.

1.5.7. Slippery Slope

Slippery slope is the argument that a small action will inevitably lead to major changes or effects (Beauchamp and Childress, 2002; 2008). It is frequently used in health care. For example, many believe that pain medication should be used sparingly because it leads to drug addiction. Some believe that if patients see their medical records, they will use the information to sue the hospital. The slippery slope argument completely overlooks the middle ground and assumes that there is an inevitability that cannot be controlled. The fear of possible drug addiction may keep people who are in real pain from either asking for medication for fear of becoming addicted or from receiving the medication they need from providers who assume they will become addicts. The slippery slope argument is best countermanded by remembering that most situations are not extreme and that the middle ground/average, is the norm.

1.5.8. Double Effect

Many times the ethical dilemma has to do with the double effect, where one act can have both a good and a bad outcome (Armstrong, 2007). The use of morphine for pain in the terminally ill has the benefit of alleviating pain but also the very real consequence of reducing respiration and hastening death. When making the decision to order or administer morphine, the nurse should consider four basic questions that can be asked of any situation when there might be a double effect and where the answer as to what to do may not be clear (Beauchamp and Childress, 2008):

1. Is the act good in and of itself and not bad? In other words, is ordering the morphine done for the reason of reducing pain and not to hasten death?
2. Is the good effect as immediate as the bad? Does the morphine reduce the pain as quickly as it might reduce respiration? If the answer is yes it is a very different decision than if you could expect the respiration to slow first followed by the reduction of pain.

3. Was only the good effect desired? Did the nurse want only to reduce pain? If the desired effect is to reduce pain than it is good.
4. Is the reason for the act as important for the good effect as for the bad? In other words, can pain reduction in the terminally ill be considered important enough to warrant its use?

1.5.9. The Active-passive Distinction

Acting in order to cause something to happen is generally held to a higher moral standard than not doing something or failing to take an action (Abronheim, Moreno, and Zuckerman, 2000). For example, giving a patient the wrong medication is often seen as 'more wrong' than failure to give a medication. Yet both may have equally dire consequences.

Nurses may argue that they are not the active decision maker but the passive recipient of a decision that they only carry out. For example, the APRN could be told by her employer physician to prescribe pain medication to a patient but not to perform the requisite pain assessment. This would be a wrong act and one that would be indefensible, as the APRN knows that prescribing pain medication without a pain assessment does not meet the acceptable standard of care. The Nuremburg Trials provided very clear guidelines on this type of thinking; all people are responsible for their actions. It is not an acceptable legal or moral excuse to say one was just following orders.

1.5.10. Ordinary and Extraordinary Care Distinction

It may be difficult to distinguish ordinary from extraordinary care, but the distinction is important because there is a moral commitment to ordinary care but not necessarily to extraordinary care (Abronheim, Moreno, and Zuckerman, 2000). Ordinary care is generally thought of as simple, low risk, routine, beneficial, and low cost care that all patients can expect. Extraordinary care, on the other hand, is high risk, expensive, complex, and may be of questionable benefit (Beauchamp and Childress, 2008), and patients do not have an absolute right to expect this level of care. Many devices and treatments that once were considered extraordinary, such as respirators and dialysis, are now considered routine, making this distinction difficult as well as ever-changing.

1.5.11. Withholding and Withdrawing Care Distinction

Withholding and withdrawing treatments provide some of the most difficult ethical decisions. On one hand, treatment is never started (withheld) and on the other, treatment that has been started is stopped (withdrawn) (Beauchamp and Childress, 2008). Withholding and withdrawing treatment decisions generally, but not always, involve the end of life. A non-end of life example of withholding treatment could be the parental decision not to have cochlear implants for a deaf child. An end of life decision might be to not start another chemotherapy regime for a child near death. Withdrawing treatment would involve stopping medication, therapies or nutrition.

Never starting a treatment or a medication can be distinguished from starting and then stopping the same. For example, beginning a course of chemotherapy and then stopping it is different than never starting it in the first place. Tube feeding provides a compelling situation. If tube feedings are never started, it can be argued that it is not necessary to interfere with the natural process of dying, but if tube feedings are started and then stopped, there may be a sense of harm. These issues may be compounded by legalities involved. To start a treatment does not usually involve the legal system, yet its discontinuance may require a court order.

Levin and Sprung (2005) write that there are important moral distinctions between withholding and withdrawing, although others, such as the AMA, do not see a difference (AMA Opinion 2.0). The AMA opinion notes that autonomy is the key ethical principle, so if a patient or the approved surrogate wants treatment not to start or to be stopped, it is within the patient's rights to do so. The AMA notes that they see no ethical difference between withholding and withdrawing treatment.

Box 1.1 - Principles of Withdrawing Life Support

1. The goal of withdrawing life-sustaining treatments is to remove treatments that are no longer desired or do not provide comfort to the patient.
2. Withholding life-sustaining treatments is morally and legally equivalent to withdrawing them.
3. Actions whose sole goal is to hasten death are morally and legally problematic.
4. Any treatment can be withheld or withdrawn.
5. Withdrawal of life-sustaining treatment is a medical procedure.
6. Corollary to 1 and 2: when circumstances justify withholding one indicated life-sustaining treatment, strong consideration should be given to withdrawing all current life-sustaining treatments.

Attributed to Rubenfeld, G.D. (2004). Principles and practices of withdrawing life-sustaining treatements. *Crit Care Clin,* 20:435–451 (used with permission from Elsivier).

1.5.12. Killing and Letting Die Distinction

Patients die every day and although it is rarely discussed, many patients die without resuscitation or extraordinary measures. In many of these cases, health care providers would say that these deaths are a good, natural and moral decision (Jackson, 2006). The patient is let to die and nature directs the time and circumstances of the death.

However, not all deaths are natural. More and more providers are contemplating the role of assisted suicide and euthanasia in health care. The discussions about assisted suicide and euthanasia are relevant to APRNs. Assisted suicide is defined as giving a person the means with which to commit suicide, such as prescriptions of pain medications or sedatives. Euthanasia means actively helping the patient to die, for example by actually administering the medications to the patient (Benedict, Peirce, and Sweeney, 1998). Giving patients prescriptions with large enough dosages to take their own life is seen as fundamentally different from administering the medication. In one, the practitioner is helping the patient hasten death, in the other there is an active sense of killing the patient. This distinction has legal precedence.

The Supreme Court has distinguished between actions that actively bring about death and those that do not (*Vacco v. Quill*, 117 S. Ct. 2293 (1997)). The judges wrote, "Everyone, regardless of physical condition, is entitled, if competent, to refuse lifesaving medical treatment; no one is permitted to assist suicide." Yet, the tide of thought about assisted suicide has been changing in this country.

As of the writing of this book, there are three states which allow limited assistance with the accumulation of prescription medications that could be used for suicide: Montana, Washington and Oregon. The Oregon Death with Dignity Act withstood a 2004 and 2006 court challenge (*Gonzales v Oregon* 368 F. 3d 1118 (2004) affirmed by 546 U.S. 243 (2006).

1.6. NURSING AND ETHICAL DECISION MAKING

Ethical decision making in the workplace may come through three primary venues: that of the individual practitioner, the ethics consultant and the ethics committee. All nurses should include themselves in bioethical discussions (see the NYSNA position paper), but this is particularly important for those with advanced preparation. Individually, advanced practice nurses make decisions on a daily basis that have ethical implications, from the simplest as to how to handle an unnecessary request for pain medications to the more complex of prescription shopping. Within teams and on ethics committees, APRNs provide a unique perspective that must be included if the goal is good decision-making.

The philosophical underpinnings of ethical thought have led to several different approaches to rational decision-making (Ahronheim, Moreno and Zuckerman, 2000; Beauchamp and Childress, 2008; Childress, 1997). Although they often are not clearly differentiated, it is helpful to consider them separately, as an individual who comes to ethics with a strong virtue-based approach may have fundamental differences with someone who is strongly rule-adherent. Determining these differences can sometimes identify the root of the disagreement and refocus the argument to the patient. The main approaches are:

1. *Rule adherence.* All ethical decisions should follow the prescribed, previously established rules. These may include policies and procedures, as well as regulations and laws.
2. *Utilitarian approach.* The ethical decision should be the one that does the least harm and brings about the greatest good.
3. *Human rights approach.* Ethical decision-making should be based upon human rights, including free will, liberty, privacy and so forth.
4. *Justice approach.* All ethical decisions should be fair and just, based upon the ideals of distributive and commutative justice.
5. *Virtue approach.* Ethical decisions should contribute to character by demonstrating or being consistent with the appropriate virtues such as kindness, loyalty, unselfishness and so forth.

1.6.1. Ethics Committees, Ethics Consultants and Ethical Decision Making Processes

Hospital Ethics Committees (HEC) evolved from suggestions of the court in the Karen Ann Quinlan case (Scheirton and Kissell, 2001). Almost all hospitals now have ethics committees as a result of state or organizational mandates, but even if they don't, JCAHO requires that all hospitals have a mechanism to resolve ethical issues. In general, HECs are composed of physicians, nurses, clergy, attorneys, social workers, hospital administrators and others (see Peirce, 2004 about the importance of diversity in committee composition). HECs provide guidance and direction about ethical dilemmas, develop policies and provide ethics education and training. The assumption underlying the work of HECs is that the focus is on the patient and not that of the institution or workers, although that is not always true, nor desirable. It should be noted that HECs have quasi-legal standing and courts often defer to their decisions (Peirce, 2004).

Ethics consultants are clinical ethics experts who can be called upon when there are ethics questions. The consultant can lead the interested parties through a decision making process, helping to clarify issues and solidify decisions. The consultant can either be an individual or sometimes a subcommittee of a larger HEC.

Common issues that are generally considered by ethics committees (Romano *et al.*, 2008):

1. Withholding or withdrawing treatment
2. Appropriateness of treatment, goals of care, or futility
3. Resuscitation
4. Legal-ethics interface
5. Competency or decisional capacity
6. Psychiatric
7. Family conflict
8. Staff or professional conflict
9. Discharge disposition
10. Allocation of resources

HECs, consultants and individuals may all use a rationally-based, step-wise process to resolve ethical dilemmas. To start with, all relevant information must be gathered—not only from the person posing the dilemma, but from those representing alternate views as well. It may be necessary to review case law, institutional policies, relevant literature or other precedent cases. Baseline ethical principles should be identified in any case. Finally, a written summary and recommendation should be provided.

Not all advanced practice registered nurses will work in places with HECs or consultants, but all nurses can use the same process by themselves or with interested others to more fully understand a dilemma before making a final decision. It also should be remembered that neuroethics may play a strong, previously unrecognized role in decision making. A generic list of rationally based questions, culled from a variety of sources, is as follows (Ahronheim, Moreno and Zuckerman, 2000; Beauchamp and Childress, 2008; Childress, 1997):

1. What is the dilemma?
   a. A clear concise articulation of the problem is the first step.

2. What are the facts of the case?
   a. If it is a question regarding a patient, what is the current medical situation, treatment ramifications if relevant, and prognosis?
   b. Is the patient competent?
      (1) What are the patient's wishes?
3. Who is concerned about the situation and why?
   a. Who else should have input into the decision?
   b. What does the family want?
   c. Are there religious considerations?
4. Are there quality of life issues?
5. What ethical principles are relevant?
6. Are there legal issues?
   a. Are there laws governing the case?
   b. Are there advanced directives, living wills, power of attorney, guardianship or other legal documents to be considered?
7. Are there institutional policy issues to be considered?
8. Are there professional standards or codes of ethics to be considered?
9. Are there undue financial or social burdens involved?
10. Is the conflict resolvable or is there an acceptable compromise?
11. What next steps are needed if no resolution is possible?

1.7. SUMMARY

Ethics and ethical decision making is important and will become even more so in the future. Advanced practice registered nurses must make decisions regarding clinical care that are ethically defensible. This chapter will provide the language and background needed to participate in discussions about ethical dilemmas. In the following chapters, specific clinical populations with their particular issues will be considered.

1.8. REFERENCES

ACOG Committee Opinion. Number 371. (July 2007). Sterilization of women including those with mental disabilities. *Obstet. Gynecol., 110*(1): 217–220.

Ad Hoc Committee of the Harvard Medical School (1968). A definition of irreversible coma—report of the Ad Hoc Committee of the Harvard Medical School to examine the definition of brain death," *Journal of the American Medical Association, 205*(6): 337–40.

Ahronheim, J.C., Moreno, J.D. and Zuckerman, C. (2000). *Ethics in Clinical Practice.* Gaithersberg, MD: Aspen.

AMA. Opinion 2.20- Withholding or withdrawing Life-Sustaining Medical Treatment. American Medical Association. http://www.ama-assn.org/ama/pub/physican-resources.

Armstrong, A.E. (2007). *Nursing Ethics: a Virtue-Based Approach.* New York: Palgrave MacMillan.

Arras, J. (2010). *Theory and Bioethics. Stanford Encyclopedia of Philosophy.* http://plato.stanford.edu/entries/theory-bioethics/

Aristotle (1980). *The Nicomachean Ethics.* Ross, D. trans. Revised by Ackrill, J.L. and Urmson, J.O. Oxford UK: Oxford University Press.

Baltzly, D. (2010, revised). Stoicism. *Stanford Encyclopedia of Philosophy.* http://plato.stanford.edu/entries/stoicism/

Bartz, R. (2000). Remembering the Hippocratics: Knowledge, practice, and ethos of ancient Greek physician-healers. In: *Bioethics: Ancient Times in Contemporary Issues.* Kuczewski, M.G. and Polansky, R.(eds). Cambridge MA: Bradford.

Beauchamp, T. (2008). The principle of beneficence in applied ethics. *Stanford Encyclopedia of Philosophy.* http://plato.stanford.edu/entries/principle-beneficence/

Beauchamp, T.L. and Childress, J.F. (2002). *Principles of Biomedical Ethics* (2nd ed.). New York: Oxford University.

Beauchamp, T.L. and Childress, J.F. (2008). *Principles of Biomedical Ethics* (6th ed.). New York: Oxford University.

Beauchamp, T., Walters, L., Kahn, J.P. and Mastroianni, A.C. (2008). *Contemporary Issues in Bioethics* (7th ed.) Belmont, CA: Thomson Wadsworth.

Benedict, S. and Kuhla, J. (1999). Nurses' participation in the euthanasia programs of Nazi Germany. *Western Journal of Nursing Research, 21*(2):246–63.

Benedict, S., Peirce, A. and Sweeney, S. (1998). Historical, ethical, and legal aspects of assisted suicide. *Journal of the Association of Nurses in AIDS Care, 9*(2): 34–44.

Bentham, J. (1961). The Principles of Morals and Legislation. Garden City: Doubleday.

Blackburn, S. (2001). *Ethics: a Very Short Introduction.* Oxford UK: Oxford University Press.

Bok, S. (1978). *Lying: Moral Choice in Public and Private Life.* New York: Vintage Books.

Bulger, R.E., Heitman, E. and Reiser, S.J. (2002). *The Ethical Dimensions of the Biological and Health Sciences* (2nd ed.). Cambridge UK: Cambridge University Press.

Childress, J.E. (1997). *Practical Reasoning in Bioethics.* Bloomington, IN: Indiana University.

Chitty, K.K. and Black, B.P. (2011). *Professional Nursing: Concepts and Challenges.* Maryland Heights MO: Saunders Elsevier.

Cicero (1914). *De Finibus et Molorum.* H. Rackham, trans. NY: Macmillan.

Cohen, A. (2010). Hume's Moral Philosophy. *Stanford Encyclopedia of Philosophy.* http://plato.stanford.edu/entries/hume-moral/

Collins, K. (2007). Maimonides and the ethics of patient autonomy. IMAJ, 9:55–58.

Daniels, N. (2008). Justice and access to health care. *Stanford Encyclopedia of Philosophy.* http:// plato.stanford.edu/entries/healthcareaccess/

Driver, J. (2009). The history of utilitarianism. *Stanford Encyclopedia of Philosophy.* http://plato.stanford,edu/entries/utilitarianism-history/

Drizis, T.J. (2008). Medical ethics in the writings of Galen. *Acta med-hist Adriat, 6*(2): 333–336.

Engel, G.L. (1977). The need for a new medical model: A challenge for biomedicine. *Science,* 196:129–136. doi: 10.1126/science.847460

Faden, R. and Shebaya, S. (2010). Public Health Ethics. *Stanford Encyclopedia of Philosophy.* http://plato.stanford.edu/entries/publichealth-ethics

Fowler, M.D.M. (2010 reissue). *Guide to the Code of Ethics for Nurses: Interpretation and Application. Silver Spring MD: American Nurses Association.*

Frankena, W. (1988). *Ethics.* Englewood Cliffs, NJ: Prentice Hall.

Fry, S.T. and Veatch, R.M. (2006). *Case Studies in Nursing Ethics* (3rd ed.). Sudbury MA: Jones and Bartlett .

Gazzaniga, M.S. (2005). *The Ethical Brain.* New York: Dana Press.

Gert, B. (2011 revised). The definition of morality. *Stanford Encyclopedia of Philosophy.* http://plato.stanford.edu/entries/morality-definition/

Gesundheit, B. (2011). Maimonides' appreciation for medicine. *RMMJ, 2*(1): 1–8.

Goarke, L. (2011 revised). Informal logic. *Stanford Encyclopedia of Philosophy.* http://plato.stanford.edu/entries/logic-informal/

Greene, J. (2003). From neural 'is' to moral 'ought': what are the moral implications of neuroscientific moral psychology? *Nature Reviews/Neuroscience, 4*(October):847–850.

Greene, J.D. (2007). Why are VMPFC patients more utilitarian? A dual process theory of moral judgment explains. *Trends in Cognitive Sciences, 11*(8): 322–323.

Greene, J.D., Cushman, F.A., Stewart, L.E., Lowenburg, K., Nystrom, L.E. and Cohen, J.D. (2009). Pushing moral buttons: The interaction between personal force and intention in moral judgment. *Cognition.* doi:10.1016/j.cognition.2009.02.001.

Greene, J.D., Morelli, S.A., Lowenberg, K, Nystrom, L.E. and Cohen, J.D. (2008). Cognitive load selectively interferes with utilitarian moral judgment. *Cognition,* doi:10.1016/j.cognition.2007.11.004.

Greene, J.D. and Paxton, J.M. (2009). Patterns of neural activity associated with honest and dishonest moral decisions. *PNAS, 106*(30): 12506–12511.

Hauser, M.D. (2008). The liver and the moral organ. *Soc. Cogn. Affect Neurosci., 1*(3):214–220.

Held, V. (2005). *The Ethics of Care.* Oxford: Oxford University Press. doi:10.1093/0195180992.001.0001.

Houchmandzadeh, B. and Vallade, M. (2012). Selection for altruism through random drift in variable size populations. *BMC Evol. Biol., 12*(1), 61.

Hursthouse, R. (2012). *Virtue Ethics. Stanford Encyclopedia of Philosophy.* http:// plato.stanford.edu/entries/ethics-virtue/

Jackson, J. (2006). *Ethics in Medicine.* Malden MA: Polity Press.

Johnson, R. (2008). Kant's moral philosophy. *Stanford Encyclopedia of Philosophy.* http:// plato.stanford.edu/entries/kant-moral/

Jones, O. (2012). The end of discussing free will. *Chronicle of Higher Education.* http:// chronicle.com/article/Is-Free-Will-An-Illusion-131159.

Kahneman, D. (2002). Maps of bounded rationality: A perspective on intuition, judgment and choice. Nobel Prize Lecture, December 8, 2002. http://www.nobelprize.org/nobel_prizes/economics/laureate/2002/kahnemann-lecture.pdf.

Kahneman, D. (2011). *Thinking Fast and Slow.* NY: Farrar, Straus and Giroux.

Kant, I. (1998) *Critique of Pure Reason.* Guyer, P. and Wood, A.W., trans-eds. Cambridge UK: Cambridge University Press.

Kant, I. (1993). *Grounding for the Metaphysics of Morals.* J.W. Ellington, trans. London UK: Hackett.

Klein, G.A. (2004). *The Power of Intuition.* NY: Currency Book.

Klein, G.A. (2009). *Streetlights and Shadows: Searching for the Keys to Adaptive Decision Making.* Cambridge, MA: MIT Press.

Kuczewski, M.G. and Polansky, R. (eds.) (2000). *Bioethics: Ancient Times in Contemporary Issues.* Cambridge MA: Bradford.

Levin, P.D. and Sprung, C.L. (2005). Withdrawing and withholding life-sustaining therapies are not the same. *Crit. Care, 9*(3):230–232.

Levy, N. (2011). Neuroethics: A new way of doing ethics. *AJOB Neurosci., 2*(2): 3–9.

Mappes,T.A. and Degrazia, D. (2001). *Biomedical Ethics* (5th ed.). New York: McGraw-Hill.

McConnell, T. (2010). Moral dilemmas. *Stanford Encyclopedia of Philosophy.* http:// plato.stanford.edu/entries/moral-dilemmas/

McIntyre, A. (2011). Doctrine of the double effect. *Stanford Encyclopedia of Philosophy.* http://plato.stanford.edu/entries/double-effect/.

Meyers, H.S. (2006). *Review of Maimonides* (2005) by S.B. Nuland. NY: Schoken. JAMA 295(2):217. doi: 10.1001/jama.295.2.217-a.

Mill, J.S. (1871). *Utilitarianism.* London UK: Longmans.

Moore, M. (2011) The natural law tradition. *Stanford Encyclopedia of Philosophy.* http:// plato.stanford.edu/entries/natural-law-ethics/

Morris, W.E. (2009, revised). David Hume. *Stanford Encyclopedia of Philosophy.* http:// plato.stanford.edu/entries/hume/

Murphy, L.B. (1993). The demands of beneficence. *Philosophy and Public Affairs, 22*: 267–92.

NYSNA. New York State Nurses Assciation. (n.d.) Role of the registered professional nurse in ethical decision-making. NYSNA Position Statement. http:// www.nysna.org/practice/positions/position6.htm

Nussbaum, M. (2003). Capabilities as fundamental entitlements: Sin and social justice. *Feminist Economics, 9*:2-3:33–59.

O'Connor, T. (2010 revised). Free will. *Stanford Encyclopedia of Philosophy.* http:// plato.stanford.edu/entries/free will/

Office of Research Integrity (ORI). (2012). Nuremberg Code. http://ori.dhhs.gov/education/products/RCRintro/ c03/b01c3html. Accessed July 2, 2012.

Paul, E.F., Miller, F.D. and Paul, J. (2002). *Bioethics.* Cambridge UK: Cambridge University.

Paxton, J.M. and Greene, J.D. (2010). Moral reasoning: Hints and allegations. *Topics in Cognitive Science,* DOI: 10.1111/j.1756-8765.2010.01096.x

Paxton, J.M., Ungar, L. and Greene, J.D. (2011). Reflection and reasoning in moral judgment. *Cognitive Science,* doi: 10:1111/j.1551-6709.2011.01210.x

Paharia, N. Kassam, K.S., Greene, J.D. and Bazerman, M.H. Dirty hands, clean work: The moral psychology of indirect agency. *Organizational Behavior and Human Decision Processes.* doi: 10.1016/jobhdp.2009.03.002.

Peirce, A.G. (2004). Some considerations about decisions and decision–makers in hospital ethics committees. *Online journal of Health Ethics,* 1:1. http://test2.ojhe.org/index.php/ojhe/article/viewarticle/14/17

Peirce, A.G. and Eckhart, P. (nd). 'Black Swan' nursing in times of evidence based practice. Unpublished manuscript.

Peirce, A.G. and Smith, J.A. (2008). The ethics curriculum for doctor of nursing practice programs. *Journal of Professional Nursing, 24*(5): 270–274.

Pellegrino, E.D. and Thomasma, D.C. (1993). *The Virtues in Medical Practice.* New York: Oxford University.

Pence, G.E. (1990). *Classic Cases in Medical Ethics* (4th ed.). New York: McGraw-Hill.

Pearlman, R.A. (2010 modified). Ethics in Medicine: Ethics Committees and Ethics. University of Washington School of Medicine. http://depts.washington.edu/bioethx/topcs/ethics.html

Prehn, K, Wartenburger, I, Mériau, K., Scheibe, C., Goodenough, O.R., Villringer, A., van der Meer, E. and Heekeren, H.R. (2007). Individual differences in moral judgment competence influence neural correlates of socio-normative judgments. *Soc. Cogn. Affect Neurosci., 3*(1):33–46.

Rawls, J. (1971). *A Theory of Justice.* Cambridge MA: Belknap Press.

Rescher, N. (2005 revised). Reductio ad absurdam. *Internet Encyclopedia of Philosophy.* www.iep.utm.edu/reductio/

Richardson, H.S. (2007 revised). Moral reasoning. *Stanford Encyclopedia of Philosophy.* http://plato.stanford.edu/entries/reasoning-moral/

Robeyns, I. (2011). The capability approach. *Stanford Encyclopedia of Philosophy.* http:// plato.stanford.edu/entries/capability-approach/

Rohlf, M. (2010). Immanuel Kant. *Stanford Encyclopedia of Philosophy.* http:// plato.stanford.edu/entries/kant/

Romano, M.E. , Wahlander, B., Lang, B.H., Li, G. and Prager, K.M. (2009). Mandatory Ethics Consultation Policy. *Mayo Clin. Proc., 84*(7): 581–585.

Ross, W.D. (1930). *The Right and the Good.* Oxford UK: Clarendon Press.

Roughgarden, J. (2012). Teamwork, pleasure and bargaining in animal social behavior. *J. of Evol. Biol., 25*(7). 1454–62.

Rubenfeld, G.D. (2004). Principles and practices of withdrawing life-sustaining treatments. *Crit. Care Clin., 20*:435–451

Scheffler, S. (1997). Relationships and responsibilities. *Philosophy and Public Affairs, 26*:189–209.

Sen, A. (2005). Human rights and capabilities. *Journal of Human Development, 6*(2): 151–66.

Singer, P. (1972). Famine, affluence, and morality. *Philosophy and Public Affairs, 1*: 229–43.

Singer, P. (2011). *Practical Ethics* (3rd ed.). Cambridge UK: Cambridge University Press.

Singer, P. (1999). Living high and letting die. *Philosophy and Phenomenological Research. 59*:183–87.

Smeltzer, S.C., Bare, B.G., Hinkle, J.L. and Cheever, K.H. (2010). Brunner and Suddarth's Textbook of Medical-Surgical Nursing (12th ed.). Philadelphia: Wolters Klower Health/Lippincott, Williams and Wilkes.

Soon, C.S., Brass, M., Heinze, H-J. and Haynes, J-D. (2008). Unconscious determinants of free decisions in the human brain. *Nature Neuroscience, 11*:543–45. doi: 10.1038/nn2112

Wilson, D.S. (2007). Rethinking the theoretical foundation of sociobiology. *The Quarterly Review of Biology, 82*(4):1–43. doi: 10.1086/522809.

Zumpano-Canto, J. (1996). Nonconsensual sterilization of mentally disabled in North Carolina: An ethics critique of the statutory standard and its judicial interpretation. *Journal of Contemporary Health Policy Law, 13*(1): 79–111.

CHAPTER 2

Research Ethics

NANCY KING REAME

"The scientific research enterprise is built on a foundation of trust. Scientists trust that the results reported by others are valid. Society trusts that the results of research reflect an honest attempt by scientists to describe the world accurately and without bias. But this trust will endure only if the scientific community devotes itself to exemplifying and transmitting the values associated with ethical scientific conduct."
—On Being a Scientist (National Academy of Sciences, 2009)

2.1. INTRODUCTION

With the rapid developments in 21st Century health care, most doctorally-educated nurses, whether DNP or PhD-prepared, will be involved in either the discovery or translation of clinical care innovation. Research ethics, defined as "the ethics of the planning, conduct and reporting of research" (National Advisory Panel on Research Integrity, http://research-ethics.net), is a necessary cornerstone of training for all clinical scholars. To develop and integrate evidence-based practice requires a working knowledge of the responsible conduct of research and the elements of scientific integrity. Specifically, a foundation in research ethics is essential for several reasons:

1. To fully comply with the legal requirements for knowledge competency about the ethical treatment of human subjects, all participants at any level of the research team, from subject recruiter to lead investigator, including students, must be certified by their sponsoring institution.
2. To ensure the safety of patients serving as research participants, including their privacy and fully-informed consent to participate.
3. To protect students and researchers themselves from unsafe or unethical practices.

4. To appropriately guide the resolution of misunderstandings, disputes or research misconduct.
5. To preserve the public's trust and support of the national research agenda.

While it is hoped that all advanced practice nurses will ultimately hold a doctorate, in the immediate future not all readers will. Clinical nurse specialists, clinical leaders, nurse navigators and others in specialty roles also require an understanding of research ethics, given their important role in patient advocacy and safety, and as valued members of the research team. Because the breadth and scope of content in research ethics has dramatically expanded in the last decade, this chapter serves as a general introduction to essential content for the ethical conduct of research involving human subjects. Additional readings and resources are provided for advanced study.

2.2. HISTORICAL CONTEXT FOR THE CONTEMPORARY MODEL OF RESEARCH ETHICS

A detailed discussion of the philosophical underpinnings of research ethics is beyond the scope of this chapter, but it is important for the doctoral-level student to understand the historical context of the rules, regulations and moral codes that define the ethical conduct of contemporary research. Sadly, many of the regulations and laws that guide the American research enterprise today came about in response to terrible acts of misconduct and unethical practices of medical researchers over the last 70 years. Most infamously, the medical experiments performed on prisoners of war by Nazi doctors in the early 1940s served as the springboard for worldwide guidelines to prevent such atrocities ever again. The Nuremberg Code in 1949 was the first international code of ethics to specify rules for the humane treatment of research subjects. Although it had no force of law, key elements included mandates that:

- Human participation must be justified, and only after animal studies show promising results.
- There has been voluntary, informed consent, with the freedom (free will) to withdraw.
- The expected outcome holds promise of benefit to society.
- Subjects are protected from unnecessary physical and mental harm or injury, without any undue risk of suffering, disability or death.
- The experimenters are qualified.

The Declaration of Helsinki, created for physicians in 1964 by the World Medical Association, amplified the principles of the Nuremberg code to specifically address the use of patients as research subjects in the context of their care. It also expanded the limits of informed consent to allow for surrogate (proxy) consent when the potential research subject is incompetent, physically or mentally incapable of consenting, or is a minor.

2.2.1. Scientific Misconduct and Ethical Abuses in the U.S.

Despite these international reforms, it wasn't until the 1970s that the U.S. government responded with its own laws and regulations, after several alarming cases of abuses involving highly vulnerable populations were disclosed in the lay press (Truog, 2012). For example, in the early 1960s, researchers at the Willowbrook State School in New York intentionally infected disabled children with hepatitis to test a gamma globulin treatment. In a separate case at the same time, elderly patients at the Brooklyn Jewish Chronic Disease Hospital were injected with liver cancer cells without their knowledge and observed for tumor growth. Dr. Henry Beecher's exposure of these and dozens of other abuse cases in the *New England Journal of Medicine* (Beecher, 1966) forced the American public health community to confront the idea that blatantly unethical research was prevalent in the U.S., even in the wards of the most prestigious academic medical centers.

Probably the most notorious and consequential case of ethical abuses in biomedical experiments occurred in the Tuskegee syphilis study, which ran for 40 years from 1932–1972. Sponsored by the U.S. Public Health Service, medical researchers studied the effects of untreated syphilis in some 400 African-American men from impoverished farming areas near Tuskegee, Alabama. Although not deliberately infected with syphilis as is sometimes reported in error (Reverby, 2001), male residents of Macon County were recruited to undergo diagnostic lumbar punctures (called "back shots"), and then told they were being medically "treated" for "bad blood", a lay term of the time referring to a non-specific medical condition. Not only were subjects unaware of their participation in a research study, but they were intentionally deceived about the nature of their illness, and offered incentives for staying in the study including free health care (for conditions other than syphilis), exemption from the military draft, and life insurance coverage for funeral costs. Most troubling, the subjects were not given counseling on how to avoid spreading the disease to their partners, nor treated with penicillin once it became widely available by the late 1940s. It wasn't until a young investigator revealed the story to the *New York Times* in 1972, that the study was forced to close down. By that time, more than 100 affected individuals (including wives and children) had died. As noted by Corby-Smith (1999), the 40-year study became "the longest non-therapeutic experiment on humans in the history of medicine, and has come to represent not only the exploitation of blacks, but the potential for exploitation for any population that may be vulnerable because of race, ethnicity, gender, disability, age or social class". Although it would take another 25 years before an official Presidential apology was issued to the surviving victims and their families (Reverby, 2000), the Tuskegee scandal spawned a series of landmark regulations and rules of conduct that remain in effect today to help protect research subjects and researchers themselves from acts of deliberate or unintentional wrong-doing.

2.3. THE U.S. GOVERNMENT RESPONDS TO RESEARCH ABUSES: THE BELMONT REPORT

In 1973, the Department of Health, Education and Welfare (now Health and Human Services) drafted the first set of federal regulations on the protection of human subjects. Foremost was the mandate that all biomedical research studies funded by the government must be reviewed, approved and overseen by a local institutional review board (IRB) composed of scientists and the lay community for the purpose of protecting the rights of research participants. In 1974, the National Research Act was passed by Congress, which authorized federal agencies to systematically formalize (codify) regulations for the protection of human research subjects. The Act also created a national commission to examine the ethics of research with human subjects. It took 5 years for this same commission to publish its famous Belmont Report (named after the building where the meetings took place in Washington, DC) in 1979 that defined the key principles that serve as the foundation for the ethical conduct of research today. The Belmont Report laid out three fundamental rules of conduct as a framework for judging professional ethical practices in all aspects of research: respect for persons, beneficence, and distributive justice (HEW, 1979).

2.3.1. Respect for Persons

Respect for persons is derived from the ethical principle of autonomy, or the right to self-determination. To be respectful of the autonomous individual, the Report's authors noted that researchers must respect the decisions that a competent person makes, including choosing not to participate in a research study, no matter how potentially worthy or beneficial to public health. Persons not capable of making a competent decision (diminished autonomy) are still entitled to participate in research, as long as special protections are in place. Individuals with diminished autonomy include children (where autonomy is not fully mature), prisoners with restricted freedoms, and persons with cognitive or emotional disabilities. The Report emphasized that autonomy can vary in different situations, such as during an incapacitating illness, and should be reevaluated over time. In the abuse cases noted above, this ethical guideline was the one most flagrantly violated.

2.3.2. Beneficence

Beneficence refers to the ethical obligation to act for the benefit of, or promote the welfare of, others. The complimentary obligation is to prevent or remove possible harms, also known as maleficence (i.e., derived from the "Do No Harm" caveat of the physician's Hippocratic Oath). Beneficence is thus accomplished when one "maximizes the benefits while minimizing possible harms" for research participants (Belmont Report, 1979). Because there is also an obligation for researchers to benefit society, the Report acknowledged that natural tensions and conflicts can arise between benefits to society and direct benefits to the individual research participant. In these cases, avoiding immediate risks to the individual subject "carries special weight" and takes priority, although the interests of others beyond the participant can be justified in some circumstances, providing the subject's rights are protected.

2.3.3. Distributive Justice

Distributive justice means that the benefits and burdens of research should be fairly distributed and equally shared. Publically-funded research that leads to new therapeutic innovations should not be made available only to those who can afford them, nor should the same research over- burden persons from groups unlikely to benefit directly from the research findings. It is worth noting the special emphasis placed on the need to prevent exploitation of vulnerable subjects. The authors of the Report cautioned:

> *"Certain groups, such as racial minorities, the economically disadvantaged, the very sick, and the institutionalized may continually be sought as research subjects, owing to their ready availability in settings where research is conducted. Given their dependent status and their frequently*

compromised capacity for free consent, they should be protected against the danger of being involved in research solely for administrative convenience, or because they are easy to manipulate as a result of their illness or socioeconomic condition." (HEW, 1979).

The Belmont Report also provided examples of how the three ethical rules of conduct should be applied to the consent process and other research procedures (Table 2.1).

TABLE 2.1. Translating the Belmont Report's Ethical Rules of Conduct into "Best Practices in Research" (modified from sections of the Belmont Report, HEW, 1979).

Ethical Principle	Research Procedure Safeguards
Respect for Persons	Valid Consent Safeguards • adequate information to make an informed decision as to the purpose, procedures, full disclosure of risks and possible benefits, rights and responsibilities as a participant • understandable in lay terms • without undue pressure or inducement to diminish the voluntary nature of participation
Beneficence	Assessment of the Balance of Risks and Benefits: There must be a favorable balance in the nature and scope of the likelihood (risk) for harm vs. expected benefits (i.e., the risk-benefit ratio). • Important role for the IRB. • Risks and benefits to families and larger society must also be considered. All categories of risk must be assessed including: psychological, physical (e.g., pain or injury), legal, social, economic • Other options for using human subjects or alternative procedures for reducing risks have been considered • The use of vulnerable populations must be especially justified
Justice	Equitable Selection of Subjects: • Selection methods should be fair to ensure an equitable distribution of burdens and benefits so as not to over-burden some populations vulnerable to coercion with the riskiest or least beneficial studies. • Social justice requires that special populations such as children, institutionalized adults and prisoners are only selected under certain conditions.

2.4. THE U.S. CODE OF FEDERAL REGULATIONS: THE COMMON RULE

Using the Belmont Report as the foundation, the Department of Health and Human Services (HHS) expanded and systematically organized (codified) a set of policy guidelines into the Code of Federal Regulations (CFR) in 1981. CFR Title 45 (Public Welfare), part 46 (Protection of Human Subjects) protects research participants involved in all types of research conducted or supported by the HHS. In another section of the CFR (Title 21, parts 51, 56), the Food and Drug Administration adopted similar rules for pharmaceutical and medical device research. In 1991, Subpart A of "45 CFR 46" was adopted by 14 other federal agencies (e.g., Department of Defense) as the common Federal Policy for the Protection of Human Subjects, and became known as "The Common Rule". The Common Rule for the first time defined and operationalized key functions and procedures of IRBs, and general requirements for informed consent for human subjects involved in all types of medical and behavioral research. These regulations remain in place today with additional revisions developed over time as new issues emerge.

2.4.1. Composition of Institutional Review Boards (IRBs)

All US organizations engaged in human subjects' research, whether in the public or private domain, must operate under the ongoing oversight of an objective and unbiased IRB. According to the Common Rule, an IRB committee must be composed of at least five regular members with the following characteristics:

- Sufficient scientific expertise and knowledge to "promote complete and adequate review of research activities commonly conducted by the institution";
- Relevant experience and diverse make-up in terms of gender, racial and ethnic diversity, and representativeness of community cultural attitudes;
- More than one discipline represented among committee members;
- Research experience or professional knowledge of the special needs of vulnerable populations, such as children and cognitively impaired persons, depending on the research focus of the institution;
- At least one member whose primary concerns are in nonscientific areas;
- At least one member who is not otherwise affiliated with the

Box 2.1 - HHS Policy for Protection of Human Research Subjects: Definition of Terms

(adapted from Protection of human subjects, 45 CFR 46 Subpart A; http://www.hhs.gov/ohrp/humansubjects/guidance/45cfr46.html#46.102)

Research means a systematic investigation, including research development, testing and evaluation, designed to develop or contribute to generalizable knowledge

Human subject means a living individual about whom an investigator (whether professional or student) conducting research obtains

(1) Data through intervention or interaction with the individual, or
(2) Identifiable private information.

Investigator is an individual performing various tasks related to the conduct of human subjects research activities, such as obtaining informed consent from subjects, interacting with subjects, and communicating with the IRB.

Intervention includes both physical procedures by which data are gathered (for example, venipuncture) and manipulations of the subject or the subject's environment that are performed for research purposes.

Interaction includes communication or interpersonal contact between investigator and subject.

Private information includes information about behavior that occurs in a context in which an individual can reasonably expect that no observation or recording is taking place, and information which has been provided for specific purposes by an individual and which the individual can reasonably expect will not be made public (for example, a medical record). Private information must be individually identifiable (i.e., the identity of the subject is or may readily be ascertained by the investigator or associated with the information) in order for obtaining the information to constitute research involving human subjects.

***Clinical Research** includes:

- Patient-oriented research. Research conducted with human subjects (or on material of human origin such as tissues, specimens and cognitive phenomena) for which an investigator (or colleague) directly interacts with human subjects. Excluded from this definition are in vitro studies that utilize human tissues that cannot be linked to a living individual. Patient-oriented research includes: a. mechanisms of disease; b. therapeutic interventions; c. clinical trials, or d. development of new technologies.
- Epidemiologic and behavioral studies
- Outcomes research and health services research

***Clinical Trial** is a prospective biomedical or behavioral research study of human subjects that is designed to answer specific questions about biomedical or behavioral interventions (drugs, treatments, devices, or new ways of using known drugs, treatments, or devices)

*http://grants.nih.gov/grants/policy/hs/glossary.htm

institution and who has an immediate family member affiliated with the institution; Ad-hoc members to provide specific knowledge or expertise, but who are not allowed to vote. (adapted from 45 CFR 46.202 at: http://www.hhs.gov/ohrp/humansubjects/guidance/45cfr46.html#46.202)

2.4.2. Quality Improvement\Evaluation Projects: A Subtype Of Research?

In the past, quality improvement activities were typically exempt from IRB review as there was no expectation of publication or generalization to larger groups beyond the local hospital unit or agency. However, as clinical data management techniques and corresponding regulations have increased in complexity for most health care organizations, more quality improvement activities are considered a subtype of research and rise to the threshold of IRB review. To help distinguish research from quality control studies, Hauser (2008) recommends that IRB approval should be requested when the proposed activity meets any of the following conditions:

- Assigns people or lab specimens to groups for systematic comparison;

Box 2.2 - When is Practice Really Research and in Need of IRB Approval? From: Boundaries Between Practice & Research (page 5.8 BELMONT REPORT, HEW 1979) http://science.education.nih.gov/supplements/nih9/bioethics/guide/teacher/Mod5_Belmont.pdf

"The distinction between research and practice is blurred partly because both often occur together (as in research designed to evaluate a therapy) and partly because notable departures from standard practice are often called "experimental" when the terms "experimental" and "research" are not carefully defined. For the most part, the term "practice" refers to interventions that are designed solely to enhance the well-being of an individual patient or client and that have a reasonable expectation of success. The purpose of medical or behavioral practice is to provide diagnosis, preventive treatment or therapy to particular individuals. By contrast, the term "research" designates an activity designed to test an hypothesis, permit conclusions to be drawn, and thereby to develop or contribute to generalizable knowledge (expressed, for example, in theories, principles, and statements of relationships). Research is usually described in a formal protocol that sets forth an objective and a set of procedures designed to reach that objective . . . the general rule is that if there is any element of research in an activity, that activity should undergo review for the protection of human subjects."

- Is being conducted in hopes of contributing to generalizable knowledge (and not for the sole purpose of improving a clinical process);
- Intentionally leads to publishable results or findings;
- Involves clinical procedures, interactions or observations (if patients) or work activities (if employees) that are not part of routine standard of care or employment;
- Involves increased burden to the participants;
- Involves releasing protected health information or personal information to individuals other than for regulatory/accreditation purposes (adapted from Houser, page 86).

2.5. INFORMED CONSENT

Regulations governing the informed consent process are a cornerstone of the Common Rule and remain today at the heart of ethical research practices. Investigators may not ask individuals to participate as research subjects before obtaining (usually in writing) the legally effective, informed consent of the subject or a legally authorized representative. Specific types of information in understandable language (free of medical jargon) must be included that cover an essential set of elements about the study and risks, and any other relevant types of information as required by the approving IRB (Table 2.2). Other information that the IRB will often require includes the total number of subjects in the study, any costs to the subject, reasons why a subject might be withdrawn from the study by the investigators, and the subject's right to learn of any new findings while participating that might alter the decision to participate. Importantly, researchers must never ask subjects to waive their rights or release the investigators from liability for negligence.

In addition to the Common Rule (subpart A), added protections for specific vulnerable groups of subjects were defined in subparts B, C, and D of the code: pregnant women, human fetuses, and neonates (subpart B); prisoners (subpart C); and children (subpart D).

To help implement the Common Rule, the Office for Human Research Protections (OHRP) was created within HHS to maintain regulatory oversight and provide guidance to IRBs and researchers on ethical and regulatory issues in biomedical and social-behavioral research funded by HHS. Over the years, the office has issued interpretative statements to help operationalize sections of the code. For example, OHRP interprets an "investigator" to be anyone involved in conducting human subjects research studies, including any individual who assists

TABLE 2.2. *Basic Elements of Informed Consent for the Protection of Human Subjects involved in Research. (http://www.hhs.gov/ohrp/humansubjects/guidance/45cfr46.html#46.116)*

- A statement that the study involves research
- An explanation of the purposes of the research
- The expected duration of the subject's participation
- A description of the procedures to be followed
- Identification of any procedures which are experimental
- A description of any reasonably foreseeable risks or discomforts to the subject
- A description of any benefits to the subject or to others which may reasonably be expected from the research
- A disclosure of appropriate alternative procedures or courses of treatment, if any, that might be advantageous to the subject
- A statement describing the extent, if any, to which confidentiality of records identifying the subject will be maintained
- For research involving more than minimal risk, an explanation as to whether any compensation, and an explanation as to whether any medical treatments, are available, if injury occurs and, if so, what they consist of, or where further information may be obtained
- An explanation of whom to contact for answers to pertinent questions about the research and research subjects' rights, and whom to contact in the event of a research-related injury to the subject
- A statement that participation is voluntary, refusal to participate will involve no penalty or loss of benefits to which the subject is otherwise entitled, and the subject may discontinue participation at any time without penalty or loss of benefits, to which the subject is otherwise entitled

the principle (lead) investigator, such as "physicians, scientists, nurses, administrative staff, teachers, and students, among others". This means that individuals considered to be investigators would also include any staff member who: obtains information about living individuals by intervening or interacting with them for research purposes; obtains identifiable private information about living individuals for research purposes; or studies, interprets, or analyzes identifiable private information or data for research purposes. In essence, all members of the research team (including students) share in the obligations and accountability for protecting research subjects.

2.5.1. Consent as a Dynamic, Continuing Process

Because so much emphasis is placed on the content of the written consent form, the idea that valid consent is a process, not just a signed document, sometimes gets forgotten. OHRP has developed a series of

TABLE 2.3. Added Protections for Vulnerable Research Populations in 45 CFR 46, Subparts B-D. (summarized from http://www.hhs.gov/ohrp/humansubjects/guidance/45cfr46.html#46.102).

Vulnerable Group	Key Safeguards and Requirements
Subpart B: Pregnant Women or Fetuses	All of the following must be met: (1) Where scientifically appropriate, preclinical studies on pregnant animals, and clinical studies on non-pregnant women, have been conducted and provide data for assessing potential risks to pregnant women and fetuses; (2) The risk to the fetus is caused solely by interventions or procedures that hold out the prospect of direct benefit for the woman or the fetus; or, if there is no such prospect of benefit, the risk to the fetus is not greater than minimal and the purpose of the research is the development of important biomedical knowledge which cannot be obtained by any other means; (3) Any risk is the least possible for achieving the objectives of the research; (4) If the research holds out the prospect of direct benefit to the pregnant woman, the prospect of a direct benefit both to the pregnant woman and the fetus, or no prospect of benefit for the woman nor the fetus when risk to the fetus is not greater than minimal and the purpose of the research is the development of important biomedical knowledge that cannot be obtained by any other means, her consent is obtained in accord with the informed consent provisions of subpart A of this part; (5) If the research holds out the prospect of direct benefit solely to the fetus then the consent of the pregnant woman and the father is obtained in accord with the informed consent provisions of subpart A of this part, except that the father's consent need not be obtained if he is unable to consent because of unavailability, incompetence, or temporary incapacity or the pregnancy resulted from rape or incest. (6) No inducements, monetary or otherwise, will be offered to terminate a pregnancy; (7) Individuals engaged in the research will have no part in any decisions as to the timing, method, or procedures used to terminate a pregnancy; and (8) Individuals engaged in the research will have no part in determining the viability of a neonate. **Viable neonates.** A neonate, after delivery, that has been determined to be viable may be included in research only to the extent permitted by and in accord with the requirements of subparts A and D.

(continued)

TABLE 2.3 (continued). Added Protections for Vulnerable Research Populations in 45 CFR 46, Subparts B-D. (summarized from http://www.hhs.gov/ohrp/humansubjects/guidance/45cfr46.html#46.102).

Vulnerable Group	Key Safeguards and Requirements
Research involving neonates	Additional safeguards for neonates of uncertain viability and nonviable may be found at §46.205 (www.hhs.gov/ohrp/humansubjects/guidance/45cfr46.html#46.102)
Subpart C: Prisoners	**Approved categories of Research involving Prisoners:** A. A study of criminal behavior and of the possible causes, effects, and processes of incarceration that presents no more than minimal risk and no more than inconvenience to the subjects B. A study of prisons as institutional structures or of prisoners as incarcerated persons that presents no more than minimal risk and no more than inconvenience to the subjects C. Research on conditions particularly affecting prisoners as a class (for example, vaccine trials and other research on hepatitis which is much more prevalent in prisons than elsewhere; and research on social and psychological problems such as alcoholism, drug addiction, and sexual assaults). D. Research on practices, both innovative and accepted, which have the intent and reasonable probability of improving the health or well-being of the subject. http://grants.nih.gov/grants/policy/hs/prisoners_categories_research.htm
Subpart D: Children	**In most cases, parents must provide permission for children under age 18 (varies by State) to participate in research** **When capable, a child's assent (agreement) is needed** **Research can be approved when these categories apply:** • where there is no greater than minimal risk (no greater than what is encountered in daily life or in routine medical practice) • greater than minimal risk is permitted, if there is a favorable benefit equal to that of alternative treatments • if there is no direct benefit, but the risk represents only a minor increase over minimal risk and the research can yield vital information about the child's specific condition/disorder • when not otherwise approvable but determined by the IRB and the HHS Secretory to hold promise of new findings about a serious health problem

web-based educational materials, tips and FAQs designed to clarify and interpret the Common Rule's regulations for informed consent. Importantly, it emphasizes the prospective, dynamic, ongoing nature of the consent process that begins with the initial recruitment activities, and doesn't end until the study is completed. Much more than a piece of paper, "the informed consent process is an ongoing exchange of information between the investigator and the subject and could include, for example, use of question-and-answer sessions, community meetings, and videotape presentations. In all circumstances individuals should be provided with an opportunity to have their questions and concerns addressed on an individual basis." (Informed Consent, FAQs, OHRP: http://answers.hhs.gov/ohrp/categories/1566).

2.5.2. Other Vulnerable Groups

In addition to pregnant women, fetuses, children and prisoners, the Common Rule also identifies mentally disabled persons and those who are "economically or educationally disadvantaged" as likely to be vulnerable to coercion or undue influence and thus in need of special safeguards to protect their rights and welfare when participating as research subjects. In 2009, the NIH commented on the special challenges to involving volunteers with questionable capacity to consent (Table 2.4).

Students and employees of the research organization are also considered "vulnerable" groups, whether justified or not, due to the potential

TABLE 2.4. Research Participants with Questionable Capacity to Provide Informed Consent: Issues to Consider. (Office of Extramural Research, 2009; adapted from http://grants.nih.gov/grants/policy/questionablecapacity.htm#_ftn9).

- A wide variety of mental disorders, neurologic diseases (dementia, stroke), metabolic impairments, psychoactive medications, substance abuse, and injuries (head trauma) can impair a person's ability to understand and make an informed decision about research participation.
- Consent capacity in the same individual can vary depending on the complexity and nature of the research study.
- The ethical principle of equitable subject selection requires that persons with impaired cognition not be excluded from research, in order to advance the knowledge base in neurologic disease and brain injury. Indeed, those with the most severe impairments may be the most important participants.
- Rather than specific HHS requirements, each IRB can recommend on a case by case basis the nature of any additional safeguards, as well as state and local laws.

of undue gains for research participation (e.g., pay raise for employees, or higher grades for students), or conversely, retaliation from supervisors in the case of refusal to volunteer.

2.6. OTHER SOCIAL INFLUENCES ON HUMAN SUBJECTS' PROTECTIONS

Beyond human subject abuses, another important force shaping the evolution of research ethics has been the huge societal shifts in attitudes and values about the individual's rights. As noted by Truog (2012), the patients' rights movement in the U.S. was spawned from the consumers' rights movement and the social gains for women and ethnic minority groups beginning in the 1960s. After a government audit revealed that most NIH research grants were singularly focused on men or used male animal models to study disease mechanisms, Congress passed the NIH Revitalization Act (PL103-43) in 1993, which mandated that women and ethnic minorities be included in all clinical research studies. Critics of the bill argued that such action was unnecessary and costly, believing (erroneously) that most scientific findings observed in white men could be directly applied to women and men of non-white ethnicities. Moreover, they viewed studies using women as too complex because of the issue of menstrual cycle hormones. At the same time, many researchers still believed that women of childbearing potential should be automatically excluded from medical studies because of possible harm to the fetus. As a result of the collective reforms over the last few decades of the twentieth century, medical paternalism was slowly replaced with a shared decision-making model that re-positioned the locus of authority from the physician to the patient. In turn, this paradigm shift has also transformed the relationship between investigator and research volunteer. Increasingly, with the advent of community-based, participatory research, where the community is actively engaged in all aspects of the research process including identification of the study question and design, research participants and the community itself are viewed as co-researchers or research partners.

2.6.1. Role Conflict

Sometimes tensions and conflicts are created for the clinician-researcher who must occupy two distinct roles: clinician and scientist. As noted by Resnick (2009), "As a clinician, the investigator has duties to provide the patient with optimal care and undivided loyalty. As a scientist, the investigator has duties to follow the rules, procedures and methods described in the protocol." (page 1). Consider the following real case concerning pregnant women as a vulnerable research population.

> *A clinical investigator writes a NIH grant application for the study of perinatal stress effects on maternal-fetal/newborn health outcomes in a sample of low SES minority patients. The application receives an outstanding score, but the NIH reviewers request the addition of a urine toxicology test to the prenatal screening assessment of the eligible research participants. The grant is funded and the investigator presents the revised research proposal for final approval to the local Institutional Review Board (IRB) where the study will be conducted. Before approving, the Committee wants to know from the investigator, "What will be done if the urine toxicology is positive?" The investigator would like to simply withdraw anyone from the study with a positive result without disclosing to the volunteer the true reason for the protocol failure. In that way, the subject's confidentiality would be protected, but the researcher worries about the potential harm to the fetus, if there was no follow-up referral to the obstetrical care provider. She wonders if the IRB will approve this strategy.*

In the end, an acceptable plan for handling a positive drug screen was approved by the IRB, which provided for an alert in the consent form that urine drug screens will be conducted during the study and the provision for follow-up disclosure of a positive test to the volunteer's provider. The case also prompted a collaborative commentary on the ethical challenges of clinical care studies (Rohan *et al.*, 2011).

2.7. THE HIPAA "PRIVACY RULE"

The HIPAA Privacy Rule is the common term for the federal regulation that protects the privacy of personal health information (PHI) of individuals either living or deceased. It was established as law under the Health Insurance Portability and Accountability Act (HIPAA) of 1996, became effective in 2003 for most "covered entities" (see definitions below, Box 3) and continues to undergo refinements in scope. In terms of research, the "Privacy Rule" specifies the conditions under which researchers can gain access to PHI. Its goal is to balance an individual's interest in keeping health information confidential with other social benefits, including health care research. According to the NIH website http://privacyruleandresearch.nih.gov/clin_research.asp, covered entities are "health plans, health care clearinghouses, and health care providers that transmit health information electronically in connection with certain defined HIPAA transactions, such as claims or eligibility inquiries". Researchers are not themselves covered entities, unless they are also health care providers and engage in any of the covered electronic transactions. Nonetheless, investigators may be indirectly affected by the" Privacy Rule" if covered entities (e.g., hospitals) supply their data.

2.7.1. Impact of HIPAA on Research

Because researchers frequently make use of medical records and other types of personal health information, HIPAA permits access to these important data sources under specific conditions explained in the following box.

Box 2.3 - HIPAA Privacy Rule: Relevant Definitions for Research (http://privacyruleandresearch.nih.gov/dictionary.asp)

Research—A systematic investigation, including research development, testing, and evaluation, designed to develop or contribute to generalizable knowledge. This includes the development of research repositories and databases for research.

Covered Entity—A health plan, a health care clearinghouse, or a health care provider who transmits health information in electronic form in connection with a transaction for which HHS has adopted a standard.

Health Information—Any information, whether oral or recorded in any form or medium, that (1) is created or received by a health care provider, health plan, public health authority, employer, life insurer, school or university, or health care clearinghouse; and (2) relates to the past, present, or future physical or mental health or condition of an individual; the provision of health care to an individual; or the past, present, or future payment for the provision of health care to an individual.

Individually Identifiable Health Information—Information that is a subset of health information, including demographic information collected from an individual, and (1) is created or received by a health care provider, health plan, employer, or health care clearinghouse; and (2) relates to the past, present, or future physical or mental health or condition of an individual; the provision of health care to an individual; or the past, present, or future payment for the provision of health care to an individual; and (a) that identifies the individual; or (b) with respect to which there is a reasonable basis to believe the information can be used to identify the individual.

Protected Health Information—PHI is individually identifiable health information transmitted by electronic media, maintained in electronic media, or transmitted or maintained in any other form or medium. PHI excludes education records covered by the Family Educational Rights and Privacy Act, as amended, 20 U.S.C. 1232g, records described at 20 U.S.C. 1232g(a)(4)(B)(iv), and employment records held by a covered entity in its role as employer.

Box 2.4 - How can Researchers Obtain PHI?

The Privacy Rule allows access to patient data as long as the information is uncoupled to the individual in any identifying manner, and written authorization has been obtained from the individual. Required authorization can be waived in the following circumstances:

- for the creation of a limited data set with a data use agreement;
- to conduct a preliminary feasibility assessment (but not the actual removal of records) in preparation for research;
- when individuals are deceased.

In all three instances, documented approval by an IRB must be obtained.

(modified from: How Can Covered Entities Use and Disclose Protected Health Information for Research and Comply with the Privacy Rule? http://privacyruleandresearch.nih.gov/pr_08.asp#8i) accessed June 16, 2012)

2.7.2. De-identifying Protected Health Information Under the Privacy Rule

The "Privacy Rule" specifies 18 types of information that must be removed from a patient/medical record before PHI can be used for research (Table 2.5).

All investigators are required to undergo periodic institutional training in order to make their research HIPAA-compliant. In general, researchers should assume that anytime a patient participates as a research subject in an IRB-approved study protocol, a signed HIPAA authorization to release medical information must also be obtained. As noted on the website of Columbia University Medical Center's HIPAA Training Program, "Consent is permission to participate in a research protocol. Authorization is permission to use the data collected during the study". (https://www.rascal.columbia.edu/servlet/edu.columbia.rascal.presentation.tc.servlets.TCMainServlet?targetCourse=19)

Table 2.6 lists the 8 key elements that must be included in a HIPAA Clinical Research Authorization form. Once signed by the research participant, it must be kept by the lead investigator for 6 years.

2.7.3. HIPAA HITECH

In response to the massive expansion of the use and exchange of electronic data and the increasing potential for confidentiality and privacy breaches, the Health Information Technology for Economic and Clinical Health (HITECH) Act was signed into law as part of the sweeping reforms of the American Recovery and Reinvestment Act in

2009 (http://www.hhs.gov/news/press/2009pres/10/20091030a.html). Part D of the Act dramatically increased the penalties and fines for privacy violations (up to $1.5 million) as a way to encourage institutions, both public and private, to develop their own internal set of strict compliance programs. It also mandated that entities report data breaches involving 500 or more individuals to HHS and the media as well as to the affected individuals. In response, health care and research institutions have amplified the security training of their employees, students and faculty members. Most now require that all investigators use only

TABLE 2.5. The 18 HIPAA-Mandated Data Elements that Must be Removed from an Individual's PHI Record Prior to Research Use http://privacyruleandresearch.nih.gov/pr_08.asp#8i, accessed June 26, 2012.

1. Names.
2. All geographic subdivisions smaller than a state, including street address, city, county, precinct, ZIP Code, and their equivalent geographical codes, except for the initial three digits of a ZIP Code if, according to the current publicly available data from the Bureau of the Census:
   - The geographic unit formed by combining all ZIP Codes with the same three initial digits contains more than 20,000 people.
   - The initial three digits of a ZIP Code for all such geographic units containing 20,000 or fewer people are changed to 000.
3. All elements of dates (except year) directly related to an individual, including birth date, admission date, discharge date, and date of death; and all ages over 89 and all elements of dates (including year) indicative of such age, except that such ages and elements may be aggregated into a single category of age 90 or older.
4. Telephone numbers.
5. Facsimile numbers.
6. Electronic mail addresses.
7. Social security numbers.
8. Medical record numbers.
9. Health plan beneficiary numbers.
10. Account numbers.
11. Certificate/license numbers.
12. Vehicle identifiers and serial numbers, including license plate numbers.
13. Device identifiers and serial numbers.
14. Web universal resource locators (URLs).
15. Internet protocol (IP) address numbers.
16. Biometric identifiers, including fingerprints and voiceprints.
17. Full-face photographic images and any comparable images.
18. Any other unique identifying number, characteristic, or code, unless otherwise permitted by the Privacy Rule.

TABLE 2.6. Required Elements of the HIPAA Clinical Research Authorization Form (Form A). (From HIPAA Training for Columbia University Medical Center Faculty and Staff Engaged in Human Subjects Research. (https://www.rascal.columbia.edu/servlet/edu.columbia.rascal.presentation.tc.servlets.TCMainServlet?targetCourse=19).

1. The information you intend to use.

   The authorization must include all the health information needed. This includes standard PHI, as well as subjects' history, physical findings, reports and laboratory test results.
2. The people/organizations that may use or disclose the information (e.g., the PI and research team).
3. The people/organizations who will receive the information (e.g., study sponsor, central laboratories, IRB, FDA).
4. The purpose of the use or disclosure (study description).
5. Expiration date (e.g., anticipated end of study).
6. Right to refuse to sign the authorization.
7. Right to revoke the authorization.

   (Researchers are now required to inform subjects that they must withdraw in writing in order to revoke permission for subsequent use or disclosure of their PHI).
8. The individual's signature and date (HIPAA requires subjects be provided with a signed copy of the HIPAA authorization).
9. Re-disclosure

   If PHI will be disclosed to another party—such as the external sponsor— a statement is required informing the subject that the external sponsor may make subsequent disclosures, which will not be covered under the HIPAA privacy regulations.

encrypted (password-protected) desktop and portable devices (laptops, cell phones, USB drives) for storing, sending and retrieving clinical data. Institutional email systems should only be used to send PHI internally within the institution, and never used to send data external to the organization. External document storage sites, Wikis, blogs, or web-based calendars should never be used to store research subject files.

Two case studies relevant to doctoral-prepared nurses are presented below.

2.7.4. HIPAA Case Studies

2.7.4.1. HIPAA Case Scenario #1: Converting Patient Records to a Clinical Database

Dr. Jenna Smith, DNP is a nurse-midwife who also occasionally engages in clinical research. Dr. Smith has kept all of the outcome data from her obstetrical patients for the last 20 years and frequently consults the database for interesting trends that could form the basis of research. Since Dr. Smith has documentation on all of the postpartum patients' consents granting their permission to use their PHI for research, she assumes she has the right to keep her own research database of her patient's data. When she queries the University's HIPAA compliance officer, she is told she may keep a separate research database providing certain measures are taken. Dr. Smith will need to submit a protocol and obtain IRB approval to maintain a research database. The protocol must indicate that all of Dr. Smith's patients contributing data after April 14, 2003 (when HIPAA went into effect) will sign an IRB-approved HIPAA authorization which gives her permission to use their medical information for her research. (Modified from a case scenario presented on the website of Columbia University Medical Center's HIPAA Training for Columbia University Medical Center Faculty and Staff Engaged in Human Subjects Research [https://www.rascal.columbia.edu/servlet/edu.columbia.rascal.presentation.tc.servlets.TCMainServlet?targetCourse=19] accessed Aug 12, 1012).

2.7.4.2. Case Scenario #2: Data Management and the Use of Electronic Records

You are the study coordinator for an NIH-funded trial of the effects of exercise on morbidly obese women. The project is still in the screening phase and your recruitment goal is 100 participants meeting all eligibility criteria. The PI has asked you on Friday to prepare a preliminary report of the demographics for the first 60 respondents to the study flier placed in a weight loss clinic. She needs them by Monday to add to an abstract for a poster presentation which is due at midnight. Because you will be recruiting on Saturday morning at the weight loss clinic and will be entering data directly into an electronic spreadsheet on your laptop, you can work at home on Sunday to develop the preliminary data tables. You send the raw data at 6 PM Sunday evening by email attachment to the PI's home email address to make sure she gets them in time. About a month later, one of the research volunteers reports that her son "Googled" her name for a 4th grade class project and discovered that all of her identifying information, including her reproductive history and other sensitive information, were posted on the world-wide web as part of the study file. You wonder how this could have happened. (from the files of N. Reame, Columbia University School of Nursing)

2.8. INTERNATIONAL RESEARCH: ABUSES, REGULATIONS AND GUIDELINES FOR GOOD CLINICAL PRACTICES

Unfortunately, cases of exploitation and ethical abuses of vulnerable populations are still coming to light and prompting additional protections for participants in medical research (Friedan and Collins, 2010). As recently as 2010, the Obama administration issued a formal apology for an international scandal dating back to the 1940s. In a two-year study conducted in Guatemala of the effects of different penicillin regimens as treatment for venereal diseases, the U.S. Public Health Service deliberately infected some 700 individuals. Funded by grants from the NIH, and approved by the U.S. Surgeon General, the researchers used female sex workers, institutionalized mentally-disabled patients, prisoners and soldiers as research subjects (http://www.hhs.gov/1946inoculationstudy/).

In response to the disclosure by Wellesley College Professor Susan Reverby, a Presidentially-appointed bioethics commission conducted an investigation and issued a set of 14 recommendations in 2011 to enhance accountability and study ways to compensate subjects injured during research (Presidential Commission for the Study of Bioethical Issues, 2011). Currently, the U.S. is one of the few developed nations that does not require researchers or sponsors to provide treatment, or compensation for treatment, for injuries suffered by research subjects. The commission also cited the lack of a unified federal research database or cohesive system of documentation. In closing remarks, the lead commissioner noted that "our nation vigorously and rigorously protects people who volunteer for research studies. However, the Guatemala experiments remind us to never take ethics for granted. We must never confuse ethical principles with burdensome obstacles to be overcome or evaded. Good science requires good ethics, and vice versa." (Gutmann, 2011). In 2013, it is expected that new laws will mandate a change in the U.S. policy permitting compensation for research subjects injured while participating in research. The time line of some of the most serious cases of human subject abuses and subsequent legislative reforms in U.S. research policies are summarized in Table 2.7. As emphasized by Beauchamp and Childress in their epic text, *Principles of Biomedical Ethics* (2009), the utilitarian principle that "the end justifies the means" should never take precedence over autonomy to rationalize the mis-treatment of research participants.

TABLE 2.7. The Time Course of US Federal Government Actions and Policies in the context of Human Subject Abuses (adapted from Friedan and Collins, 2010, page 264).

Year	Event
1932–1971	Tuskegee Syphilis Study
1946–1948	Guatemalan STD inoculation studies
1956–1971	Hepatitis studies at Willowbrook State School for the Retarded
1963	Jewish Hospital cancer study
1964	Declaration of Helsinki
1966	U.S. Surgeon General policy on human subject oversight by IRB
1971	NIH Office for Protection from Research Risks
1974–1978	National Commission for the Protection of Human Subjects
1974	National Research Act
1979	Belmont Report
1981	HHS 45 CFR and FDA 21 CFR 50, 56 regulations enacted
1991	45 CFR 46 becomes "Common Rule" across agencies
1993	NIH Guidelines for inclusion of women and minorities in clinical research
1995	WHO Guidelines for Good Clinical Practice
1996	Health Information Portability & Accountability Act (HIPAA)
1997	Presidential apology for Tuskegee syphilis study
1997	HIV drug studies in pregnant women in Africa
2010	Presidential apology for Guatemala inoculation study
2011	Presidential Commission to Study Bioethics recommends 14 safeguards

2.8.1. A Global Agreement for Good Clinical Practices

Rules and regulations for global protections of human subjects have also continued to evolve as the international research enterprise has expanded to include the conduct of multi-site clinical trials that transcend national borders. A number of leading medical organizations have developed standards for good clinical practices. In 1990, the International Conference for Harmonization of Technical Requirements for Registration for Pharmaceuticals was launched by the U.S., Japan and countries of the European Union. Composed of members of both regulatory agencies and pharmaceutical industries of each country, its mission is to better "harmonize" (standardize) the approval and authorization procedures needed to ensure quality, safety and efficacy of new medicinal products across countries (http://www.ich.org/). The E6 guideline for

Good Clinical Practice (GCP), finalized in 1996, is "... an international and scientific quality standard for designing, conducting, recording, and reporting trials that involve the participation of human subjects" (ICH report, 1996, (http://www.ich.org/fileadmin/Public_Web_Site/ICH_Products/Guidelines/Efficacy/E6_R1/Step4/E6_R1__Guideline.pdf.) Based on 14 ethical principles of the World Health Organization, The GCP guideline describes procedures for the monitoring, reporting and conduct of clinical trials, including the roles of the IRB, sponsor, and investigator (http://whqlibdoc.who.int/publications/2005/924159392X_eng.pdf) accessed Aug 10, 2012). As noted in the introduction, "Compliance with this standard provides public assurance that the rights, safety, and well-being of the trial participants are protected ... and that the data are credible." (page 1). The U.S. Food and Drug Administration collaborated on the development of the document and has adopted the GCP guidelines as official FDA guidance.

2.8.2. Special Protections for Vulnerable International Populations

In 1992, the Council for International Organizations of Medical Sciences (CIOMS), in partnership with the World Health Organization (WHO), published guidelines for the rights and welfare of research subjects from "underdeveloped communities" as a way to minimize their exploitation in international clinical trials. The most important sanction developed was against the use of subjects from underdeveloped/developing countries if the research could be carried out reasonably well in developed countries. A related guideline was that international studies must offer the potential of actual benefit to the residents of the developing country involved in the research. Specifically, inhabitants of the country where the research was carried out must have access to any products or interventions developed, even if the cost is substantial.

2.8.3. The AZT Trials in Africa

Despite these international safeguards, controversial clinical trials continue to be carried out seemingly at odds with the spirit of the existing international guidelines. As described on the website of the Kennedy Institute of Ethics at Georgetown University, the AZT studies in Africa in 1997 is one such example.

> *"The AZT studies in South Africa in 1997 created a public outcry when American and African researchers, funded by a grant from the Centers*

for Disease Control (CDC), gave a placebo, rather than the effective agent AZT, as a control treatment to pregnant women who were infected with HIV and were participating in clinical trials. The researchers argued that "standard" treatments for AIDS for these women were no treatments at all. (The AZT regimen studied in the U.S., for example, was too expensive for women and governments in poor countries, costing between $800–$1000 per person.) The researchers were evaluating lower and fewer doses of AZT in the African studies to see if low doses might be effective. Such doses might be affordable and accessible for the African women (and other poor women around the world). The researchers argued that placebo controls were appropriate, that they constituted the local "standard" therapy, and that they would provide answers faster than would other types of controls.

Some people argue that it is unethical to use different standard treatments for rich and poor women. Others say that western researchers should not impose "ethical imperialism" on women in other countries and that each country should determine its own standards for what is ethical in research. Still others argue that, because placebo trials end more quickly than do trials in which different doses of AZT are compared and because placebo trials use fewer subjects than do other trials, in the long run, more children would be saved through placebo trials. Still others counter that no person should be a means to an end, however positive that end might be." (adapted from Kennedy Institute of Ethics, Georgetown University http://highschoolbioethics.georgetown.edu/units/cases/unit3_8.html)

2.9. THE CONCEPT OF CLINICAL EQUIPOISE

An essential ethical condition for comparing two drugs or treatments in a randomized controlled trial is that there is no evidence that one is more effective than the other. Known as clinical equipoise, investigators must be in a state of genuine clinical uncertainty about differences in therapeutic benefit when deliberately exposing study participants to experimental interventions. Although investigators may hope or even expect one agent may be safer, more effective or even just faster-acting, there should be no solid or well-accepted evidence one way or the other of a superior benefit. If that was the case, some of the research subjects would be intentionally assigned to receive the less effective intervention. Moreover, if evidence already existed of a known benefit, then repeating the same comparisons would be wasteful and of little scientific merit.

In the case of the AZT trials in South Africa, the concern that fewer children would be saved without the efficient use of placebo-controlled trials created an ethical dilemma for worldwide policy makers. In 2002, the Declaration of Helsinki language was revised to clarify the justified use of placebo control groups: 1) on a case-by-case basis for compelling scientific reasons to determine a drug's efficacy or safety; or 2) for minor conditions when no further harm is anticipated. In 2004, a further revision added the mandate that research subjects have post-trial access to procedures identified as new or alternative medical care. Now in its 6th edition, the current version was ratified by the WMA's General Assembly in 2008 and replaces all earlier versions (http://www.wma.net/en/20activities/10ethics/10helsinki/ (accessed June 29, 2012).

2.10. THERAPEUTIC MISPERCEPTION

According to the Alliance for Human Research Protection, a national citizens' watchdog organization, some 15 million Americans are recruited every year into clinical trials (www.ahrp.org). Despite the many safeguards now in place to protect research subjects from harm, a large body of evidence has demonstrated a variety of flaws in the process to ensure truly informed consent in clinical research. For example, subjects often misunderstand the purpose of the research, and its true risks and benefits, or fail to make unbiased decisions due to illness, emotional duress, or socioeconomic and cultural barriers (Resnick, 2009). One of the most common ethical challenges to gaining valid consent is the widespread misperception that participation in a research study guarantees benefit for the patient-volunteer. As noted by Resnick (2009), "patients/subjects who are under the influence of the therapeutic misconception tend to overestimate the potential benefits of research and underestimate risks. . . . (it) is difficult to dispel, even when patients/subjects receive ample information about the research and are well-educated, because many patients enter clinical studies hoping to find a cure for their disease" (pg. 4).

2.11. ETHICAL CODES GUIDING NURSES INVOLVED IN RESEARCH

2.11.1. ANA Code Of Ethics: The Moral Framework for the Nurse's Role In Research

The *ANA Code of Ethics for Nurses* (Fowler, 2008) is the 45-yr-old set of guidelines that provides the fundamental ethical guidelines for all members of the nursing profession, regardless of level of education. Because the Code of Ethics is a living document, provisions are revised and re-interpreted regularly by ANA committees in response to emerging ethical issues in health care. It currently has nine provisions and serves as both a general guide for the profession's members and as a social contract with the public. By virtue of the advanced training and expanded roles in contributing to the generation of evidence-based practice, the doctorally-prepared nurse carries special obligations to adhere to its rules of conduct.

2.11.2. Evolution of Nursing Guidelines for Research Practice

As far back as the "Nightingale Pledge", nursing practice codes have made mention of the expected behaviors of the nurse when involved in research-related activities. More recently, the ANA's Commission on Nursing Research published *Human Rights Guidelines for Nursing in Clinical and Other Research* in 1985 for the protection of research subjects. It included for the first time a dedicated guideline to the nurse's participation on institutional review boards. As the role of the nurse in research further evolved, these codes of conduct were integrated into contemporary provisions of the ANA Code, and were accompanied by relevant interpretative statements.

As described in the latest guide for applying the ANA Code to contemporary dilemmas (Fowler, 2008), both Provision # 3 and # 7 specifically include explanatory statements that outline the expected ethical behaviors for nurses involved in research. These expectations derive not only from the central role of the nurse as the patient's advocate (Provision 3), but also from the nurse's duty to develop the profession (Provision 7). As noted in the accompanying guide (Twomey, 2008), the participation by nurses in research has increased dramatically in recent years—not only as providers of care for research volunteers, but as members of research teams, and as scientific investigators. Moreover, the expanded research activity across all health care settings now demands a greater role for the primary nurse in the informed consent process for patients under their care who may be exposed to research opportunities. The relevant guidelines for research, summarized in Table 2.8, provide a moral framework for nurses at all levels of professional education, and across all patient care settings. Importantly, they specially address the rights of research subjects to privacy, dignity and protections from harm. Notably, they emphasize the nurse's duty to

TABLE 2.8. ANA Code of Ethics Provisions and Interpretations for Research Conduct and Practices (modified from Guide to the Code of Ethics for Nurses: Interpretation and Application, 2010). http://www.nursingworld.org/MainMenuCategories/EthicsStandards/CodeofEthicsforNurses/Code-of-Ethics.pdf.

Provision 3. The nurse promotes, advocates for, and strives to protect the health, safety and rights of the patient.

Statement 3.1. The nurse safeguards the patient's right to privacy

- The nurse advocates for a physical environment that promotes privacy to disclose personal information
- The nurse advocates for policies and practices that protect the confidentially of information

Statement 3.2. The nurse has a duty to maintain confidentiality of all patient information

- The rights, well-being, and safety of the patient should be the primary factors when deciding whether to disclose confidential information received from or about the patient, whether oral, written or electronic.
- Relevant data should be shared only with those members of the health care team who have a need to know to avoid unnecessary access to data or the inappropriate disclosure of identifiable patient information.
- Duties of confidentiality are not absolute and may need to be modified in order to protect the patient, or set aside in circumstances of mandatory disclosure for public health reasons.
- When using electronic communications, special effort should be made to maintain data security.

Statement 3.3. Protection of participants in research

- Each individual has the right to choose whether or not to participate in research.
- There must be no adverse consequences or penalty for refusing to participate or withdrawing after one agrees to participate.
- The patient or legally-authorized surrogate must receive sufficient information at a comprehendible level in order to achieve an informed consent.
- Adequately-informed consent must include information about:
  - The nature of participation.
  - Potential harms and benefits.
  - Relevant alternatives to taking part in the research.
  - How the data will be protected from breach of confidentiality.
- Only qualified persons should direct and conduct research with patients.
- Prior to implementation, research must be approved by a qualified review board.

(continued)

TABLE 2.8 (continued). ANA Code of Ethics Provisions and Interpretations for Research Conduct and Practices (modified from Guide to the Code of Ethics for Nurses: Interpretation and Application, 2010). http://www.nursingworld.org/MainMenuCategories/EthicsStandards/CodeofEthicsforNurses/Code-of-Ethics.pdf.

- Nurses should recognize the special needs of vulnerable groups involved in research, such as children, prisoners, students, the elderly, and the poor.
- The nurse who participates in research in any capacity should be fully informed about the rights and obligations of both the subject and the nurse.
- Nurses have the duty to question, and if necessary, to report and refuse to participate in research they deem morally objectionable.

Provision 7. The nurse participates in the development of the profession through contributions to practice, education, administration, and knowledge development.

Statement 7.3. Advancing the profession through knowledge development, dissemination, and application to practice.

- As an obligation to society, the nursing profession should engage in scholarly inquiry to identify, evaluate, refine and expand the body of knowledge foundational to the discipline and its practice.
- The evolving knowledge base is appropriately derived from the sciences and humanities.
- All nurses working alone or in collaboration can participate in the advancement of the profession through the development, evaluation, dissemination and application of knowledge in practice.
- This level of nursing knowledge development requires an organizational climate and infrastructure that values and implements such scholarly inquiry.

question, to report and to refuse to participate in research deemed morally objectionable.

Grady and Edgerly (2009) present a case study of how the nurse as patient advocate can play an important role in resolving the ethical dilemma of therapeutic misconception.

2.11.3. Nursing Code of Ethics Case Study

"Alice is a 42-year-old woman with an aggressive cancer that has not responded to previous therapy. She is offered participation in a phase one clinical trial with a promising new investigational agent. Alice's nurse knows that the purpose of the trial is to evaluate the safety of the drug and that the possibility that Alice might benefit in terms of tumor shrinkage or an increase in the length or quality of her life is very small. The nurse is concerned that the principal investigator (PI) has not made this clear enough to Alice, and is concerned that Alice is not well informed about what alternatives are available to her. Respecting Alice's right to make her own decision about study participation, the nurse feels strongly that Alice's informed consent may be compromised. When the nurse raises these concerns, the PI expresses apprehension about confusing Alice. The nurse suggests that a multidisciplinary discussion of the options available for Alice and a plan for assuring she understands the options would be helpful for everyone. The PI agrees. The nurse organizes a patient care conference to include the PI, medical fellow, relevant nursing staff, social worker, spiritual counselor, and bioethicist. All agree that it would be helpful if the nurse spent additional time reviewing information about the study with Alice. After a lengthy and engaging discussion with Alice about the study and her options, the nurse asks Alice to explain in her own words what the study is about, what is likely to happen during the study, and what other choices she has besides participation. Much more confident that Alice has a better understanding of the study and is making an informed choice about participation, the nurse offers continued discussion with Alice throughout the study." (Grady, C. and Edgerly, M. (2009) Science, technology and innovation: nursing responsibilities in clinical research. *Nurs. Clin. North Am. 44*: 472.)

2.12. INTERNATIONAL NURSING RESEARCH

In 1999 at the University of Surrey in the UK, a cohort of international nursing scholars established a worldwide association of university research and teaching centers to address issues of morality, professional ethics, philosophy of care, cultural and religious values, law and accountability (www.surrey.ac.u/fhms/research/centres/ic). Known as the International Centre for Nursing Ethics (ICNE), it empanelled a working group to identify key ethical principles that should guide international nursing research (Olsen, 2003). Beyond the conventional bioethical principles of respect for persons, beneficence, and justice, the ICNE panel also emphasized respect for community, and contextual caring (not just professional obligation) as especially relevant for research across national boundaries. Based on these five principles, ICNE proposed three fundamental conditions and related assumptions under which international nursing research would be ethical (Box 2.5).

Box 2.5 - Conditions for the Ethical Conduct of International Nursing Research. (adapted from Olsen, 2003, pp 127–129)

- "the local community has an early opportunity and an ongoing mechanism to provide input into the purposes, goals and methods of the research;
- the research design generates knowledge that has the potential to benefit the community or population providing the participants*;
- there is an ethically justifiable reason to target the population from which participants will be recruited**.

*This implies that any intervention that may be shown to be successful is affordable and practical in the local milieu. Although this stipulation is often applied to drug research, much nursing research involves testing person-to-person interventions, which can also be economically costly and may need to be implemented or administered by personnel with training that is largely unavailable in the local community.

** One of the following justifications should apply:

(1) the phenomenon under consideration is biologically unique to that group or relates to a phenomenon that is biologically unique to that group (e.g., thalassemia, sickle cell anemia);

(2) the phenomenon, although culturally mediated, is widely known to be group specific (e.g., the effect of local diet or sexual practices);

(3) there is an empirically demonstrated rationale for targeting a specific group (e.g. there is a demonstrated difference in incidence rate of detection or recovery);

(4) extensive normative data exist that do not include the targeted population—if it is reasonable to believe that the targeted population may vary from the general population described by the data;

(5) comparative data between groups would be helpful to mutual understanding or in designing treatment, service delivery or education (e.g., efforts to understand differences in ethical concepts cross-culturally)."

2.13. SPECIAL ETHICAL CHALLENGES FOR NURSES IN RESEARCH

It has been argued that nurse researchers face distinct ethical considerations compared to scientists from other disciplines because of their key role as patient advocate and status as a developing academic science (Table 2.9). According to Fouka and Mantzorou (2011) the very nature of nursing may create heightened role conflict for the nurse investigator/practitioner who must protect the best interests of the patient while adhering to sound research practices. For example, to maintain scientific rigor of an intervention trial, the nurse researcher must exclude willing participants who do not meet eligibility criteria from potentially beneficial therapies, or assign some volunteers to a "wait list" control group, potentially delaying optimum patient care. Although a common circumstance faced by all types of clinical investigators, nurses in research may feel especially compelled to resolve such dilemmas with the best interests of the patient in mind. In addition, Grady and Edgerly (2009) note that patients may have difficulty distinguishing between the nurse's role as caregiver versus researcher, given the nurse's more direct contact with individual research participants than other members of the research staff. This role confusion for patients may be confounded by the three distinct nursing roles in clinical research:

> *"(a) the clinical nurse as caregiver of patient-participants before, during, or after participation in clinical research; (b) the nurse as study coordinator or clinical trial nurse who works closely with the principal investigator to coordinate all aspects of a study, and who may function as a kind of case manager for research participants in the study; and (c) the nurse as principal investigator on a research study responsible for designing, planning, and conducting clinical research. Each of these roles has its own set of particular ethical challenges." Grady, C. and Edgerly, M. (2009) Science, technology, and innovation: nursing responsibilities in clinical research. Nurs. Clin. North Am. 44:473.*

2.13.1. Qualitative Methods and Internet Research Approaches

As noted by several nurse scholars (Robley, 1995; Morse, 2007, Grady and Edgerly, 2009), ethical guidelines established for the traditional scientific method are not adequate for qualitative research methods, in which unintended consequences and unanticipated implications for research participants emerge spontaneously as the data are collected. There is greater risk for the development of a therapeutic relationship during the interview and role confusion for both parties. Because human protection guidelines for qualitative research may be less prescriptive, there is more need for ongoing ethical audits beyond annual progress updates. Moreover, the common use of verbal agreements rather than formalized written consent procedures may pose documentation challenges. Robley (1995) noted that the use of case studies as data points makes it difficult to ensure findings are anonymous, thus increasing the vulnerability of subjects to breaches of confidentiality, privacy and psychological or social harms. With the expanding use of the Internet for on-line focus groups, interviews and analysis of social network electronic conversations, the United Kingdom's Royal College of Nursing (RCN), in its research ethics guide, recommends special

TABLE 2.9. Do Nurse Researchers have Special Ethical Challenges? Food for Thought. (Adapted from the Statement on Ethics of Nursing Research, Nursing research section, New Zealand Nurses' Organization. http://www.nursingresearch.co.nz/about/etics.php3?Nurses_Session=049da11c91fd745d9839496a84c490f2 accessed June 10, 2012.

1. Because patient advocacy is central to nursing's code of ethics, the general research population at large—and not just special groups such as the mentally ill or children—should be considered vulnerable.
2. Because the potential for physical harm resulting from nursing research is generally small, there may be a tendency to underestimate other forms of risk, such as the chance of psychological harm.
3. Because of the trust and intimacy inherent in the nurse-patient relationship, nurses have privileged access to multiple sources of formal and informal personal information, which may place them at special risk for breach of confidentiality.
4. As a relatively young academic discipline, there is a critical need to develop the science, yet the pool of experienced nurse researchers is still relatively small, making optimal training not always readily accessible.
5. In the public arena, the professional status of nursing has been ambiguous, and nursing research is still in the process of developing a distinct identity. Thus, the public may not yet have clear expectations for nurses in the researcher role.
6. While the future of nursing research depends upon its success in attracting funding, obtaining research grants is increasingly competitive. Given the current practice to adopt the same strategies which have been successful for other disciplines, nurse investigators may be exposed to the same social pressures and incentives for breaches in scientific integrity and ethical abuses.

protections for maintaining confidentiality, gaining informed consent and determining the identify of research participants when "using cyberspace as a research environment" (Royal College of Nursing, 2009). The RCN report notes that no policies for Internet research currently exist, but recommends that nurses follow the ethical guidelines of the Association of Internet Researchers (http://aoir.org). The two case studies below emphasize different issues relevant to decisions regarding the need for research consent.

2.13.2. Case Studies in Consent: When to Seek IRB Approval

2.13.2.1. Case study #1: Is Pilot Testing a Simple Online Tool OK without IRB approval?

You are a PhD student who is designing a new web-based risk assessment tool to prevent falls in the elderly. Your study population will be community-dwelling home-owners, age 65 and older and living alone. From the adult learning literature and in consultation with your advisor, you have devised a set of audiovisual and graphic tools that requires the user to make appropriate responses using a desktop computer. A focus group of research volunteers will first be tested for overall user acceptability, comprehension of the instructions, and voice preferences. Before you launch the focus group, you plan to ask your 74-yr-old grandfather and 3 of his friends who live on the same floor in an assisted living facility to try out the software and work out any "kinks' in the system to help fine-tune the study protocol. You simply want to see if they can understand the audio commands, read the screen accurately and follow the instructions written at the 6th grade reading level. Because you do not plan to actually assess their fall risk level or use any of their data, you assume that you do not need IRB approval for this pre-pilot test.

2.13.2.2. Case Study #2: Consent to Study Identified Bio-banked Samples

Your first assignment as a part-time research assistant is to obtain 500 donated blood samples from the hospital bio-bank for a genetic biomarkers study. The samples are coded with identifiers to allow future contact and matching with clinical information. You know that your hospital includes standardized language on the admission form that says, "This is a teaching and research institution, and any specimens remaining after your care is complete may be used for teaching and research purposes". When you arrive at the bio-bank facility, the technician tells you that even though the desired blood samples are coded so as to make them unidentifiable to you, you still must have the express permission of each patient in order to gain access to the samples. This seems like a "Catch 22". Is he correct?

2.14. SCIENTIFIC INTEGRITY AND RESPONSIBLE CONDUCT OF RESEARCH

Although scientific integrity is fundamental to the ethical practice of research, it has only been since the 1980s that professional standards for the responsible conduct of research have been comprehensively promulgated by the scientific community. *On Being a Scientist*, now in its third edition (2009), describes the essential behaviors and values for fostering research integrity in early career researchers. First published by the National Academies Press (www.nap.edu) in 1989, the goal of these guidelines are to keep up with the ethical challenges faced by researchers that arise from the pace and complexity of 21st Century science. At the heart of the guidelines, however, are the same moral values that serve as the ethical foundation of everyday life: honesty, fairness, objectivity, openness, trustworthiness, and respect for others. In the context of research, these values translate to practices such as sharing research materials, fairness in reviewing grant proposals and manuscripts, respect for one's colleagues and students, honesty in reporting research results, and the disclosure of potential conflicts of interest.

2.14.1. Research Misconduct

In the 1980s, cases of scientific fraud and negligence in data acquisition, management and reporting prompted the federal government to establish policies for the investigation, review and punishment of the most serious violations of professional standards known as "research misconduct." Overseen by the HHS Office of Research Integrity (ORI), research misconduct includes the intentional or reckless acts of "fabrication, falsification, and plagiarism in proposing, performing, or reviewing research, or in reporting research results." (Box 2.6). Other types of standards violations are considered to be "questionable research practices" such as mistakes caused by negligence due to haste, carelessness or inattention. In keeping with ORI policies, all research institutions that receive federal funds must have policies and procedures in place to investigate, report and manage research misconduct, and anyone who is aware of a potential act of misconduct must follow these policies and procedures. Although primarily emphasizing ethi-

Box 2.6 - Definitions of Research Misconduct

- **Fabrication** is making up data or results and recording or reporting them.
- **Falsification** is manipulating research materials, equipment or processes or changing or omitting data or results such that the research is not accurately represented in the research record.
- **Plagiarism** is the appropriation of another person's ideas, processes, results or words without giving appropriate credit.

As expressly noted in the CFR, Research misconduct does not include honest error or differences of opinion (minutes of the Secretary's Advisory Committee on Human Research Protections, July 19, 2011,pg 20, http://www.hhs.gov/ohrp/sachrp/mtgings/mtg07-11/july2011minutes.pdf.pdf).

cal dilemmas confronted by "bench scientists", the ORI has become increasingly active in the education and training of students in avoiding research misconduct, offering on-line video case studies for resolving ethical challenges and clarifying responsible conduct (http://ori.hhs.gov/thelab).

2.15. MENTORSHIP IN ETHICAL RESEARCH PRACTICES

The NIH places special emphasis on the importance of mentorship as part of the obligation to train the next generation of responsible scientists. The NIH specifically recommends that all research fellows and trainees receive both formal and informal instruction in the responsible conduct of research that involves a variety of formats throughout the entire training experience. "While online courses can be a valuable supplement to instruction in responsible conduct of research, online instruction is not considered adequate as the sole means of instruction." http://grants1.nih.gov/grants/guide/notice-files/NOT-OD-10-019.html In addition, other federal requirements regarding training for investigators must be met, such as the National Institute of Health's (NIH) requirement for the training of key personnel in NIH-sponsored or -conducted human subjects research. Ultimately, it is the principle or lead investigator who is accountable for the training of the research team in ethical practices. Topics covered typically include data acquisition and management, research misconduct, responsible authorship and avoiding conflicts of interest.

2.15.1. Case Study: Mentorship and Responsibilities of the Investigator

You're a DNP student who has just been hired as a part-time research assistant to help start up a new clinical study. The study is designed to identify early cancer bio-markers in individuals considered healthy and without overt clinical evidence of disease. The Principle Investigator, a molecular biologist, has already demonstrated elevated concentrations of a plasma protein produced in the liver in mice who develop spontaneous hepatomas. The animals with a specific genetic polymorphism in the protein's DNA remain healthy. This polymorphism is also present in humans in approximately 20% of the population. The next phase of the study will be to retrieve archived blood samples from the hospital's bio-bank to conduct research assays, DNA genotyping and characterize patient samples with and without the polymorphism. In the last phase of the project, a subset of the former patients in both groups will be contacted to participate in a detailed work-up of liver function. The PI is not a clinician and is relying on your clinical expertise and training to help carry out the recruitment and conduct of the clinical protocol, once patients are involved. You tell him you have already completed all the online training required by your university, and therefore can proceed with the studies.

In addition to going against the NIH recommendation to include more than online web-based training in research ethics, what's wrong with this approach?

2.16. CONFLICTS OF INTEREST IN RESEARCH

"In academic research, the relationships between researchers and industry are critically important for the healthy exchange of ideas, opportunities and resources. These relationships can give rise to significant discoveries and to the translation of those discoveries into useful products. . . . The financial incentives that accompany such relationships, however, may lead to financial conflicts of interest that have the potential to create real or apparent bias in research. Conflicts of interest may affect research integrity, and in the case of human subjects research, may place research subjects at additional risk . . . even the appearance of the conflict of interest may reduce confidence in the research enterprise generally, and in Columbia in particular." (slide 3, Training Course TC0091, Financial Conflicts of Interest, Office of Research Compliance and Training, Columbia University).

As noted on Columbia University's website on research compliance and training (http://www.columbia.edu/cu/compliance/docs/conflict_interest/index.html), a conflict of interest (COI) exists when a researcher's outside employment or personal activities could improperly affect, or give the appearance of affecting, the researcher's primary responsibilities supported by her academic institution and research sponsor(s). Due to a growing concern that academic scientists were being unduly influenced by the pharmaceutical industry and other for-profit business opportunities, the Public Health Service issued the regulation "Responsibility of Applicants for Promoting Objectivity in Research for which PHS Funding is Sought" in 1995 (42 C.F.R. Part 50, Subpart F). Its purpose was to provide transparency to the public about potential and real conflicting financial interests of individuals and institutions applying for federal grants. Such interests were defined as stocks or other interests in companies, royalties or license fees, or directorships and management roles. The rule defined the nature of financial interests to be disclosed, and called for each institution to develop a management plan, including public disclosure procedures, enforcement mechanisms and sanctions. (An example of a public access website for COI disclosures used by the Columbia University Medical Center can be found at: https://www.rascal.columbia.edu/public/coi).

Investigators are responsible for updating their financial disclosures annually and within 30 days when circumstances change substantially. Typically, a special Conflict of Interest Review Committee, separate from the IRB, oversees and reviews disclosures. Because the relevance of financial interest may vary with research proposals, investigators must also submit an updated, protocol-specific COI disclosure each time a new or continuing application to the IRB for human subjects research is submitted. In 2011, the PHS rule was amended to expand disclosure rules to cover financial interests of investigators, including student-investigators (and their immediate families) related to all "institutional responsibilities" (clinical care, education, committees), in addition to research. The level of "significant" financial interest was lowered from $10,000 to $5,000, and now covers payments for travel, as well as consulting and honoraria. Although the rule extends to relationships with non-profit groups, investigators do not have to include (1) salary paid by the institution or (2) income from seminars, lectures, teaching, service on advisory committees or review panels sponsored by a Federal, state or local government agency, a U.S. institution of higher education, an academic teaching hospital, a medical center, or a research institute affiliated with a U.S. institution of higher education (HHS Office of Extramural Research http://grants.nih.gov/grants/policy/coi/index.htm).

2.17. THE NURSE EXPERT AS CONSULTANT

As doctoral students launch their practice and research careers, they will participate in a variety of scientific meetings, continuing education programs and consultancies to report on research findings or provide expert opinion and knowledge on best practices. Most professional organizations, hospitals and other public or private institutions now require that speakers/consultants disclose in advance any potential or real conflicts of interest, including financial, professional or personal relationships that could influence or bias their remarks. An example in Box 2.7 provides a typical Speaker Disclosure Form for information about the nature and management of potential conflicts.

Box 2.7 - Example of a Statement of Speaker's Disclosure and Resolution of Vested Interests. (modified from a Speaker's Form for Disclosure of Potential Conflicts of Interest, Montefiore Hospital Nursing Research Committee/Nursing Department, New York, NY, 2012.)

A. Is there a financial, professional, or personal relationship that could potentially bias the content of the educational activity?

If yes, please list the companies and type of relationship (e.g., Research Support, Speaker's Bureau, Consultant, Shareholder, Other Support, Other):

If yes, you must disclose this information during your presentation. How will you do this? (e.g., Information provided in handouts, audiovisuals (slides, overhead, etc.)

If verbal disclosure is made, there must be a written verification on the part of the sponsor who was in attendance, which attests that a verbal disclosure did occur and that identifies the contents of the verbal disclosure).

B. How have you resolved this potential conflict of interest?

- The conflict has been discussed with the individual who is now aware of and agrees to our policy.
- Presenter has signed a statement that says s/he will present information fairly and without bias.
- An RN with minimum of a baccalaureate degree will monitor session to ensure conflict does not arise.
- Other. Please describe:

C. Disclosure of Unlabeled Use

Is there intent to discuss the use of a product/medication for a purpose other than that for which it was approved by the FDA? If yes, you must disclose this information during your presentation. How will you do this?

The signature is required (faxed, scanned, handwritten, or a digitally verified signature are acceptable)

Signature Date

2.18. ETHICAL PRACTICES FOR SCIENTIFIC WRITING

Because of the weight given to academic publishing as a measure of investigator success, peer recognition, and worthiness for promotion and tenure, beginning scholars may need specific training in professional writing standards. The HHS Office of Scientific Integrity has developed a web-based tutorial for recognizing and avoiding questionable writing practices ("Avoiding plagiarism, self-plagiarism, and other questionable writing practices: A guide to ethical writing" by Miguel Roig at http://ori.hhs.gov/plagiarism-0). The resource offers a set of definitions, guidelines and training exercises for the practice of ethical scientific writing. Of Professor Roig's 26 guidelines, those most relevant for the doctorally-prepared nurse writing data-based, research reports are the following:

- Plans for authorship (including order of authors) should be in place at the start of research collaborations with the designated contributors aware of their roles and responsibilities that are based on well-accepted guidelines.
- In the spirit of honesty and openness, researchers have an ethical obligation to disclose sufficient details of the study design and methodologies so that others can independently replicate the findings.
- To avoid the appearance of misrepresentation of the quality and volume of data-based papers, authors should avoid publishing complex research findings in serial publications or publishing reports that contain primarily old data with a few new data points included.
- Study results should be published in the context of the originally proposed data analysis plans; alternative statistical approaches used in the course of data analysis (e.g., the elimination of outliers) must be well-described and justified.
- Investigators have an obligation to consider alternative interpretations of their findings, to report and reconcile evidence that contradicts their hypotheses, and alternatively, to use only methodologically sound evidence to support their findings.

2.18.1. Unacceptable Writing Practices

Professor Roig also notes a series of unethical writing practices including: " assignment of authorship as a courtesy to administrators/employers or study funders with no other role; use of professional "ghost" authors where the work is credited solely to the investigator; (and the) inappropriate assignment by mentors of credit to students or (alternatively) failure to acknowledge student work" (These ethical guidelines have been modified from M. Roig, 26 Guidelines at a Glance at: http://ori.hhs.gov/plagiarism-0).

It is important to read carefully the author's instructions prior to submitting a research study to a particular journal, as required content varies from journal to journal. For example, the authors' guidelines for the journal, Nursing Research, (http://edmgr.ovid.com/nres/accounts/ifauth.htm) recommends the use of the following scientific standards and ethical practices for the submission of manuscripts for publication:

- De-identification of authors in the body of the manuscript to aid the reviewers in an anonymous review.
- Guidelines for avoiding plagiarism (e.g., see the AJN plagiarism policy on the AJN Web site (http://www.editorialmanager.com/ajn/).
- The CONSORT guidelines for reporting randomized controlled trial (RCT) (http://www.consort-statement.org).
- The PRISMA (Preferred Reporting Items for Systematic Reviews and Meta-Analyses) guideline (http://www.prisma-statement.org/) for reporting a systematic review and meta-analysis.
- An explicit statement in the manuscript affirming the status for institutional review of human or animal subjects.

2.18.2. Authorship and the Allocation of Credit

For beginning nurse researchers, determining the composition and order of authorship in academic work is perhaps one of the thorniest issues to manage. Although students' scholarship may reflect their own independent work in collaboration with their advisor, in general, other individuals should be included as a co-author if they "make a substantial intellectual contribution to the design of the research, the interpretation of the data, and the drafting of the paper" (Committee of the NAS, NAE, IOM, 2009).

As pointed out by the authors of the well-respected report, *On Being A Scientist* (Committee of the NAS, NAE, IOM, 2009), there are two reasons for determining authorship: fairness in recognition, and responsibility for the content. However, as more and more research is conducted in multidisciplinary teams, with diverse research perspectives and journal policies, the level of incongruity and disagreement about authorship rules may rise. The report's authors go on to observe that "the distribution of accountability can be especially difficult in interdisciplinary research. Authors from one discipline may say that they are not responsible for the accuracy of material provided by authors from another discipline. A contrasting view is that each author must be confident of the accuracy of everything in the paper—perhaps by having a trusted colleague read the parts of the paper outside one's own discipline. One obvious but often overlooked solution to this problem is to add a footnote accompanying the list of authors that apportions responsibility for different parts of the paper."

The International Committee of Medical Journal Editors is the rec-

TABLE 2.10. Definitions for Determining Level of Contributor Role in Data-based Reports (from: Uniform Requirements for Manuscripts Submitted to Biomedical Journals: Ethical Considerations in the Conduct and Reporting of Research: Authorship and Contributorship at: http://www.icmje.org/ethical_1author.html).

Authors must fulfill all 3 criteria:
• Contributed substantially to the conception and design of the study, the acquisition of data, or the analysis and interpretation; • Drafted or provided critical revision of the article; • Provided final approval of the version to be published.
Acknowledged contributors:
Individuals contributing to the manuscript but who do not meet the criteria for authorship *Note:* Because readers may infer their endorsement of the data and conclusions, these persons must give written permission to be acknowledged.

ognized body that sets the standard requirements for manuscripts submitted to biomedical journals (http://www.icmje.org/about.html). Most journals, including those in nursing, follow their suggested guidelines for distinguishing recognized authors from acknowledged contributors (Table 2.10).

A suggested format for the content and language of the acknowledgements section of a research report is provided in Box 2.8.

Box 2.8 - Example of Language and Content for the Acknowledgments Section of a Research Report.

Authors' contributions

NN led the study, developed initial interpretations of the data and drafted and revised the manuscript. MG reviewed initial data analysis summaries and made substantial revisions to draft versions of the manuscript. CA conducted the interviews, assisted with the data analysis and reviewed versions of the manuscript. All authors read and approved the final manuscript.

Acknowledgements

We are indebted to the patients who served as research volunteers. We also thank the Institutes of Health Research (grant number) for funding for this project. Staff member X kindly provided assistance with subject recruitment and the IRB approvals. Professor Y served as scientific advisor and critically reviewed the study proposal. Nurse Colleague collected clinical data and cared for study patients. First Author is supported by a New Investigator Award from the Institute of Health Policy Research. The sponsors' support of this work should not imply endorsement of the conclusions, for which the authors retain sole responsibility.

Box 2.9 - Case study on Authorship and the Allocation of Credit

Dr. Ima Leader, PhD is a nationally-known nurse-scientist who directs the Biobehavioral Nursing Research Laboratory, an NIH-funded research center, at Renowned University School of Nursing. Her program has its own policy about authorship, which Leader discusses with each new member who joins her lab: (1) only those who have made a significant intellectual contribution to a project will be included on any paper; and (2) Leader is the final authority, should a disagreement arise, on what is defined as a significant intellectual contribution. Although not explicitly stated, it is common knowledge that Leader will be included as last (senior) author on any paper that results from research done in her program.

You are a third-year PhD nursing student being mentored by Dr. Leader. Your dissertation study aims to adapt a novel self-management approach for menopause symptoms in Hispanic breast cancer survivors that applies biobehavioral stress concepts using social networking. The project is funded as a small pilot study from several federal funding sources, including an RO1 (investigator initiated project), a Training Grant to support pre- and postdoctoral fellows, and pilot studies funds from the NIH Center program grant to Dr. Leader, who is the principal investigator on all projects. You work with several other trainees more senior to you, a postdoctoral fellow, and several junior nursing faculty, all involved in varying ways with the project.

Based on social networking principles, you have adapted an "off-the-shelf" model of a healthy lifestyle program for an intervention protocol in a way that has never been done (to your knowledge). Your dissertation study is a pilot test of the feasibility of the design and protocol in the target population.

In the weekly lab meetings you meet with the entire Center personnel to discuss your project, along with the other projects under Dr. Leader's direction. The discussions tend to be informal, with opportunities to trouble shoot problems with study design or challenges to progress. Two individuals are particularly encouraging with ideas on how to proceed in your research. Assistant Professor Dr. Colab Orator, PhD, an informatician, has sent you three articles on informatics, with lengthy emails from which you have gleaned a number of insights about alternative interpretations of the data that ultimately made it into the discussion section of your first poster presentation. Dr. Pearla Wisdom, RN, MS, PhD , is a 2nd year postdoctoral fellow who understands the research planning process. She usually gives you insights on how to navigate the system to complete the IRB applications, progress reports, and get to the right people for quick answers. This is always in hallway discussions after the meeting or during open dialogue on the agenda items.

Dr. Nancy Nurse, DNP directs a community nursing practice where patients will be recruited. She is a seasoned clinician who has worked with Dr. Leader for many years as a consultant on clinical issues. She has worked very closely with you on facilitating recruitment of study participants, doing most of the troubleshooting and optimization of procedures for your intervention protocol.

(continued)

Box 2.9 (continued) - Case study on Authorship and the Allocation of Credit

Ms. Bea Quik, BSN is a first year graduate student who is currently doing a six-week rotation through Leader's lab. She assists you in a highly focused, state-of-the-science literature review of data mining applications for cell phone-delivered health care interventions. While conducting the review, she uncovers new insights from the literature that suggested that this approach would be a good model for protocol testing.

Dr Leader encourages you to submit the systematic review for publication as quickly as possible. You do the writing, give the paper to Leader for review, and then present the findings at the lab meeting the following week. Following the meeting, Dr Orator sends an email to you, asking if she can be the "senior" author on your paper, as it would strengthen her CV in a needed area of expertise in time for her upcoming promotion review. You are a bit surprised as you had not planned on including her at all as a co-author. Your plan was to include Ms Quick as second author and Dr Leader as the last author on the paper since the work was done in her lab and supported by funds from her program.

(This hypothetical vignette is adapted from a case study for engineers by Daniel Vallero found at the website http://www.onlineethics.org/Resources/Cases/Chaos.aspx . It has been tailored to authorship practices relevant to those encountered by practice and research faculty in schools of nursing, students and other research team members).

Discussion Questions:

1. What should be the order of authorship for this manuscript?
2. Who should receive an acknowledgment? Omitted completely?
3. To whom or where would you go to seek authorship advice?

2.19. GENERAL RESOURCES

Belmont Report: Ethical Principles and Guidelines for the Protection of Human Subjects of Research. The National Commission for the Protection of Human Subjects of Biomedical and Behavioral Research, HEW, 1979 http://www.hhs.gov/ohrp/humansubjects/guidance/belmont.html

TRAINING IN RESEARCH ETHICS Collaborative Institutional Training Initiative. CITI is a subscription service providing research ethics education to all members of the research community. To participate fully, learners must be affiliated with a CITI participating organization.

Committee on Science, Engineering, and Public Policy, National Academy of Sciences, National Academy of Engineering, and Institute of Medicine. *On Being a Scientist: A Guide to Responsible Conduct in Research,* 3rd Edition. 2009. Washington DC: National Academies Press. www.nap.edu accessed July 3, 2012.

Informed Consent – FAQs. http://answers.hhs.gov/ohrp/categories/1566

The International Committee of Medical Journal Editors. Uniform Requirements for Manuscripts Submitted to Biomedical Journals, http://www.icmje.org/about.html

Resources for Research Ethics Education. Website of the National Advisory Panel on Research Integrity (http://research-ethics.net/)

2.20. REFERENCES

American Nurses' Association (ANA). (1985). *Human Rights Guidelines for Nurses in Clinical and Other Research.* Kansas City, MO.

Anderson, E. E. (2010). The role of community-based organizations in the recruitment of human subjects: ethical considerations. *The American Journal of Bioethics*, 20–21.

Appelbaum, P.S., Lidz, C.W. and Grisso, T. (2004) Therapeutic misconception in clinical research: frequency and risk factors. *IRB: Ethics and Human Research 26*: 1–8.

Beauchamp, T.L. and Childress, J.F. (2009) *Principles of Biomedical Ethics,* 6th Edition. New York: Oxford University Press.

Corbie-Smith, G. (1999) The continuing legacy of the Tuskegee Syphilis study: Considerations for clinical investigation. *Am. J. Med. Science* 317: 5–8.

Fowler, M.D.M. (2010) *Guide to the Code of Ethics for Nurses: Interpretation and Application.* Silver Spring, MD: American Nurses Association.

Friedan, T.R. and Collins, F.S. (2010) Intentional infection of vulnerable populations in 1946-1948: another tragic history lesson. *JAMA 304*: 2063–64.

Fouka, G. and Mantzorou, M. (2011). What are the major ethical issues in conducting research? Is there a conflict between research ethics and the nature of nursing? *Health Science J. 5*(1): 3–14.

Grady, C. and Edgerly, M. (2009). Science, technology and innovation: nursing responsibilities in clinical research. *Nurs. Clin. North Am. 44*: 471–481.

Guttman, Amy. "Ethically Impossible" The Blog, for The Huffington Post, posted 9/14/2011. http://www.huffingtonpost.com/amy-gutmann/guatemala-syphilis_b_963035.html, accessed 8/272012.

Haigh, C. and Jones, N. (2005). An overview of the ethics of cyberspace research and the implication for nurse educators. *Nurse Education Today 25*: 3–8.

Hauser, J. (2011) Legal and regulatory considerations in research. In: *Nursing Research: Reading, Using and Creating Evidence,* Second Ed., pp. 53–99. Jones and Bartlett Publishers.

Morse, J.M. (2007) Ethics in action: ethical principles for doing qualitative health research. *Qual Health Research 17*: 1003–05.

National Advisory Panel on Research Integrity (NAPRI) http://research-ethics.net/introduction/NAPRI/#overview

Noble-Adams, R. (1999) Ethics and nursing research. 1: Development, theories and principles. *Br. J. Nurs. 8*(13):888–92.

NOH. (2003) Protecting Personal Health Information in Research: Understanding the HIPAA Privacy Rule. NOH Publ # 03-5388. http://privacyruleandresearch.nih.gov/HIPAA_Booklet_4-14-2003.rtf; accessed June 26, 2012

Olson, D.P., for the Working Group for the Study of Ethical Issues in International Nursing research. (2003) Ethical considerations for international nursing research: A report from the international centre for nursing ethics. *Nursing Ethics 10*: 122–137.

Presidential Commission for the Study of Bioethical Issues. (2011) "Ethically Impossible" STD Research in Guatemala from 1946 to 1948. Washington, DC, September, 2011. www.bioethics.gov

Resnik, D.B. (2009) The clinical investigator-subject relationship: a contextual approach. *Philosophy, Ethics, and Humanities in Medicine 4*:16.

Reverby, S. (2001) More than fact and fiction: Cultural memory and the Tuskegee Syphilis Study. *Hastings Center Report* 2001; Sept/October: 22–28.

Reverby, S. (2011) The art of medicine: listening to narratives of the Tuskegee Syphilis Study. *Lancet 377*:1646–47.

Robley, L.R. (1995) The ethics of qualitative nursing research. *J. Prof. Nursing 11*:45–48. http://www.sciencedirect.com/science/article/pii/S8755722395800727. Accessed June 10, 2012.

Rohan, A., Monk, K., Marder, K. and Reame, N.E. (2011) Prenatal toxicology substance abuse screening in research: codes and consequences. *Substance Abuse 32*:159–164.

Truog, R.D. (2012) Patients and doctors: the evolution of a relationship. *New Eng. J. Med. 366*:581–85.

Twomey, J.G. (2010) *Provision Three. In: Guide to the Code of Ethics for Nurses: Interpretation and Application.* Silver Spring, MD: American Nurses Association, pp. 24–39.

U.S. Dept of HHS Office of Scientific Integrity. Guidelines for Avoiding Plagiarism and Other Questionable Writing Practices. http://ori.hhs.gov/plagiarism-0

World Medical Association General Assembly. (2008) Declaration of Helsinki, Ethical Principles for Medical Research Involving Human Subjects. 6th revision, October 2008. http://www.wma.net/en/20activities/10ethics/10helsinki/. Accessed Aug 21, 2012.

CHAPTER 3

Ethical Guidelines Particular to Practice

COURTNEY REINISCH

Clinical patient care is guided by knowledge, competency, and the maintenance of ethical standards. Maintenance of ethical standards is one area shared by all care providers. Attention should be paid to the following ethical tenets: autonomy, beneficence, non-malfeasance, justice, veracity, and confidentiality. Paternalism is an ethical concern to providers. Providers who demonstrate a thorough understanding of ethical principles serve both the patient and themselves and strengthen the patient's trust with adherence to ethical standards.

3.1. AUTONOMY

Autonomy allows a patient to make decisions that affect their needs: free from deceit, duress, constraint or coercion. Patients are to be informed participants in the decision-making process. Autonomy respects personal freedom for both the patient and clinician. This respect enhances professionalism within the clinical encounter.

Inherent to the principle of autonomy is the concept of informed consent. Patients have the right to be properly informed of their state of health, be it illness or wellness. Risks and benefits of any procedures that will be used to assess and treat them should be clearly described in order to facilitate patient decision-making regarding their own care. Discussions regarding treatment options and the decision to treat or not to treat are necessary to allow the patient to be thoroughly informed prior to consent.

When discussing risk and benefits of treatment, the APRN should speak in a manner which is understandable to the patient. This may present a challenge when patients' native languages are different from the APRN's or when patients' literacy levels are limited. Efforts must be employed to ensure the patient understands what is being discussed. Interpretation services should be used to confirm consent is truly informed.

Additionally, when providing written information to patients, forms must be written at an appropriate literacy level. When dealing with patients with literacy issues, written informed consent may be challenging to obtain. In these cases, the form should be read to the individual to ensure their comprehension. Again, forms for consent should be available in the patient's native language to ensure understanding.

Another challenge in obtaining informed consent is the concept of health literacy. Individuals may be able to read and write above the fourth grade level; however, how literate are they regarding their health, the concepts, and language used by health care providers? When discussing a procedure or treatment, the APRN must be cautious about the language and terminology used when speaking with patients. What is common knowledge and easily understood by providers may be unclear to the patient. Therefore, the patient may give consent without a true understanding of what was presented.

The APRN who respects the principle of autonomy respects the individual's freedom to make their own decisions. For example, an 89 year old female presents to her internist as she is preparing to travel with her family. The patient lives in the community with an aide due to Alzheimer's dementia. She is forgetful at times regarding appointments, keys, and pots on the stove. She no longer drives or cooks, as these tasks are completed by the assistant. The patient is oriented to person, place, location, and time. She knows the names of all her family members.

The patient advises the provider she will be traveling with her daughter's family to a location at 5000 feet elevation. The internist advises the patient and her daughter that he would not advise this patient to travel due to the risks associated with air travel and being at high altitudes. The internist is acting paternalistically although he believes he is working from the standpoint of beneficence.

The patient and her daughter consult the APRN for a second opinion. The APRN understands the concern for the effects of altitude and possible anxiety associated with air travel. However, the APRN respects the patient's autonomy. She asks the patient, "Do you want to go on this trip?" The 89 year old patient confirms that she really wants to travel with her family. Although this patient has Alzheimer's dementia, she is able to articulate her desires. Understanding the risks, the APRN develops a plan for the patient to travel with her family.

3.2. BENEFICENCE

Beneficence is defined as the principle of doing "good". It involves doing as much good as possible in order to benefit another. It may consist of a positive action which removes or prevents the patient's problem. Beneficence strives to promote the very best.

Doing "good" sounds like a reasonable charge; however, this may be a challenge for the practicing APRN. When evaluating a 69 year old obese male patient for right leg pain who presents to the emergency department due to a fall, the APRN determines that the patient has no fractures or thrombosis, a history of chronic back pain, and recurrent lower extremity cellulitis. This patient is unable to ambulate during this evaluation and the APRN calls the patient's primary care provider to discuss possible admission to the hospital for physical therapy evaluation and potential sub-acute placement. In the APRN's opinion, it is not safe to discharge this patient to home as he lives alone and is unable to care for himself. The APRN is acting utilizing the principle of beneficence.

The APRN respects the patient's autonomy and discusses the proposed plan with the patient. The patient verbalizes understanding of the issues and the reasons for admission. He agrees that this seems like a reasonable plan. However, when the APRN speaks to the patient's primary care physician, she is met with resistance. The PCP suggests that the APRN is not telling the truth, and that the patient could walk if he so chose. The APRN advocates for the patient and the patient was admitted. Although doing "good" seems a reasonable goal for the APRN, it may be a challenge.

3.3. NONMALEFICENCE

Nonmaleficence is defined as "do no harm nor inflict damage to another". Nonmalficence is embodied in the principle of Primum Non Nocere. It is reflected in the Hippocratic Oath as "physician—do no harm". Treatment for a particular patient's diagnosis may not balance the risks associated with the treatment when a risk-benefit analysis is considered. Ergo, a provider may choose to not perform a procedure or intervention if there is an increased risk of doing harm.

When considering any treatment, the prudent APRN will consider both the risks and the benefits to the patient. For example, a 29 year old patient with end-stage leukemia requests to enroll in a clinical trial to appease her parents' request for her to not resign herself to hospice and palliative care. In the parents' view, accepting hospice care would be "giving up." The APRN is challenged to accept this patient's request. The risks associated with the clinical trial include side effects of the medications and possibly no effect of the treatment to slow or stop the progression of the patient's disease. The risk of death is inherent in the case, as the patient is already dying. The benefits for the patient could be a possible improvement in her condition to the point of (although highly unlikely) possible eradication of her disease.

When considering care for this patient the concepts of autonomy, veracity, and beneficence must be considered in this type of decision making. The APRN wants to respect the autonomy of the 29 year old patient with leukemia to make her own decisions. The APRN is truthful about the risks and benefits of the treatment being considered and the APRN wants the patient to benefit from a proposed treatment.

Evidence-based treatment guidelines may also be employed when considering a risk benefit analysis. The acceptance and treatment within guidelines provides benefit to the majority of the patients, not the exceptions to the rule. Providers use guidelines to provide benefit to the average patient.

3.4. JUSTICE

Justice includes the concepts of fairness and entitlement. Fairness encompasses the distribution of goods and services as well as equitability amongst a society. Fairness evaluates who receives benefits and to what degree. Patients are entitled to be treated in a fair and equal manner regardless of ethnicity, social status, religious beliefs, or any other social or personal uniqueness.

The APRN may serve justice in the system by utilizing evidence-based guidelines which have been shown to provide positive patient outcomes. By following guideline-based care for patients with diabetes, the APRN may optimize the patient's glucose levels. This may then prevent future, costly complications to the patient and the health care system at large.

The APRN who respects health care resources as limited and valuable understands distributive justice. Distributive justice is an important concept when considering health care services as a right for all or when considering a social system of health care services. The APRN who is able to deliver high quality care at an affordable price will be a key player in restricting healthcare costs for the U.S.

3.5. VERACITY

Veracity refers to truth telling. It involves comprehensive, accurate and objective communication of information between the practitioner and patient. The obligation of veracity is closely linked with fidelity. Fidelity requires an agreement and kept promise. Veracity and fidelity prohibit deceit. These ethical tenets protect trust. Patients cannot be expected to trust a care provider if they are not provided the truth. Truth telling is at the core of the provider-patient relationship and is required for the establishment of a trusting relationship.

Developing a strong patient-provider relationship may be difficult due to today's practice environment. APRNs may be pushed to see a high volume of patients which may reduce time spent with each individual patient. APRNs may be part of a large multi-provider practice where patients are seen by a different provider at each visit. Patients may research their diagnoses on the Internet prior to accessing care. Their research may result in a different diagnosis than the APRN reaches and they may challenge the APRN's decision. These factors may limit the APRN's opportunity to establish a relationship.

Truth telling seems straight forward, but there are times when this may be a challenge for the APRN. When the APRN must deliver news of a difficult diagnosis, the APRN must be straightforward, but not overwhelming. Culture may influence truth telling. In certain cultures and religions, it is not acceptable to plan for end of life. The APRN may also be asked by family members to not tell the truth to a patient with a terminal diagnosis. The APRN may have to speak to a patient without family present in order to have an honest discussion.

There are times when the APRN may be instructed not to tell the patient the truth. An example is when a nurse advises the APRN that she will need to repeat a phlebotomy procedure due to improper labeling of the tubes by another nurse who is now off duty. The nurse wants to tell the patient that the specimen was hemolysed and therefore needs to be re-drawn. This is not the truth, but told to the patient rather than telling them the specimen was not properly labeled. The nurse's intentions are not to harm the patient, but what does the APRN do in this situation? Should she support this lie?

An attending physician may instruct an APRN not to tell a patient about a mass seen on a chest radiograph. Rather, the physician may advise the APRN to tell the patient that an admission is required due to an abnormality seen on the radiograph. The plan is to advise the patients of the mass when it is confirmed after further imaging studies are complete. This is not exactly lying, but the truth is withheld until a later time. The APRN may advise the attending physician that she sees withholding information as morally wrong and will therefore advise the patient the truth.

3.6. CONFIDENTIALITY

Confidentiality protects patient's privileged information and guards a care provider's trustworthiness. Patients surrender some privacy by divulging privileged information to a health care provider. It is important to note that in this process, they do not surrender control over how the information is used. Confidentiality obligates the provider to not share privileged information without permission from the patient. Trust is weakened if the patient fears unauthorized disclosure and will impede the provider's ability to care for the patient.

Federal guidelines have been enacted to protect patient confidentiality. The Health Insurance Portability and Accountability Act (HIPAA) is a federal law intended to protect patient privacy by limiting identifiable data and establishing how this information may be used. Information includes anything related to the past, present or future of that patient's physical or mental health where there is an identifiable piece. Since the Health Information Technology for Economic and Clinical Health (HITECH) Act was passed in 2009, the scope of Health Insurance and Portability and Accountability Act's (HIPAA) privacy and security protections has expanded to notifying patients of privacy breaches (Fisher & Clayton, 2012).

The consequences of violating HIPAA may result in both civil and criminal penalties, including fines and possible jail time. A health care provider may be individually sued for defamation, invasion of privacy or harassment and face personal liability. APRNs must use caution to protect patient confidentiality and avoid HIPAA violations.

Social media is a growing technology with potential for unintentional HIPAA violations. Misconduct on social media websites may raise liability under state or federal regulations focused on preventing patient abuse or exploitation. If the health care provider's conduct violates the policies of the employer, the provider may face employment consequences, including termination. The reputation of the health care organization may be at stake when a HIPAA violation occurs (NCSBN, 2011).

APRNs now face new challenges in protecting patient confidentiality. The majority of patients, family, and providers use smart phones in their daily lives. These phones have Internet capability at the touch of the fingertip. An APRN may see a patient while the patient is posting on a social media site about the visit. The patient may wish to photograph a procedure being performed by the APRN during the visit. The patient being an autonomous individual may choose to do this; however, the APRN must be careful when using a social media website not to post patient identifying information.

When consulting a specialist, the APRN may wish to share information with the other provider. The APRN may want to email a picture of a wound or a radiograph to the specialist. Sharing information with another provider involved in the care of a patient is not a violation of privacy. However, using an unsecure means to deliver this information may be a violation of HIPAA. APRNs need to use caution when sharing information with other providers to avoid HIPAA and institutional violations.

3.7. PATERNALISM

Paternalism permits health care professionals to act on behalf of the patient if the patient is not able to choose or act for him or herself. Paternalism, when utilized in conjunction with autonomy and veracity, allows the practitioner to assist the patient in care related decisions. The provider must act in the fiduciary relationship, placing the needs of the patient above their own personal needs, and the needs of others. This may prove challenging when there are opposing views on the particular treatment of a patient.

Paternalistic decisions may occur in the emergency or surgical setting. The APRN in anesthesia may make a decision to provide additional pain relief during a surgical procedure based on vital sign changes. The patient under anesthesia care is unable to verbalize the need for additional pain relief, but the provider will make that decision.

If any of these seven ethical tenets—autonomy, beneficence, nonmalfeasance, justice, veracity, and paternalism—are challenged, a provider will face an ethical dilemma. Understanding these tenets will guide the provider to resolve the dilemma. This may still prove difficult and result in moral uncertainty and distress.

3.8. MORAL UNCERTAINTY, DILEMMAS, DISTRESS, FATIGUE—JUSTICE

The term moral certainty is associated with probability. Moral certainty is achieved with a very high degree of probability, sufficient for action, but short of absolute or mathematical certainty (Cohen and Erikson, 2006). Thus moral uncertainty lacks certainty or probability, and makes action questionable. When the resolution is not transparent, it is difficult for the health care provider to act. The APRN may choose to enlist the opinion of an expert and utilize a group to decrease uncertainty.

Bart Kosko is a writer, researcher, and professor of electrical engineering and law. He is known for popularizing fuzzy logic. Kosko (1993) advises, "The more information we have about a fact, the less we tend to blame the fact on probability or 'luck'" and, he asserts, "Total information leaves little room for probability." (p. 45). Complete and accurate records vastly reduce the probability of waste, fraud, and abuse. According to Kosko, the fuzzy principle means that everything is a matter of degree. In science, he notes that fuzziness is formally known by the term multi-valence and its opposite is bivalence. Fuzziness means that three or more options occur and perhaps an infinite number of them exist. The difference between truth and falsehood is defined on a continuum, rather than as an either/or choice. (pp. 18,19)

Kosko says adaptive fuzzy systems "suck the brains" of experts. Experts are not required to tell the system what makes them experts. The merely need to "act like experts." Doing so provides the data the neural nets needed to "find and tune the rules." (pp. 39,40). It is assumed the meaning derived from the records created by "experts" will be of higher quality, value, and utility than those created by those who are less skillful in the discipline in question.

In *The Wisdom of Crowds,* James Surowiecki (2005) argues that "under the right circumstances, groups are remarkably intelligent, and are often smarter than the smartest people in them." According to Surowiecki, if four basic conditions are met, a crowd's "collective intelligence" will produce better outcomes than a small group of experts. Crowd wisdom needs: (1) diversity of opinion; (2) independence of members from one another; (3) decentralization; and (4) a good method for aggregating opinions (p. 10). The diversity brings in different information; independence keeps people from being swayed by a leader with a single opinion; people's errors balance each other out; and including all opinions guarantees that the results are "smarter" than if a single expert had been in charge (p. 22).

Thinking Fast and Slow, by economist Daniel Kahneman (2011), proposes a brain governed by two clashing decision-making processes. The largely unconscious brain makes intuitive snap judgments based on emotion, memory, and hard-wired rules of thumb. The painfully conscious brain checks the facts and does the math, but is so "lazy" and distractible that it usually defers to the system which utilizes snap judgments. This is important for the practicing APRN to consider in order to avoid making snap decisions.

Cohen and Erikson (2006) advise that nurses are challenged to fulfill every professional core duty and responsibility in their everyday practice. Nurses commonly encounter clinical situations that contain ethical conflicts. Examples include administering futile care to an end of life patient against their expressed wishes because the family insists. Another nurse reports that while a surgeon is operating, she was asked to push the button on his Bluetooth so he may talk on the phone. A nurse may be involved in administering CPR to an elderly patient with terminal cancer whose family has just rescinded the do not resuscitate order. Unresolved conflicts may cause feelings of frustration and powerlessness, especially when nurses are faced with circumstances associated with moral uncertainty or distress (Cohen and Erikson, 2006).

APRNs may face similar challenges in their practices. Additional education in biomedical ethics provided in doctoral level education will assist these providers in resolving these challenging situations and ultimately minimize job dissatisfaction. APRNs, due to the nature of their practices, may have more autonomy than nurses. Nurses by scope of practice often work based on the orders of a physician or face employment loss or punishment by an institution for the act of insubordination.

APRNs may educate patients and families and engage in the practice of shared decision making to help to resolve ethical conflicts in their practice. The APRN may consult the institution's bioethics team when a challenging conflict arises. Additionally, the APRN may wish to consider Surowiecki's opinion that wise groups will make smart decisions and utilize this concept when faced with an expert's opinion which is contrary to their own.

Justice is the principle of fair and equal treatment for all. Due reward and honor are shared by all members of a provider or research team. In research, justice also includes equitable distribution of benefits and burdens of research. Additionally, justice represents treating people without prejudice. The APRN must apply the principle of justice to any role in which they act: researcher, educator, clinician, and scholar.

In the role of the researcher, the APRN must apply ethical guidelines to authorship. Authorship is defined as having substantial participation in the conception and design of the research study or intervention, or in the analysis and interpretation of data or results. Authorship must include substantial participation in the drafting or editing of the manuscript. The author provides final approval of the version of the manuscript to be published. The author has the ability to explain and defend the study or intervention in scholarly settings (International Committee of Medical Editors, 2009).

The APRN participating in research will likely be a member of a team. In these cases, the order of authorship is determined by the output from each of the contributing authors. The researcher who makes the largest contribution is entitled to appear as the lead author, or may choose to assume any other position of his or her choice. The lead author should generate the original concept of the work, perform the actual research study, and be identified as the Primary Investigator. Additionally, the lead author analyzes and interprets the data, and the writing of all or most of the manuscript. In cases where two or more authors equally meet the above requirements, the authors should resolve the dilemma in a collegial manner. The designation of lead author should be assigned to the person who either played the more significant role in the implementation of the research study or wrote the largest portion of the manuscript text (International Committee of Medical Editors, 2009).

Most institutions will have set guidelines for the ethical conduct of research and this will be discussed in another chapter in this book. The purpose of these guidelines is to avoid research misconduct. Research misconduct is defined as deliberate fabrication, falsification, or plagiarism in reporting research results (American Psychological Association, 2012). It does not include honest error or differences of opinion. The APRN engaged in research wants to avoid research misconduct as this may result in sanctions from employers, professional associations, and by agencies funding research. The APRN should consult the institutional guidelines to be certain to engage in ethical research.

3.9. INFORMED CONSENT—SURROGACY

The term informed consent was first used in 1957 by Paul G. Gebhard during a medical malpractice case (Princeton University, 2012). Health care providers are challenged to obtain informed consent from patients who are truly informed. Impairments to reasoning and judgment may make it impossible for an individual to give informed consent. Intellectual or emotional immaturity, high levels of stress, mental retardation, severe mental illness, intoxication, severe sleep deprivation, Alzheimer's disease, or unconsciousness are examples of conditions in which an individual may not be able to provide informed consent. Providers must find other acceptable sources (family members, surrogates, legal guardians, etc.) to provide consent in the aforementioned cases.

Patients may not fully understand the meaning of a procedure or treatment as described by a provider. Informed consent requires a clear appreciation and understanding of the facts, implications, and future consequences of an action. To give informed consent, the individual must have adequate reasoning faculties and have all relevant facts before consent can be given.

The APRN must consider the notion of competency when seeking consent. Is a patient competent to understand the question in context of the circumstance in order to provide consent? This is often a challenge for health care providers. What is competence? A legal definition of competence is provided in another chapter of this text.

Healthcare providers must be aware that individuals may be competent to perform a task at one point in time and not be competent at a later time due to a change in their health status. In some cases, the APRN must evaluate a patient's capacity to make a decision if the individual experiences periods of confusion requiring admission to the hospital. The APRN would need to assess the patient's orientation to person, place and time when determining capacity for decision making. The APRN may have to return at a later time to reassess the patient's condition and ability to make decisions, if the initial evaluation revealed a level of confusion. Any discussion requires documentation.

In other cases, an individual may have the capacity for judgment except in the reference to their health state. An example would be a patient who has become accustomed to using opioids to treat chronic pain. Because of the side effects of these medications, this individual may lack the capacity to consider other options. The APRN must always completely and accurately document the individual's state when discussing options for care.

Laws regarding competence were created to protect property rather than individuals (Beauchamp and Childress, 2009, p. 71). Unfortunately, the law does not aid the APRN, as laws regarding competence are not well suited for medical decision making. As competence may vary depending on context, it is not appropriate to globally judge competence. An individual may not have the capacity to make a decision while suffering through an acute migraine headache or a transient ischemic attack, but this does not mean the individual is globally incompetent. The APRN must document any discussion with patients and note if they are pain free or oriented at the time of the discussion.

A lack of informed consent makes it legally impossible to act. When an individual is unable to give informed consent, another person may be authorized to give consent on his behalf. In the case of minors, parents or legal guardians may give consent. Caregivers for the mentally ill may give consent. In cases of individuals who are critically injured or unconscious, physicians, advanced practice registered nurses and other members on the healthcare team will administer life-saving treatment. They will act with implied, emergent consent.

If an unconscious or incapacitated individual cannot express consent, the law assumes that the individual consented to treatment for the emergency situation. Implied legal consent is based on two principles: (1) Duty to obtain informed consent is excused if death or irreparable harm may result if the physician delays providing treatment. (2) The law presumes that a reasonable, competent, lucid adult would consent to lifesaving treatment. (Canterberry v Spence, 1972).

Courts differ on the definition of a "true emergency." Courts generally will allow the doctrine to protect physicians who act in good faith in caring for a patient with a perceived emergency condition (Thomson v Sun City Community Hospital, 1984). If emergency physicians have doubt regarding the legality of a situation, "they should do what they believe to be in the patient's best interest and worry about the legal consequences later" (Monico, 2009). It is clear there is protection for physicians' decisions in an emergency situation. Nurses are judged based on doing what another prudent nurse would do in that situation. APRNs are likely to be held to similar standards.

In circumstances where an individual is unable to provide consent, a surrogate may be appointed to act on the behalf of an individual. The surrogate has the power to act on behalf of the patient, as long as there is reason to believe that the surrogate is making decisions based on the patient's wishes, values, or interests. Whenever possible, the APRN must keep in mind that all patients have a right to decide and their choices must be considered even when a surrogate has been assigned. The APRN must assess that the surrogate is indeed acting in the patient's best interest and is respecting the individual's autonomy.

Surrogate decision makers must uphold three standards. The substituted judgment standard requires the surrogate decision maker to make the decision the incompetent individual would have made if competent (Beauchamp and Childress, 2009, p. 99). The pure autonomy standard respects prior autonomous judgments regardless of the existence of a formal advance directive (Beauchamp and Childress, 2009, p. 101). Without written advance directives, a surrogate decision maker may make decisions based on their own values and selectively consider events from the patient's life which may not be relevant to the decision at hand.

The final standard is the "best interest" standard, which holds that a surrogate decision maker must weigh options and maximize benefit through a comparative assessment of options—while discounting inherent risks or cost (Beauchamp and Childress, 2009, p. 102). The best interest standard is open to interpretation and is dependent upon who is making the decision. Parents may choose to volunteer a child to donate an organ for a sibling, although the child refuses. The best interest of the patient may override the desire of the donor. The prudent APRN would consider an ethics committee evaluation in such a case.

According to the American Medical Association (AMA) code of ethics (1996), if there is no advance directive that designates a proxy, the patient's family should become the surrogate decision maker. Although the term family is not exact, it includes persons with whom the patient is closely associated. Typically the patient's closest family member is the first choice as surrogate. Family may include partners, spouses, and very close friends.

In cases where there is no one closely associated with the patient, but there are persons who both care about the patient and have sufficient relevant knowledge of the patient, such persons may be appropriate surrogates. APRNs must familiarize themselves with specific state and institutional rules and regulations regarding surrogates. The APRN must be sensitive to possible multiple conflicting views of family members in these circumstances. In the case of a comatose married woman, her husband became her surrogate. However, conflict arose when the patient's mother wanted care withdrawn. The patient's mother petitioned the courts and lost. In this situation, the husband's status as closest family member won out.

3.10. WITHDRAWING AND WITHHOLDING TREATMENT

End of life decisions are viewed as complex and are often instilled with uncertainty. Each person experiences health decision-making uniquely. In the context of end of life situations, both patients and their families are challenged with complex decision-making. These situations involve questioning, and uncertainty intersects with a struggle to do the right thing. Families and care providers also struggle with the possibilities of failing to do the right thing according to the expectations of self and others (Milton, 2010).

Withholding and withdrawal of life support is a process through which various medical interventions are either not given to patients or removed from them with the expectation that the patients will die from their underlying illnesses. The withholding and withdrawal of life support is legally justified primarily by the principles of informed consent and informed refusal, both of which have strong roots in the common law. The principles hold that treatment may not be initiated without the approval of patients or their surrogates except in emergency situations, and that patients or surrogates may refuse any or all therapies.

End of life decisions are often made using a shared decision-making model. Under this model, clinicians attempt to clarify a patient's values and reach consensus about treatment courses consistent with them (Luce, 2010). Most critically ill patients are decisionally-impaired, leaving family members and other surrogates to make end-of-life decisions, in accord with a substituted judgment standard (Luce, 2010). Health care providers often make decisions for patients who lack families or other surrogates and have no advance directives, based on a best interests standard (Luce, 2010).

What may seem the right thing to do to one individual may seem cruel and unjustified to another. Patients and families may elect to withhold feeding and hydration, and allow death to occur "naturally." However, as the patient is dying, a family member may question if they are causing death by not feeding or hydrating the patient. The goal of nonmaleficence should be at the forefront when challenges arise. It may be reasonable for the family to provide a dying patient a small amount of water as this is not likely to neither cause harm nor change the outcome. Providing pain relief may be acceptable for the same reason.

Just as some health care providers may have mixed motives in caring for dying patients, some family members may want to ease their loved ones' pain while possibly hastening death. Family members may disagree on the chosen approach and may try to alter the plan by having the patient treated emergently in an acute care facility. They may be challenged to respect the patient's autonomy and decision to withhold treatment. APRNs may provide education and support to patients and family members when the decision to withhold further treatment is made in an attempt to ensure the patient is spared additional, unwanted medical intervention.

APRNs are often key members of a palliative care team. Palliative care is the prevention or treatment of pain, dyspnea, and suffering in terminally ill patients (Luce, J.M. and Alpers, 2000). The withholding and withdrawal of life support and the administration of palliative care usually involve a multidisciplinary approach, and all involved parties, including the APRN, should participate in planning how such care is realized. The APRN may work to achieve the goal of palliative care, which is to provide comfort. Measures that do not relieve suffering but merely hasten death should be avoided.

To minimize conflict, the goal of palliative care and the means of achieving that goal should be clearly spelled out in the health record. The health care team must document the process to forego life-sustaining treatment and how the plan of achieving patient comfort will be conducted (Luce, J.M. and Alpers, 2000). Orders for sedatives and analgesics should be written to provide proper dosage boundaries while also allowing nurses to use some discretion in drug administration so that patient comfort can be achieved. Nurses should describe how the goal of palliative care was reached and what steps they took to achieve it, including an indication of all sedatives and analgesics they administer to the patient (Luce, J.M. & Alpers, 2000).

All documentation must reflect the goal of palliative care to avoid ethical and perhaps legal conflict. Opportunity exists for APRNs to assist in the process of shared decision making regarding end of life planning, withholding, and withdrawing of treatment. APRNs in community settings can assist the process by engaging in meaningful discussion with patients long before they are critically ill. The APRN should work with patients to clarify end of life desires in advance, utilizing clearly written advance directives which could minimize the need for surrogates.

3.11. ORDINARY vs. EXTRAORDINARY TREATMENT

Patients may be eligible for medical treatment, regardless of whether the treatment is viewed as extraordinary or ordinary. The APRN should not confuse the term ordinary with usual or customary. Ordinary care implies any treatment modality which offers reasonable hope of benefit, and can be used without excessive expense, pain or other inconvenience for the patient (Beauchamp and Childress, 2009, pp. 123–124).

Extraordinary care, if used, would not offer a reasonable hope of benefit. Any treatment which is excessively expensive, excessively painful, or is inconvenient may be considered extraordinary (Beauchamp and Childress, 2009, pp. 123–124). Employing this definition of care would imply that any treatment which offers no reasonable hope or benefit should be avoided, as this would be considered harmful to the patient. The APRN may be challenged to reconsider the notion of ordinary and extraordinary care with the concept of optional management. The following example illustrates this distinction. Treating pneumonia in an elderly community residing female is usual and prudent care. In the case of an 88 year old female with advanced Alzheimer's, COPD, and alcoholism, the family and primary care provider agreed to forego treating this patient's acute pneumonia. Instead, this patient was provided comfort measures in her home where she died within 48 hours of diagnosis.

Opting not to treat the patient's pneumonia seems reasonable utilizing a shared decision making model. Treating the patient's pneumonia could ultimately have prolonged her life; however, the question of benefit should be examined. Treatment in this cause would require an inpatient admission, as the patient was not lucid. She would have required ventilator support and invasive management in an intensive care setting. This would make the treatment of pneumonia in this case extraordinary care as it would be expensive, painful, and inconvenient. The APRN well versed in shared decision making can assist patients in choosing the best options for care.

Health care providers may make sound moral judgments by examining the type of treatment to be used. Consideration must be given to the degree of complexity or risk, the cost and availability of the treatment. Payment should not influence treatment decisions of the moral provider. By comparing the risks of a particular treatment with the potential for benefit, and accounting for patient's base line health status and the current acuity of the situation, prudent decisions regarding care can be made.

When deciding to employ an extraordinary treatment, a health care provider must consider the patient's desires, condition, the likelihood of survival and the cost. Employing a costly and limitedly available therapy may be appropriate if there is significant long term benefit. The availability of organs for transplantation can be scarce. This modality is therefore not readily available to all patients. Teams are typically involved in the decision making for who should obtain this limited resource. APRNs may be members of these teams.

APRNs should encourage patients to accept those treatments which they believe are reasonable and beneficial, while considering the burdens of a particular treatment will vary from person to person. Ultimately the APRN must respect that it is the patient's responsibility to accept or decline treatments. The APRN should exercise best judgment in cases in which a patient's motives may be questionable.

3.12. MEDICAL NUTRITION

Medical nutrition refers to nutritional procedures including assessment and interventions in the treatment of an illness, injury or disease condition. A specially tailored diet is planned based upon the patient's medical, psychosocial history, physical examination, and dietary history. Medical nutrition may reduce the risk of developing complications in conditions such as diabetes, or it may ameliorate the effects of conditions such as hyperlipidemia. Many medical conditions may either develop or worsen due to improper (or lack of) nutrition.

Invasive interventions such as feeding tubes may be employed to improve a patient's nutritional status when a patient is unable to eat or swallow. The use of feeding tubes in nursing home residents with advanced dementia is a well-known example. In this patient population, the nutritional need is evident. However, providing forced nutrition will not reverse the patient's dementia and the disease will progress. The APRN should remember that patients ultimately have the right to accept or decline a therapy.

Nurses play a vital role in providing information and guiding family members through difficult nutrition decisions. Lopez, Amella, Mitchell, and Strumpf (2010) found that nurses believe family members would benefit from guidance in decisions regarding the placement of feeding tubes. However, their findings also indicate that nurses were reluctant to become involved in these difficult decisions. For nurses to guide family members about the use of feeding tubes, they require education about the rationale for doing so utilizing evidence-based research, as well as support in exercising their nursing diagnosis and care plan responsibilities. APRNs may be key members of the health care team to support education of patients, staff nurses and families and enable all to reach decisions which are beneficial to the patient with optimum quality of life.

Feeding tubes have associated risks and complications, including obstruction and site infection. They require daily maintenance. The demands of this therapy may be more than a family can provide and this in turn may infringe upon the patient and family's quality of life. APRNs must weigh the benefits of nutritional therapy with the associated risks when considering this option for a patient. APRNs may provide recommendations for nasal gastric feeding tube placement on an as needed basis as opposed to a more invasive procedure.

When a patient requires more nutritional support, the APRN can request a consultation with a gastroenterologist for placement of a percutaneous feeding tube. The APRN should engage in the process of shared decision making with the family and other members of the health care team. The APRN should support the patient's wishes in the process of determining what the best nutritional therapy is for the patient.

3.13. MEDICAL FUTILITY

Futile medical care exists when there is no hope for improvement in an incapacitating condition. Futile care fails to offer benefit (Khatcheressian, Harrington, Lyckholm, and Smith, 2008). Futile care has no possibility of achieving a good outcome and serves only to prolong life

(Appeal, 2009). There is no known physical or spiritual benefit derived from such care. Futile care may prolong grieving and give false hope. Caregivers may see themselves as forced to act against the best interests of their patient in cases of futile medical treatment.

In a setting of limited resources, futile care involves the expenditure of resources that could be used by other patients who have a likelihood of achieving a positive outcome (Appeal, 2009). The utilitarian will argue that a just society should spend and ration its resources sensibly in order to save as many lives as possible (Appeal, 2009). A grim prognosis does not justify an end to care, but a truly futile prognosis requires further consideration by the APRN and members of the healthcare team.

For example, Baby K was born anencephalic with only the brainstem having developed during pregnancy (Ascension Health, 2012). The baby's mother had been notified of her condition following ultrasound and had been advised to terminate the pregnancy by her obstetrician and neonatologist. The mother chose to carry the child to term because of her religious beliefs. The mother and the hospital in which she delivered had opposing views on care for this child.

The hospital physicians strongly advised a Do Not Resuscitate (DNR) order for the child, which the mother refused. Baby K remained on ventilator support for six weeks while a search for another hospital was done. No other facility would accept Baby K. Finally, the child was transferred to a long term care nursing facility after being weaned from a ventilator, but the baby returned to the hospital many times for respiratory problems. Many critics of this case insist that the medical expenses used to keep Baby K on life support for over two years could have been better spent on awareness and prevention efforts of her condition (Ascension Health, 2012).

Some argue that futile clinical care should be a market commodity able to be purchased (Appeal, 2009). If the purchaser of the clinical services has the necessary funds, and as long as other patients are not being denied access to clinical resources as a result, it may be reasonable to utilize this commodity. In this scenario, Baby K would be able to receive ICU care until funding vanished.

In the case of extremely costly new chemotherapies, the issues of equity often arise in treatment of end-stage cancer (Khatcheressian, Harrington, Lyckholm, and Smith, 2008). Khatcheressian, Harrington, Lyckholm and Smith (2008) report lack of provider-patient communication regarding prognosis, goals of therapy, and benefits of aggressive symptom management contribute to the delivery of futile chemotherapy. APRNs should engage in open communications to avoid subjecting patients to futile care.

The purchasing of care is a questionable option. If the goal of nursing practice is to do no harm and to benefit a patient, is futile care providing the patient benefit? If the patient or family has the resources to provide the necessary care to keep a patient alive and not tax the system at large, is it reasonable to allow for this type of care? Is it really beneficial to the patient?

When caring for an infant who survives an anoxic brain injury and requires home ventilator support, this question is a difficult one. These children require expensive, daily multidisciplinary therapies, including speech therapy, physical therapy, occupational therapy, and nursing care. They require care from primary pediatric services, as well as subspecialty services, such as pulmonary medicine. The parents require education and support in caring for a technology dependent child. As these children grow, they will continue to require services and durable medical equipment.

Resuscitating infants who suffer anoxic brain injuries at birth may result in lifelong care. It is a difficult decision for health care providers and parents to allow a neonate to die without intervention. The parents may choose to have every intervention done to save their infant even after being given a poor prognosis. It may be satisfying to the parent to have the baby in their care regardless of the outcome. Truly informed consent is necessary in these circumstances because of the high level of emotions involved.

APRNs should communicate openly with parents in these challenging situations. The APRN must thoroughly explain the process of resuscitation and that successful resuscitation does not negate brain injury. The dilemma is who is obtaining benefit from care in this situation—the parent or the child. There may be a role for ethics committees to determine if some patients are beyond medical hope and if care would be futile (Appeal, 2009).

3.14. ETHICS COMMITTEES

Ethics committees typically include members from diverse backgrounds who support health care institutions with three major functions: providing ethics consultation, developing and/or revising select policies pertaining to clinical ethics, and facilitating education about topical issues in clinical ethics. These committees may assist with interpreting advance directives, withholding and withdrawing life-sustaining treatments, informed consent, and decisions surrounding organ procurement.

Ethics committee members may represent major clinical services and other stakeholders in health care delivery such as clinicians from medicine, surgery, psychiatry, nursing, social work, a chaplain, and a community representative. APRNs may serve as committee members. These committees often include a quality improvement manager, an educator employed by the facility, a lawyer, and at least one individual with advanced training in ethics. The individual with advanced training in ethics may come from philosophy, law, medicine, theology, or anthropology.

A clinician faced with an ethical dilemma should consider asking for an ethics consultation when two conditions are met: there is an ethical problem in the care of a patient, and the resolution does not occur after bringing this to the attention of the team responsible for the care of the patient. A true ethical dilemma occurs because there is a conflict between principles of autonomy, beneficence, and justice, or between principles and outcomes.

Clinical ethics consultations are interventions by trained members of a bioethics advisory committee to help resolve an ethical dilemma or answer an ethical question that arises in the course of patient care. The consultation is purely advisory. Bioethics committee members and consultants have no authority to make patient care decisions. Patients and their insurers are typically not charged for ethics consultations.

The process of an ethics consultation consists of several steps. Consultants review medical records and interview the patient, physicians, nurses, family members, surrogate decision makers, and other relevant parties. The consultants provide an analysis of the ethical issue and suggest means to resolve it. This may include a face-to-face meeting with all parties. The case may be presented to a full bioethics advisory committee meeting and discussed. Follow-up is often performed.

The most common issues prompting clinical ethics consultations are conflicts between the medical and nursing staffs over the best care of the patient. Other reasons may include a conflict between the medical-nursing staff and the family over the best care of the patient, evidence that the medical staff is not following the wishes of the patient or surrogate, or evidence that the family or surrogate decision maker is making a decision that is not in the patient's best interest.

3.15. CASE STUDIES

The APRN may face multiple ethical challenges while engaging in clinical practice. The following scenarios are examples of situations that may arise.

3.15.1. Case One

A nineteen year old female patient presents to the urgent care center with her mother and with a 10 day history of right lower quadrant pain. Both are feeling frustrated due to lack of a diagnosis. Patient was seen 10 days ago in an emergency department and discharged being told she had a hernia which would require evaluation as an outpatient. She then saw her family physician three days later and was referred to a surgeon who would be seeing her in two weeks. She presents this evening due to continuation of the pain and her mother's pressuring her to "find out what is wrong." Patient denies any loss of appetite, nausea, vomiting or diarrhea. She reports dysuria with frequency. She denies that movement or lifting increases her pain. She also denies any bulges to her abdominal wall, just a small "bump" to the right lower abdominal region that is not painful. It is difficult to obtain a history directly from the patient because her mother continually interrupts and answers the questions for the patient.

On further questioning, the patient admits to a vaginal discharge, burning with urination, and sexual activity without barrier protection. She had a boyfriend for the past year with whom she recently ended the relationship. She is uncertain as to whether he had other sexual partners. She reports that he had been her only partner. Her last gynecologic visit was one year ago. She denies a history of previous sexually transmitted infections (STI). Her last menstrual period was two weeks prior and was normal.

After examination, the patient was diagnosed with a sexually transmitted disease. She did not wish to share this information with her mother. The patient's mother pressured the provider for answers and a diagnosis. The provider was challenged to maintain the patient's confidentiality. What principle would guide this provider's decision making? How should she handle the missed diagnosis by the family physician? Are there legal ramifications? What if the patient loses fertility because of the delay in diagnosis? If the mother of the patient was paying for the patient's medical bills, would that change what information she should be given?

3.15.2. Case Two

A 78 year old male patient was admitted to the hospital with a brain injury after a fall. He has a history of diabetes mellitus, hypertension, anemia and dementia. He presented with areas of ecchymosis to his forehead. His computerized tomography (CT) scan showed hemorrhagic contusions of the bilateral frontal lobes, left temporal lobe, and small subdural hematomas on the frontal lobes. During his hospitalization he was oriented to person, place, and time and dates for a portion of his stay. The nursing staff reports the patient suffers from occasional confusion, mild short term memory loss, and intermittent agitation. At times he was aggressive to the nursing staff and often refused medications, including insulin and antihypertensive prescription drugs. The APRN managing this patient's care is faced with a dilemma. Can this patient with a documented brain injury and history of dementia refuse his medical therapy? Can he be forced to take his medications? How should the practitioner proceed? Is an ethics committee consult necessary?

3.15.3. Case Three

An 82 year old female is admitted from the nursing home for an acute exacerbation of congestive heart failure (CHF) and hypernatremia. The patient suffers from advanced Alzheimer's dementia. The patient required diuresis with intravenous furosemide (Lasix) and over the next four days, the CHF symptoms and sodium levels improved. Two days later, the sodium levels decreased and a nephrology consultation was obtained. The patient was started on tolvaptan (Samsca) to treat the hypernatremia. This improved the sodium levels, but the patient became hypokalemic, requiring treatment for the elevated potassium. The patient then experienced an episode of syncope resulting in a fall, from which she recovered. The following day, she had an episode of staring off into space which was suspected to be a seizure. The patient was evaluated for a cerebral vascular accident and no acute bleeding was identified. The patient continued to experience a complicated hospitalization and worsening of her dementia.

How does the APRN approach an elderly frail patient with multiple complex conditions? Was admission for the CHF and resulting complications worth the risk of worsening the patient's dementia? How could this situation be avoided? When is palliative care appropriate for this patient?

3.15.4. Case Four

A sixteen year old female comes to the office with her mother for an annual physical examination including a pelvic examination. During the exam, when she is alone with the practitioner, the patient advises the

APRN that she has been sexually active for the past year. The APRN completes the examination and during the follow-up office time, recommends the vaccination for human papilloma virus (HPV). The patient's mother refuses this vaccination as she states her daughter is not sexually active. The patient's mother is concerned that by vaccinating her daughter, she is encouraging early sexual debut. The patient is not vaccinated on this visit and the APRN recommends a follow up visit in two weeks. At the next visit, the patient arrives without her mother and she requests the HPV vaccination and oral contraceptives. The APRN agrees to both treatments and the patient gives assent. What principles are guiding the APRN's decision to vaccinate this patient and provide contraceptive therapy without parental consent? Are there legal issues involved? Does the provider have a duty to tell the patient's mother? Is the provider obligated to counsel the patient to tell her mother?

3.16. REFERENCES

American Medical Association (1996). Opinion 2.20—*Withholding or Withdrawing Life-Sustaining Medical Treatment.* AMA Code of Ethics http://www.ama-assn.org/ama/pub/physician-resources/medical-ethics/code-medical-ethics/opinion220.page

American Medical Association (1992). Decisions near the end of life. *JAMA 267*: 2229–2233.

American Psychological Association (2012). Research Misconduct. http://www.apa.org/research/responsible/misconduct/index.aspx

Appeal, J. (2009). *What's So Wrong with "Death Panels"*? Huffpost politics. http://www.huffingtonpost.com/jacob-m-appel/whats-so-wrong-with-death_b_366804.html

Aristotle. (1958). Nicomachean ethics (W.D. Ross, Trans.) In: *The Pocket Aristotle,* pp. 158–274. J.D. Kaplan (Ed.). New York: Washington Square Press.

Ascention Health (2012). Baby K. Retrieved from http://www.ascensionhealth.org/index.php?option=com_content&view=article&id=237&Itemid=173.

Beauchamp, T.L. and Childress, J.F. (2009). *Principles of Biomedical Ethics Sixth Edition.* New York: Oxford University Press.

Canterberry v Spence, 464 F2d 772 (DC Cir), cert denied 409 US 1064 (1972).

Cohen, J.S. and Erickson, J.M. (2006). Ethical dilemmas and moral distress in oncology nursing practice. *Clinical Journal of Oncology Nursing* (6):775–80.

Emnett, J., Byock, I. and Twohig, J.S. (2002). Promoting Excellence in End-of-Life Care, a National Program Office of The Robert Wood Johnson Foundation. http://www.promotingexcellence.org/downloads/apn_report.pdf

Fisher, J. and Clayton, M. (2012). Who gives a tweet: Assessing patients' interest in the use of social media for healthcare. *Worldviews on Evidence Based Nursing 9*: 100–108.

Havighurst, C.C. and Richman, B.D. (2008). *Fairness in Health Care: Who Pays? Who Benefits?* ExpressO. http://works.bepress.com/clark_havighurst/1

International Committee of Medical Editors (2009). Uniform Requirements for Manuscripts Submitted to Biomedical Journals: Ethical Considerations in the Conduct and Reporting of Research: Authorship and Contributorship. http://www.icmje.org/ethical_1author.html

Khatcheressian, J., Harrington, S.B., Lyckholm, L.J. and Smith, T.J. (2008). *"Futile care": What to do when your patient insists on chemotherapy that likely won't help.* Oncology (8). http://www.cancernetwork.com/cme/article/10165/1168027?pageNumber=1.

Kahneman, D. (2011). *Thinking Fast and Slow.* New York: Farrar, Straus and Giroux.

Kosko, B. (1993). *Fuzzy Thinking: The New Science of Fuzzy Logic.* New York: Hyperion.

Lopez, R.P., Amella, E.J., Mitchell, S.L. and Strumpf, N.E. (2010). Nurses' perspectives on feeding decisions for nursing home residents with advanced dementia. *Journal of Clinical Nursing 19*(5–6):632–8.

Luce, J.M. and Alpers, A. (2000). Legal aspects of withholding and withdrawing life supportfrom critically ill patients in the united states and providing palliative care to them. *American Journal of Respiratory and Critical Care Medicine 162*(6): 2029–2032.

Luce, J.M. (2010). End-of-Life Decision Making in the Intensive Care Unit. American *Journal of Respiratory and Critical Care Medicine 182*: 6–11.

Milton CL. (2010). Failing to do the right thing: nurse practice and the family experience. *Nursing Science Quarterly 23*(3):206–8.

Monico, E.P. (2009) "When in Doubt" rule. *Emerg. Dept. Legal Letter 20*:61–65.

National Council of State Boards of Nursing. (2011). White paper: A nurse's guide to the use of social media. Available at : https://www.ncsbn.org/Social_Media.pdf.

Princeton University (2012). Informed Consent. Retrieved from http://www.princeton.edu/~achaney/tmve/wiki100k/docs/Informed_consent.html

Surowiecki, J. (2005). *The Wisdom of Crowds: Why the Many Are Smarter Than the Few and How Collective Wisdom Shapes Business, Economies, Societies and Nations.* New York: Random House.

Thomson v Sun City Community Hospital, 668 P2d 605 (1984).

University of Washington Department of Bioethics and Humanities. (2010). *Ethics Committees and Ethics Consultation.* http://depts.washington.edu/bioethx/topics/ethics.html

CHAPTER 4

Ethical Considerations in the Care of Vulnerable Adult Populations

JOAN VALAS

4.1. INTRODUCTION

According to the ANA Code of Ethics, nurses are held to "high standards of compassion and respect for all—especially those most vulnerable" (Taylor 2010, p. 3) and recognize that the injustice of unequal health care is the result of many factors. The vulnerable may be frail, homeless, and disenfranchised. They may be poor or marginalized, often living on the periphery and in the shadows of society. These inequalities and disparities of health are what make them so vulnerable. Federal guidance, covered in the Code of Federal Regulations, Title 45 Part 46—Protection of Human Subjects for the conduct of human subject research for vulnerable populations, includes children, pregnant women, mentally disabled persons, or economically or educationally disadvantaged persons; several of these groups will be discussed in this chapter.

As they are often not "visible"—which can result in inequalities or disparities of health— these persons enter our health care systems with more acute illnesses that might have been prevented if adequate preventive care had been available. Recognition of those that are vulnerable and at risk is an essential primary preventive measure for the practice of advanced practice nursing.

4.2. VULNERABLE POPULATIONS (DEFINITION/DESCRIPTION)

An elderly female was brought in to the hospital by EMS and was admitted because of an altered mental status. Until recently, she had been able to care for herself and lived alone, according to her neighbors. She is unable to communicate her health history and it is unclear if she has any family members to contact. Her health care needs must be considered as well as the ethical concerns for her care. This vignette is an example of the problems facing the nurse practitioner dealing with vulnerable populations. So who are the most vulnerable?

Aday (2001) reminds us that the "origins and remedies" arise from the bonded human community and as such all humans have the potential to be vulnerable (p. 1). Humans share the universal condition of vulnerability as well as that of human strength (Nyamathi and Koniak-Griffin 2007 p. xiv). However, most research and policies concerning vulnerable populations focus on subpopulations (Aday 2001) such as ethnic and racial minorities, women and children, the elderly, the poor, the chronically and mentally ill, disabled, imprisoned, the homeless, and substance abusers. These groups are at risk for poor physical, psychological and social health (Aday 1994; 2001) and have an increased risk to adverse health outcomes, as evidenced by increased morbidity and mortality (Flaskerud and Winslow, 1998; Flaskerud *et al.*, 2002; IOM, 2002). Shi and Stevens (2010) have put forth five reasons to focus national attention on vulnerable populations: they have greater health needs; their numbers are increasing; vulnerability is a social issue resolved through social means; it is intertwined with the nation's health; and there is a growing emphasis on the equality of health, particularly among racial and ethnic minorities.

It is important to distinguish between the terms "vulnerable populations" and "at-risk individuals", as they are often used interchangeably and grouped collectively. Categorizations and use of standardized lists used to describe vulnerable groups should not be used exclusively to describe these populations. Moreover, "a focus on misery, poverty, and crisis alone, [may] contribute to the objectification of a population" (Susser, 2001) and only serve to marginalize people in need, creating barriers to care and service. DeBruin (2001) suggests that vulnerability "ought not to be considered as a characteristic of groups . . . rather certain traits may render certain persons vulnerable in certain situations". Often included in these categories are the specific groups detailed above in federal regulations; however, it may be necessary to cast a broader net to ensure inclusion to those who need care the most in consideration of ethics and the concept of health disparities. Nurse practitioners should not limit their understanding of vulnerable populations to a list or a category, but rather look more widely and assess their patients more fully for their vulnerability.

However, Gutherie (2005) has noted that there has been a growing need to understand the relationship between health disparities and vulnerable populations among racial and ethnic minorities in the United

States. Health disparities may be defined as inequalities of health status as well as the provision, access and quality of care. Health inequalities are particularly apparent when comparing vulnerable populations to non-vulnerable populations (Nyamthi, Koniak-Griffin and Greengold, 2007). Disparity of health care, a core representation of social injustice, has raised national attention on vulnerable groups (Nyamthi, Koniak-Griffin, and Greengold, 2007; p. 6). As a result of a Congress-commissioned study, the Institute of Medicine's (IOM) report entitled *Unequal Treatment* (2003) concluded that racial and ethnic minorities are less likely to receive needed health services, creating disparities of health and making them more vulnerable and at risk for poor health outcomes. In this report, the IOM also looked at other factors that contributed to these health disparities, such as cultural and linguistic barriers, costs, care delivery sites, health care provider prejudice and stereotyping against racial and ethnic minorities. Nurse practitioners should consider all of these factors and not limit assessments of their patients to medical needs alone. Nurse practitioners can help to "close the gap in community health" in working with diverse vulnerable populations, not only by having an understanding and first-hand knowledge of the communities (*The Future of Nursing 2010*) where they work, but also in recognizing the vulnerability of those who live in these communities. The IOM *Future of Nursing* (2010) report recommended that nurses be able to critique the ethical aspects of health policy in terms of vulnerable populations (p. 518).

There is no checklist of questions in order to assess for vulnerability just as there is no checklist to assess the culture of our clients; however, the nurse should consider further inquiry and assessment into their clients' economic status and geographic location, health, age, functional or developmental status, and identification of communication barriers and be cognizant of obscure vulnerability associated with race, ethnicity, and gender. Furthermore, assessments and inquiry of vulnerability and culture of clients, populations and communities served by the nurse practitioner in practice or PhD nurse conducting research have many similarities that are helpful to understand. Cultural competence has "emerged as the mantra of contemporary practice", with an abundance of books and journal articles describing "formulas and instructions for students, educators, and clinicians" on how to become culturally competent which is "difficult to measure as well as to teach" (Dreher, Shapiro and Assesselin, 2006, p. 5). The discussion of research guidelines and conceptual models of vulnerability offered below aim to clarify this assessment and its ethical implications on practice and research.

4.3. ETHICAL GUIDELINES AND REGULATIONS FOR THE PROTECTION OF HUMAN SUBJECTS IN RESEARCH

It is important for nurse practitioners to be familiar with federal regulations and ethical guidelines for the protection of human subjects research. After the World War II War Crime Trials, the Nuremberg Code was established in 1947 as a set of standards to assure research was carried out in an ethical manner. The Office of Human Research and Protection (OHRP) operationally sits within the Office of the Deputy Director for Human Research (DDIR), the National Institutes of Health (NIH) which is part of the U.S. Public Health Service within the Department of Health and Human Services (DHHS). OHPR has published a variety of policy and regulatory guidance materials to assist the research community in conducting ethical research that is in compliance with DHHS regulations. A full historical description of the development of the federal regulations for human subject research is found elsewhere in this book. The ethical guidelines as they relate to vulnerable populations are described here. The National Commission for the Protection of Human Subjects of Biomedical and Behavioral Research was created on July 12, 1974 by the National Research Act (Pub. L. 93-348). The Commission identified the basic ethical principles and developed guidelines that would underlie the conduct of biomedical and behavioral research involving human subjects. *The Belmont Report—Ethical Principles and Guidelines for the Protection of Human Subjects (1979)* summarizes these basic ethical principles. The three basic principles—respect of persons, beneficence and justice—have relevance to the ethics of research involving human subjects and serve as an analytical framework to guide research. Respect for persons implies that individuals are autonomous agents and that persons without autonomy have the right to protections. Beneficence is the obligation of the practitioner to do no harm and to maximize possible benefits and minimize harm to their subjects and patients. Justice implies fair and equal distribution of benefits and burdens among people, meaning that each person has an equal share. While they are important in their application to research, The Belmont Report does not always provide clear resolutions to the ethical dilemmas faced in research (NIH 2004).

Research involving vulnerable populations is covered in the Code of Federal Regulations, Title 45 Part 46—Protection of Human Subjects. This regulation requires that institutional review boards (IRB) take into account the purpose of the research and mandates that research pay particular attention to the special needs and problems of vulnerable populations. This regulation lists children, prisoners, pregnant women, mentally disabled persons, and economically or educationally disadvantaged persons as vulnerable groups.

Nurse practitioners involved in research and care of vulnerable populations must consider the special needs of their patients who fall into these vulnerable groups, keeping in mind that inequalities and disparities of health are part of what makes them so vulnerable. The concept of vulnerability is complex and the literature from numerous disciplines is replete with attempts to describe the effects on health care and health outcomes. Several conceptual models exist which describe the relationships among factors associated with vulnerability.

4.4. CONCEPTUAL MODELS OF VULNERABLE POPULATIONS

Conceptual models and frameworks for studying the vulnerable examine why they are more at risk for poor health and experience inferior health care. While several theoretical frameworks have guided vulnerable populations studies (social cognitive theory, theory of reasoned action and health beliefs model), they are not specific to address these risks and experiences (Nyamathi, Koniak-Griffin and Greengold, 2007). Traditional ethical principles focus on the individual and do not cover the wider population.

4.4.1. Aday: Model of Vulnerability

The underlying concept of Lu Ann Aday's conceptual model is risk. Risk assumes that everyone has an equal chance of an adverse health related event. However, certain individuals and groups have more risks than others and these are described as vulnerable populations. They have greater multifaceted health needs that may be debilitating or life threatening and require more extensive health services (Aday 1994, p. 490). The origins of poor health traditionally focus on the individual, highlighting autonomy and personal responsibility for health. These include age, race, ethnicity and gender. However, a community or societal and environmental or macro perspective of health needs focuses on risks that exist "as a function of the availability of opportunities and resources for maximizing health" (Aday, 1994, p. 490). There is a relationship between the individual and this community perspective. According to this model, vulnerability can be predicted by social status, social capital and human capital. Social status incorporates a person's age, sex, race and ethnicity. Social capital status incorporates an individual's family structure, social networks, marital status, and voluntary organizations. Human capital includes schools attended, jobs held, income and housing of the individual. The availability of these resources has a direct impact on the health outcomes of those who are vulnerable. Ultimately, "vulnerability reflects the interactions of many factors over which individuals have little control" (Nyamathi, Koniak-Griffin, Greengold, 2007, p. 7).

4.4.2. Flaskerud and Winslow's Vulnerable Populations Conceptual Model (VPCM)

The VPCM was built upon the work of Aday and others. This model proposes that links exist between resource availability, risk, and health status of vulnerable populations. These resources are similar to Aday's and are described as human capital, social connection and environmental resources. Relative risks are factored into this model and are either behavioral or biological in nature. An increased exposure to risk and limited access to resources results in poorer health status and increased morbidity and mortality. This model was "designed for clinical practice, research and policy interventions aimed at impacting links" between resource limitations and the effect on risk and health outcomes (Nyamathi, Koniak-Griffin, Greengold, 2007, p. 7).

4.4.3. Shi and Stevens—Vulnerability Model

Shi and Stevens' model is comprehensive, multi-level, and emphasizes both the individual and the community and environmental or ecological risk factors associated with vulnerability. This model highlights a broad range of risk factors that together lead to poor health and health outcomes. Individuals' risk factors are not determined by their individual characteristics alone. This comprehensive model "more accurately reflects realities and avoids . . . blaming the victims" (Shi and Stevens 2010, p. 17). Access to health services, poor quality of care and health status as well as marginalization are reflective of these risk factors. Predisposing risk factors include demographics, personal and cultural belief systems, social structure and social status (i.e., race, ethnicity, gender). Socioeconomic status, human capital and other factors including health insurance and access to care may also influence risk vulnerability. Individual risk factors are categorized as predisposing, enabling, or need, and may influence the community and ecological risk factors that interact with each other and cumulatively influence vulnerability. Predisposing risk factors include individual risk factors of age, race, ethnicity, culture and gender. At the community or ecological level, geographical setting, physical environment and sociocultural norms of the community are factors. Enabling factors socially and materially enhance individual risk factors and include income, education, health insurance coverage and community factors such as the availability of jobs, school and health services. Need risk factors are the existing health problems of the individual, including mental health issues, disabilities and disease rates. The community's risk factors include communicable disease rates and illicit drug availability.

4.4.4. Kachingwe-Huff Model of Culturally Proficient and Ethical Practice

Health care providers should provide proficient care with the necessary cultural knowledge, understand the ethical implications of working with culturally diverse vulnerable populations, and understand that ethical dilemmas may occur as a result of a dichotomy between cultural beliefs/practices of the patient and the health care provider (Kachingwe and Huff, 2007). The Kachingwe-Huff Model of Culturally Proficient and Ethical Practice contends that cultural care can be fostered by incorporating these five components: cultural awareness, cultural knowledge, interpersonal communication skills, cultural collaboration and cultural experiences (Kachingwe and Huff, 2007, pp. 46–47). Most people, including health care providers, innately view others from an ethnocentric perspective leading to distorted perceptions of their patients' health behaviors (Campinha-Bacote and Padgett, 1995; Dowd, Giger and Davidhizar, 1998; Huff and Kline, 2007; Kachingwe and Huff, 2007). Clearly, this is to be avoided in order to provide culturally and ethically proficient care. The five components of this model provide a framework for health care practitioners "to solve ethical problems, issues and dilemmas that may be encountered during a transcultural client-practitioner relationship" (Kachingwe and Huff, 2007, p. 51).

In consideration of any conceptual model that assists in understanding vulnerability, an advanced practice registered nurse must have cultural knowledge of the clients, populations and communities they serve when applying ethical principles to practice and research. Cultural knowledge requires an understanding and respect of the diversity of cultural groups and incorporating its importance "in an unbiased manner to meet the client's needs" (Kachingwe and Huff, 2007, p. 46), which is addressed in the ANA code of Ethics.

4.5. ETHICAL CONSIDERATIONS IN CARE AND RESEARCH OF ILLEGAL ALIENS, INCOMPETENT PATIENTS, PRISONERS, AND THE ARMED FORCES

4.5.1. Unauthorized Residents: Illegal Immigrants

Those born outside of the United States represent an ever-growing portion of the U.S. population. In 2009, more than 12 percent of the U.S. population (approximately 39 million) were foreign born individuals living in the United States, according to a report from the Congressional Budget Office (CBO) which included data though 2009 (CBO, 2011). Of this 39 million (Pew Hispanic Center 2010), 38 percent were from Mexico or Central America and another 27 percent were from Asia (CBO, 2011). In California, 1 in 4 persons were foreign-born and 1 in 5 were foreign-born in New York and New Jersey. These three states contain the highest percentages of foreign-born individuals in the country. The CBO definition of foreign born is a person born outside of the United States or territories to parents who are not U.S. citizens. This definition of foreign-born is further categorized. Foreign-born or immigrants may have legal permanent status because of a family-sponsored application; they may be refugees or asylum seekers. These residents are issued a "green card" which serves as identification of their legal status. Foreign-born individuals can also hold legal temporary status as a visitor with or without a visa, which grants them a time-limited stay. According to the CBO, an unauthorized resident is a noncitizen residing in the United States without legal authorization; thus the term used—illegal immigrant (CBO 2011). Of the 39 million in 2009, 22 million foreign-born did not have legal status to reside in the United States.

In 2009, an unauthorized resident with a family (3.4 members) earned an average annual income of $36,000. In the same year, fourteen percent of all foreign-born families earned an income below the poverty threshold of about $22,000 and twenty-five percent of these families were unauthorized residents. Many U.S. employers do not provide health care insurance to their low-income employees and past and present federal regulations do not provide Medicaid coverage to unauthorized residents. Provision Eight of the ANA Code of Ethics states that as nurses provide health care to culturally diverse populations, they must avoid imposing their own cultural values upon others (ANA, 2001, p. 24). The respect for other life styles and values of persons from diverse cultures requires that healthcare providers look introspectively and exam their own values and beliefs. APRNs must also understand and reflect upon their own personal beliefs and values, as there are instances where their values may conflict with their clients' and they find themselves unable to provide care that is in harmony with that of the clients. Using the example of the well-known book and author, Ann Fadaman's *The Spirit Catches You And You Fall Down,* demonstrates a cultural collision between a physician's and Hmong family's understanding of epilepsy, which resulted in the possibly preventable death of a child. In situations of unresolved conflicts between client and provider beliefs, they may be best handled by referring the case to the institution's ethics committee. However, an understanding of one's own personal beliefs and values, cultural knowledge and ethical principles should be used as a guide to APRN practice in similar situations, particularly involving immigrant populations. When conflicts between the culture of patients and those of the provider exist, the nurse practitioner is best served by bringing in other practitioners for consultation or bringing the issue before the institutional ethics boards to resolve the ethical dilemmas of these conflicts.

Persons without authorized residency or legal citizenship are referred to by many terms in the United States and other countries that have large immigrant populations. In the U.S., the politically correct terminology is highly contested (Dwyer, 2004). Some of the terms used are: unauthorized residents, illegal immigrants, undocumented immigrants and illegal aliens. Whatever the term used, it does not change the fact that these persons have health care needs. In 1965, the U.S. Immigration and Nationality Act eliminated quotas of national origin, allowing only close relatives, refugees and persons of certain professions and skill sets, yet illegal immigration remains a highly contested social and politically polarizing issue. Despite laws and rules against it, immigrants are working and living in every country (Dwyer, 2004). An even more contested and contentious issue is whether these illegal immigrants are entitled to publically-funded health care services. Immigrants, whether legal or illegal, are at greater risk for poor health outcomes [citations] and are therefore considered vulnerable. Illegal immigration occurs for many reasons, including the escape of war and prosecution, poverty, employment opportunities, and the chance of a better life for themselves and their families. Immigrants in the U.S. often do the jobs that Americans choose not to, and "have the worst jobs and work in the worst conditions" (Dwyer, 2004, p. 35). Certain factors put immigrants at greater risk for poor health outcomes regardless of their legal status. Those factors are not solely related to poor working conditions or language differences but are rather shaped by historical, social, cultural, political and economic factors, known as the social determinants of health. Understanding cultural differences has always been a central focus for the profession of nursing and is addressed through education, which develops cultural competency. Often under-emphasized in cultural competence education are other social factors that may contribute to immigrant vulnerability. It is also important to recognize how the status of being foreign-born or an unauthorized resident impacts the social determinants of health. There is no one definition of culture and the foreign-born are a diverse group of ethnicities and races. Culture is often confused with race or ethnicity. Culture can be defined as the "integrated patterns of human behavior including thoughts, communications, actions, beliefs, values, and institutions of racial, ethnic, religious, or social groups" (Kleinman, Eisenberg, and Good, 1978). It denotes a historically transmitted pattern of meanings embodied in symbols, a system of inherited conceptions expressed in symbolic forms by means of which men communicate, perpetuate, and develop their knowledge about and attitudes toward life . . ." (Clifford Geertz, 1973, p. 89). It is important for nurse practitioners to understand the forces of history, power and political economy in constructing the boundaries of these categories (Schulz and Mullings, 2006) as social determinants of health. It is this powerless state that may make the foreign-born more vulnerable. Health care providers must provide culturally proficient or competent care, understand the ethical implications of working with culturally diverse vulnerable populations, and understand that ethical dilemmas may occur as a result of a dichotomy between cultural beliefs/practices of the patient and the health care provider (Kachingwe and Huff, 2007).

The number of undocumented immigrants in the United States is growing, and the foreign-born and undocumented immigrants have lower rates of public or private insurance (Carrasquillo, Carasquillo and Shea, 2000; Goldman, Smith and Sood, 2005). The foreign born are more likely to live in poverty, are less educated and less likely to have health care insurance, although this varies by the country of origin and immigration status (Truman *et al.*, 2009, p. S278; U.S. Census Bureau; Current Population Survey 2010 available at http://www.census.gov/cps, and http://www.census.gov/prod/2010pubs/p60-238.pdf) and their unauthorized resident status does not preclude them from purchasing insurance in certain states (Goldman, Smith and Sood, 2005).

U.S. public policy has made those with unauthorized illegal status ineligible for publicly funded health care services in most cases. The 1996 Personal Responsibility and Work Opportunity Reconciliation Act (PRWORA, 1996) made most legal immigrants ineligible for Medicaid during the first five years of their residency. Undocumented persons were already ineligible prior to this act with certain exceptions. Federal

Medicaid funds are administered by individual states and are required by PRWORA to enact laws which establish eligibility. Federal funds under Section 1011, Federal Reimbursement of Emergency Health Services Furnished to Undocumented Aliens, are available, however, for payments to eligible providers for emergency health services provided to the undocumented related to hospital inpatient, outpatient and ambulance services (Centers for Medicare and Medicaid Services, available at http://cms.org accessed on July 5, 2010). These funds provided $250 billion to all 50 states until 2008. Some states still have funds available and others have exhausted their funds. Under the Patient Protection and Affordable Care Act (Pub. Law No. 111-148) and the Reconciliation bill (Health Care and Education Act of 2010, Pub. Law No. No. 111-152) known as the Affordable Care Act (ACA) for health reform, passed in 2010, undocumented immigrants are unable to purchase coverage or be eligible for tax credits and will receive no assistance from the federal government (available at http://whitehouse.gov/healthreform/myths-andfacts, accessed 07/05/11 and Center for Immigration Studies available at http://www.cis.org/medicaid-costs accessed on 07/05/11). This law will provide access to affordable health care coverage to legal immigrants, refugees and asylees. Undocumented immigrants will continue to receive Medicaid benefits only for emergency health services. Children and pregnant women have had access to public health care services through federal money given to the states to administrate through what is known as the Children's Health Plan (CHIP). Many states require similar eligibility of legal immigrant status, refugees, and those seeking asylum. CHIP was created by the 1997 Balanced Budget Act to allocate 20 billion dollars over ten years to help states cover low-income children in families ineligible for Medicaid but unable to purchase private insurance. Conditions of this act were restricted in 2007 by President George W. Bush. It was amended by President Barack Obama in 2009 to remove the restrictions. In 2010, the Affordable Care Act extended these funds to states until 2015 and provided states with more affordable choices (available at http://whitehouse.gov/files/documents/health_reform_for_children.pdf, accessed 07/05/11).

As undocumented immigrants are known to have poorer health outcomes, are often socio-economically disadvantaged, and have lower rates of public and private insurance, what ethical responsibility does society have to provide health care services for undocumented immigrants? Dwyer argues that two different answers are elicited from two polarized factions—one he calls "nationalists" and the other "humanists" (Dwyer, 2004, p. 34). Nationalists take the position that society does not have any obligation, basing this perspective on the legal rules and formal citizenship, while humanists state that society does have an obligation (Dwyer, 2004, p. 34). Humanists argue that health is a basic human right. The World Health Organization (WHO) attests that every country in the world now has a human rights treaty that addresses health as a human right and which describes health-related rights and the rights related to conditions necessary for health (http://www.who.org).

4.5.1.1. Social Determinants of Health: The Implications for Ethical Practice

Nurse practitioners working in a variety of settings, including community clinics, public health and emergency rooms, are quite likely to encounter undocumented immigrants. NPs can help and support them overcome barriers of the health care system by providing not only health care services but also providing nonjudgmental ethical and compassionate care. Immigrants often face stigma and marginalization (Derose, 2007) from the community at large and even from health care providers because of cultural differences and language barriers, making them reluctant to seek out health care services. Political debates and arguments about immigrants as economic burdens or threats to national safety occur in public spaces through newspapers, television and other media. Undocumented immigrants are not immune to the discourse and therefore do not routinely seek out health care services and only enter the health care system due to an emergency or trauma. Because only emergency medical services are available and they are without access to primary and preventive health care services, they remain vulnerable at discharge. While the Affordable Health Care Act (2010) made health care accessible to many who were previously uninsured, it did not make provisions for the undocumented. Until political differences are resolved and policies in place to address the problems of immigration, the health of undocumented immigrants remains at risk. This does not eliminate the dilemma and ethical responsibility for nurse practitioners to care for patients in need. Nurse practitioners and researchers work in ever increasingly diverse communities; many of which may be the home to undocumented immigrants. Dwyer states that the selection of patients should be on medical need alone and never on factors of residency, immigration status, or the ability to pay (2004). He also related that the "phenomena of illegal immigration" and adequate health care for them reflects the "complexity of moral thought" (p. 34). These are some of the complexities faced by health care providers working with immigrant populations. Ethical dilemmas arise for nurse practitioners when they allow the immigration status and economic status of clients to enter into their provision of care in any scenario. Similar situations can arise for nurse researchers if their research participants may not have legal residency in the United States. While federal regulations address fair access to and treatment of immigrants in research studies, they do not address their legal status. In such cases in which undocumented immigrants are enrolled in research studies, the nurse researcher must take care to inform them how any information obtained in the study would be used. They must also take care as a researcher to use pseudonyms in order to protect patient anonymity as much as possible.

Undocumented immigrants tend to underreport infectious diseases and go without routine health examinations, immunizations and screenings. Immigrant women are often victims of sexual abuse that goes unreported. Compassionate care includes linking these patients to other supportive services through the healthcare provider's own established community networks, including community social organizations, churches or schools that provide additional health services, and social and legal services for undocumented immigrants. Understanding the implications of the social, economic, and political barriers faced by undocumented immigrants is as important as understanding the cultural traditions and language in providing compassionate care.

To know that someone comes from a particular ethnicity is to know very little about that person as ethnicity "is only one marker of identity" (Turner, 2005, p. 479). Ethnic background, language, gender, socioeconomic status, education, personal and family histories and other factors all contribute to how our patients understand and experience health and illness. Immigrants, legal or illegal, come from varied ethnic backgrounds that are socially, historically and geographically based. Social customs and traditions may or may not determine their health care decisions if they have been separated from their country of origin and have become acculturated into their new homes. Ethnic groups with differing socioeconomic levels may have different perspectives (Turner, 2005, p. 479). How our patients experience health from their local perspective is more important than evaluating them or judging them based on ethnicity or their legal status. Arthur Kleinman recommends listening to the narratives of our patients or conducting mini-ethnographies to learn about their local and personal perspectives of health and illness (Kleinman, 1978; 1988).

4.5.2. Prisoners

There were over 7 million adult prisoners under correctional supervision in 2009 (Census 2010). The United States prison population accounts for one quarter of the world's prison population, with an increasing number of racial minorities, women and children. Prisons are often overcrowded and have limited access to health care programs and services despite prisoners' constitutional right to humane medical care (Gostin, 2007). Providing health care and participating in research with prisoners are of concern for the advanced practice nurse working with them. Due to their restricted autonomy, low socioeconomic status, poor educational background and poor health, prisoners are extremely vulnerable. These factors alone do not allow prisoners to "meaningfully choose" (Gostin, 2007, p. 738) if they wish to participate in medical research. They also are unable to choose their own health care providers and services when needed.

4.5.2.1. Federal Regulations Related to Research of Prisoners

The Nuremburg code (1947) was the first code of conduct for scientific human research recognized internationally. It was written in response to Nazi experiments on prisoners during World War II. It emphasized the "voluntariness" of the subject and stressed that unnecessary physical or mental suffering must be prevented.

Larkin (2011) noted that despite these regulations, unethical research involving prisoners continued through the 1970s. A wide variety of research was conducted on prisoners by the U.S. Army, several major pharmaceutical companies and other consumer products sponsors up until the early 1970s (Gostin, 2007). The research includes drugs, diet drinks, detergents, and chemical warfare agents. These declined in the mid-seventies with the formation of the National Commission for the Protection of Human Subjects of Biomedical and Behavioral Research. In 1974, prisoner coercion was revealed in the Philadelphia Prison System in the Holmesburg Prison with the research of dangerous hallucinogenic, carcinogenic and radioactive chemicals (Urbina, 2006).

The National Research Act was enacted by the National Commission for the Protection of Human Subjects of Biomedical and Behavioral Research (NCPHSBBR) in 1974. The act created the federal regulatory framework to protect human research subjects for all federal and funded research. Vulnerable populations protections specific to pregnant women was added in 1975; prisoners in 1978 and children in 1983.

In 1976, a report was published by the National Commission for the Protection of Human Subjects of Biomedical and Behavioral Research for research of prisoners called the *Report and Recommendations: Research Involving Prisoners.* This report promulgated a federal regulation enacted in 1978 as 45 CFR Part 46 Subpart C, enforced under the U.S Department of Health and Human Services, Office for Health Service Protection and known as the Common Rule, which addressed additional protections for prisoners involved in research including the requirement of informed consent.

In 2006, the Institute of Medicine (IOM), under the direction of the U.S. Department of Health and Human Services (DHHS), considered "the need for developing a new ethical framework for prisoner research and to identify regulatory safeguards" (Gostin, 2007, p. 738). Byrne (2005) notes a cultural tension that inherently exists between the prison environment and that of health services research. The restrictive nature of the prison as "custody-control-care" clashes with the "open inquiry environment" of health services research, and so present challenges for the researcher (Byrne 2005, p. 223). Similar challenges exist for advanced practice nurses working within prison health care systems.

4.5.2.2. Standards for Health Services in Prisons

Health service standards in correctional settings set the bar "to ensure the most basic human rights for prisoners, including access to health care" (Stern, Greifinger and Mellow, 2010, p. 2103). These sets of standards have been developed by the American Public Health Association (APHA 2003), the National Commission on Correctional Health Care (NCCHC, 2008) and the American Correctional Association (ACA, 2003).

4.5.2.3. Correctional Nursing

Correctional nursing, including advanced practice nursing, has emerged as a specialty to care of imprisoned adults and juveniles. A representative from the American Nurses Association (ANA) sits on the board of the National Commission of Correctional Health Care (NCCHC), which is the organization committed to improving the health care of prisons, jails and juvenile correctional facilities. The NCCHC has offered a voluntary accreditation program based on its standards since the 1970s. Separate volumes of standards give guidance to jails, prisons, juvenile detention centers, mental health and drug abuse services for correctional facilities. It also offers a certification as a Certified Correctional Health Professional for health care professionals involved with all aspects of correctional health care (NCCHC 2012). The 2007 ANA Corrections Nursing: Scope and Standards of Practice was reviewed for revisions in 2011 by the ANA and NCCHC. The 2007 principles serve as the "underpinning for corrections nursing" (Trossman, 2011, p. 13). The review will include careful attention to legal implications of practice and ensure that correctional nurses also adhere to the standards of care and the Code of Ethics for Nurses (Trossman, 2011). Advanced Practice Nurses working the within restrictive environment of the correctional system where ethical challenges exist need to understand the "culture clash" (Byrne, 2005, p. 223) between prisoner control and the caring nature of nursing to best meet the needs of their patients. Byrne offers that the strategies used in her research experience optimized ethical and continued participation of prisoners. She suggests that the researcher must have a general knowledge of the criminal justice system and specific prison systems as well as be compliant with security policies. Byrne also suggests the participatory input of the prisoners under study and " awareness of and repeated dialogue with vested individuals and groups", "constant vigilance" and having clear research goals (2005, p. 226). The nurse practitioner in the correctional system may struggle at times to provide care while maintaining prison security for inmates who are socially and culturally diverse and often socially and economically disenfranchised and disadvantaged, many who have not had access to health care before they were imprisoned. The correctional nurse practitioner must see beyond the prisoners' status to be able to clearly assess and treat their patients. For example, citing a situation where prisoners brought in inebriated were not adequately assessed for hypoglycemia and subsequently died; Trossman relates that assessments can make the difference between life and death and that correctional nurses have an "obligation to be responsive to health concerns and not arbitrarily decide someone does not have a legitimate concern" (2011, p. 13). Seeing the clients and their health care needs as separate from their crime is essential for providing ethical care. Other ethical dilemmas faced are similar to those in other settings; for example, the lack of necessary resources to provide care or not enough staff to provide adequate care for the number and acuity of patients on a hospital unit or in an overcrowded prison.

4.6. ARMED FORCES

4.6.1. Research and the Military

Military subjects are viewed as vulnerable populations, on and off the battlefield, as they are subordinate members of a hierarchical group. Due to this status, they may be unduly influenced to participate in research for fear of retaliation if they refuse (CIOMS, 2002). When conducting research with the US Military, nurse researchers must also be certain of the ability of soldiers to give informed consent to avoid coercion as they may feel compelled to "obey requests", as they are taught to obey all orders ((McManus, McClinton, Gerhardt and Morris, 2007, p. 301). Nurse researchers must recognize that military personnel as participants in research are more vulnerable due to the restrictive nature of their military status and underlying nature of military obedience to serve and obey as opposed to an informed choice to participate.

4.6.2. Physicians

Bennhaum explored the historical perspective of the role of the physician in warfare and asked if history could tell us something about the ethical dilemmas of the military physician. He believes that war teaches physicians to behave ethically, as in the Hippocratic tradition. He concluded that limiting the damage of war has been the focus of both the soldier and the physician "for as long as war has existed" (p. 355).

4.6.3. Military Nursing

Historically, nursing's role in the military has been in the care for injured and sick soldiers and often within a "dangerous environment under threats of violence" (Fry, Harvey, Hurley and Foley 2002, p. 373). According to Southby, "clinical ethics for nurses in the military versus those in the private sector, and nurses in one of the military services versus another, do not really differ" but "what is unique is the number of stressful experiences in a compressed period of time" (2003, pp. 674, 676) during wartime. The treatment of prisoners of war is ethically challenging to military health care professionals. In a post September 11 era, the controversy over the ethical treatment of prisoners and detainees has been well documented in the medical literature (Clark, 2006; Miles, 2004, 2008, 2011; Lee, Conant, Jonsen and Heileg, 2006; Holmes and Perron, 2007). Southby (2003) contends that wartime nursing does add professional strain and moral dilemmas from the exposure to casualties that include fellow military personnel, civilians, and prisoners or detainees. The ethical dilemmas are similar to those of nurse practitioners working in the U.S. prison systems noted above; however, these patients are prisoners of war as opposed to prisoners of the state and the crimes are often related to differences of philosophy and values of opposing nations engaged in war time activities.

Nurse practitioners who make decisions about the wounded during wartime utilize the triage system whose "objective is to utilize medical resources as effectively and efficiently as possible and is "a utilitarian rationale" (Beauchamp and Childress, 2009, p. 279), violates "every creed of accepted nursing practice" (Southby, 2003, p. 674). This may cause significant moral distress if the less injured are treated first over more significant or catastrophic injuries as they might be using this triage system. Significant ethical dilemmas arise for nurse practitioners working in the military due to the nature of war and in difficult decisions made during triage of who lives and who dies. The conditions of military nursing during "military crisis deployments" puts nurse practitioners especially at risk for moral distress (Fry, Harvey, Hurley and Foley, 2002, p. 379) due to austere and/or life threatening conditions, unexpected nature of deployments despite training for preparedness/ readiness, and the removal and separation from traditional support systems. "Despite this, [military nurses] are expected to provide expert nursing care under conditions that are different from those of traditional nursing practice" (Fry, Harvey, Hurley and Foley, 2002, p. 379). Upholding underlying ethical principle and "acting in the best interest of the patient" (Southby, 2003, p. 683) is the same for nurses in the military as it is for any health professional.

4.7. INCOMPETENT PATIENTS

While it has been noted previously that nurse practitioners should avoid lists to determine vulnerability, competency is something the nurse practitioner should assess in their patients in order to determine vulnerability. Being incompetent is itself an identified vulnerable group as much as the state of being incompetent leads to vulnerability. The Patient Self-Determination Act of 1990 gave patients the moral right to make their own decisions about health care and the right to accept or refuse treatments. This act came about because of several landmark right-to-die-cases and based on state laws related to end of life decisions (Grace, 2009, p. 95) and more formally known as advanced directives or living wills. Laws pertaining to legally accepted advanced directives and living wills vary from state to state and nurse practitioners must be familiar with them in the states in which they practice. What happens in circumstances when patients are determined to be incompetent or lack the capacity to make autonomous decisions about their health, and more specifically, how do we know when they are unable to do so? The Patient Determination Act and state laws exist for those purposes.

4.7.1. The Ethical Principle of Autonomy

Originating from the Greek, "autonomous" means governance of self (αυτος = self; νομος = law) and is used to describe the governance of ancient Greek city-states. The term also refers to individuals as autonomous when they are self-determining and free from control of others in accordance with their own plans (Beauchamp and Ingress, 2009, p. 99). Respect for an individual's right to autonomously make decisions "runs deep in common morality as principle" (Beauchamp and Childress, 2009, p. 99). The Code of Ethics for Nursing calls for the respect for the human dignity of the autonomous individual. Nurses that respect the individual's right to make their own decisions is "consistent with the principle of autonomy" (Fowler, 2010, p. 149). When patients are incompetent, their autonomy is challenged because they are unable to make their own decisions, which then makes them vulnerable.

4.7.2. Autonomous Choice, Competency and Vulnerability

Is a patient competent to make a decision about his or her own health? Health care determinations about competency may lead to over-riding an individual's decisions (Beauchamp and Childress, 2009, p. 111). In such cases, health professionals may turn to informal or formal means to assist them in making health care decisions for their patients. In certain cases, legal incompetence is declared by a court decision and a surrogate decision-maker is appointed. In other cases, health professionals may turn to family members or others responsible for or appointed to act on behalf of the patient, if the patient lacks the ability/capacity to understand the benefits and risks of a therapy, a procedure, or a research protocol.

Competence is the ability to perform a task or a range of tasks related to a particular decision to be made by an individual. "Competence may vary over time and may be intermittent and as such, judgments of competence may be complicated by various categories and progress of diseases". Just give the reference. The concept of competence in decision-making is closely related to the concept of autonomy. Patients must be competent to understand information given to them by their health care provider to make an autonomous decision.

4.7.3. Paternalism, Autonomy and Vulnerability

Nurse practitioners must understand their own ethical values and should rely on defined standards of practice and ethical principles in making decisions for patients with or without capacity. Many patients and research subjects "are vulnerable to a range of decisional defects or impairments that render them unable to protect their own interests" (Miller and Wertheimer, 2007). Moreover, ethical codes for research are paternalistic in that they are meant to protect subjects. However, ensuring that the patient or research subjects' voices are still heard and perspective considered during decision-making is equally as important. They must also consider any harm to the patient and others in making decisions. When one with authority restricts or limits the autonomy of a patient, this is referred to as paternalism. Paternalism refers to a parent acting in the best interest of his child by regulating and carrying out decisions on the child's behalf because he or she is not old enough nor has the capacity to make an autonomous decision. Health care providers may find themselves in situations in which a decision must be made for a patient without capacity to do so as an autonomous person. A health care provider has the knowledge, authority and power to determine the patient's best interests but, unlike "a loving parent" (Beauchamp and Childress, 2009, p. 208), must be certain to avoid paternalistic decisions. This power of information and knowledge may also limit the patient with capacity or an alternate decision-maker when patients lack capacity to do so for themselves. The health care provider can do this intentionally or unintentionally by limiting information, offering or not offering treatment options or by treating or refusing to treat without regard to the patient's wishes (Yeo, Moorehouse, Khan and Rodney, 2010, p. 165). Nurse practitioners must also be clear about how and under what circumstances someone is capable of making an autonomous decision and what is necessary to assure that an autonomous decision is made (Grace, 2009, p. 20). Health care providers have a duty to act in the best interest of the patient in an emergency or life-threatening case, or in an end-of-life situation when patients do not have the capacity to decide for themselves and their wishes are unknown.

4.7.4. The Health Care Professional as the Gatekeeper: Judging Competence

Health care professionals often find themselves as gatekeepers in the determination as to whether a patient has the capacity or competence to make a decision. Competence and capacity are often used interchangeably in health care literature. "Health professionals' judgments of a person's incompetence may lead them to override that person's decision" (Beauchamp and Childress, 2009, p. 111) about decisions of care, but they do not have the legal authority to declare patients as incompetent.

Competence may fluctuate over the course of an illness, while under the influence of a prescribed medication or illicit drug or with the progression of an illness such as Alzheimer's disease. "Decision-making capacity is specific to the task or situation that requires a decision (Tunzi, 2001). Tunzi (2001) describes four clinical scenarios that should alert clinicians that further assessment is warranted. The first is a patient with abrupt mental status change which might be due to hypoxia, medications, or acute metabolic, neurological or psychological processes. The second alert for further assessment is when a patient refuses recommended treatment and is unwilling to discuss their reasons. A third alert occurs when a patient consents too quickly to treatments that are invasive or carry high risks. The fourth alert occurs when patients may have a known risk factor for decision-making. These include the vulnerable groups described in this chapter, neurological or psychiatric conditions, education levels, language or cultural barriers, or particular age group, such as children or the elderly. Careful assessment is always warranted because anyone in these described groups should not be automatically assumed to have diminished decision-making capacity. Wong, Clare, Gunn and Holland (1999) outlined three methods of assessing capacity: by the outcome of the decision, the status or membership of the patient to a specific group and by an assessment of the patient's decision-making skills and abilities as applied to a particular decision. In the first method of assessing capacity, the provider's own views, beliefs and values may prevent the provider from seeing the decision from the patient's perspective and thus consider the patient non-compliant and therefore incompetent. Health care providers should be aware of the diversity of cultural life styles, beliefs and values and which may have an impact on patient health care decisions. The second method groups patients as infants, children, the mentally and cognitively impaired and the institutionalized (both patients and prisoners). Judging capacity based on these classifications is not sufficient. While the autonomy of these classifications may be compromised or denied, some will have the capacity to make a decision. The third approach to assessing capacity is a functional approach in which the patient's decision-making skills as they apply to a particular decision are assessed at a particular relevant time. Health care providers using this approach recognize that there are different kinds of decisions with different levels of complexity. "A doubt about capacity represents a doubt about specific tasks or decisions, and not necessarily about all decisions" (Yeo, Moorehouse, Khan and Rodney, 2010, p. 158). Nurse practitioners should follow appropriate guidelines, standards and resources for evaluating decision-making capacity. For example, The Hartford Institute for Geriatric Nursing and

The Alzheimer's Association have resources for assessing the geriatric patient with dementia (available at www.consultGeriRN.org or www.hartfordign.org). Decision making capacity is not "an all-or-nothing on-off switch, but a patient's bad decision from the health care professional's perspective is not an indicator of lack of capacity and sign of incompetence" (Mitty, 2007).

4.8. CASE STUDY

4.8.1. Case Study 1

The threat of a deadly pandemic flu and vaccine shortage has brought healthcare providers, public health professionals and local public officials together to discuss strategies for setting up the local flu clinics in the community in which you are working. This is the public health emergency preparedness-planning and response group. Given this threat and shortage, multiple sites will be needed to distribute the vaccine to the public. The plan calls for the opening of clinics throughout the municipality in public schools, churches, and municipal buildings as well as at private practitioner offices and the hospital. In the past, the flu vaccine was given to children, the elderly and those with special medical needs as a priority over other populations. The community in question is a suburb of a large metropolitan area that is ethnically diverse and is believed to have a large number of unauthorized resident/illegal immigrants, although this cannot be verified by local public officials. The healthcare providers and public health professionals have considered that due to the enormity and seriousness of this pandemic, and in light of the vaccine shortage, that another plan to determine which populations should have priority access to the vaccine will be necessary. Personnel from the local community hospital are concerned about a rush on their emergency room and have suggested that all clinics demand proof of residency as a prerequisite for obtaining the vaccine. Given the threat of this deadly pandemic and vaccine shortage, as a member of this decision-making group, how would you prioritize distribution of the vaccine? What ethical goals and standards should this group consider in the preparation of these flu clinics? What are the ethical dilemmas you might face?

4.8.2. Case Study 2

The pandemic flu has taken its toll on the community. More and more patients are requiring ventilator support. There is a shortage of ventilators in your area and a request for additional equipment has been made to the federal government, as the President has declared the epidemic a national disaster. However, decisions as to how to allocate the ventilators to those who critically need them must be made accordingly. You are working as the advanced practice nurse in the medical ICU and the policy is to use the hospital's triage protocols and the CDC's *Ethical Guidelines in Pandemic Influenza* (2007) to make these types of decisions. Your team is making rounds on the patients, as there are two intubated patients in the ER that are being manually oxygenated with bag/valve/mask devises until a ventilator becomes available. One of the ICU patients is on a ventilator after suffering a severe stroke and did not have an advanced directive on record prior to coming in to the ER via EMS last night. You know that one of the patients in the ER is a 25 year old immigrant mother of five with no health insurance and the other is a 65 year old local business man accompanied by his wife and adult children. What dilemmas would you and your team face in allocating a ventilator to only one of these patients?

4.8.3. Case Study 3

You are a co-investigator on a study with the physician in your NP practice. Many of the patients in your practice have become participants in this collaborative research study. Part of the study requires an interview with clients after the experimental procedure under study has been completed. You learn from several of these patients for whom English is their second language, that they are not sure why this procedure had been done. You also discover that in some cases the consent was signed after the procedure was done. You show those who did sign their signed consent, but they clearly do not understand what they signed or the procedure. You know the physician has been asking his resident and fellow to enroll these patients. You speak to your co-investigator about what you have learned from interviewing some of the patients. The physician does not seem concerned, saying the procedure was to their [the patient] benefit anyway. How do you proceed and what changes would you make in conducting such future collaborative research studies?

4.9. REFERENCES

Aday, L.A. (1994). Health status of vulnerable populations. *Annual Review of Public Health, 15*(1): 487–509.

Aday, L.A. (2001). *At Risk in America: The Health Care Needs of Vulnerable Populations in the United States* (Second ed.). San Francisco: Josey-Bass.

American Nursing Association. (2010). *ANA Code of Ethics for Nurses with Interpretative Statements.*

Beauchamp, T.L. and Childress, J.F. (2009). *Principles of Biomedical Ethics* (6th ed.). New York: Oxford University Press.

Campinha-Bacote, J., and Padgett, J. (1995). Cultural competence: A critical factor in nursing research. *Journal of Cultural Diversity, 2*(1): 31–34.

Carrasquillo, O., Carrasquillo, A.I., and Shea, S. (2000). Health insurance coverage of immigrants living in the United States: Differences by citizenship status and country of origin. *American Journal of Public Health, 90*(6): 917–923.

Centers for Medicare and Medicaid Services, Patient Protection and Affordable Care Act (Pub. Law No. 111-148 Health Care and Education Act of 2010, Pub. Law No. No. 111-152. Retrieved from http://cms.org.

Clark, P.A. (2006). Medical ethics at Guantanamo Bay and Abu Ghraib: The problem of dual loyalty. *The Journal of Law, Medicine and Ethics, 34*(3): 570–580.

Code of Federal Regulations, Title 45 Part 46 Protection of Human Subjects.

Committee on the Robert Wood Johnson Foundation Initiative on the Future of Nursing, Institute of Medicine (2011). *The Future of Nursing: Leading Change, Advancing Health.* The National Academies Press.

Congressional Budget Office (2011). Retrieved from http://www.cbo.gov/.

Council for International Organizations of Medical Sciences (CIOMS). (2002). International Ethical Guidelines for Biomedical Research Involving Human Subjects.

Debruin, D. (2001). Reflections on vulnerability. *Bioethics Examiner, 5*(2): 1–7.

Derose, K.P., Escarce, J.J. and Lurie, N. (2007). Immigrant and health care: sources of vulnerability. *Health Affairs, 26*(5): 1258–1268.

Dreher, M, Shapiro, D and Asselin, M. (2006) *Healthy Places Healthy People: A Handbook for Culturally Competent Community Nursing Practice.* Sigma Theta Tau International Honor Society.

Dowd, S.B., Giger, J.N., and Davidhizar, R. (1998). Use of Giger and Davidhizar's Transcultural Assessment Model by health professions. *International Nursing Review, 45*(4): 119–122.

Dwyer, J. (2004). Illegal immigrants, health care, and social responsibility. *The Hastings Center Report, 34*(1): 34-41.

Fadiman, A. (1997). *The Spriti Catches You and You Fall Down: A Hmong Child, Her American Doctors, and the Collision of Two Cultures.* New York: Farrar, Straus and Giroux.

Flaskerud, J.H., and Winslow, B.J. (1998). Conceptualizing vulnerable populations health-related research. *Nursing Research, 47*(2): 69–78.

Flaskerud, J. H., Lesser, J., Dixon, E., Anderson, N., Conde, F., Koniak-Griffin, D., et al. (2002). Health disparities among vulnerable populations: Evolution of knowledge over five decades in nursing research publications. *Nursing Research, 51*(2): 74–85.

Fowler, M. D. M. (Ed.). (2010). *Guide to the Code of Ethics for Nurses: Interpretation and Application:* American Nurses Association.

Geertz, C. (1973). Religion as a cultural system. In: *The Interpretation of Cultures,* pp. 87–125. Basic Books.

Goldman, D.P., Smith, J.P., and Sood, N. (2005). Legal status and health insurance among immigrants. *Health Affairs, 24*(6): 1640–1653.

Gostin, L.O. (2007). Biomedical research involving prisoners. *JAMA: The Journal of the American Medical Association, 297*(7): 737–740.

Grace, P.J. (2009). *Nursing Ethics and Professional Responsibility in Advanced Practice.* Boston: Jones and Bartlett Publishers.

Gutherie, G. (2005). Bridging health disparities: Addressing unmet needs of women of color. *Journal of Obstetric, Gynecological, and Neonatoal Nursing, 5*: 385.

Holmes, D., and Perron, A. (2007). Violating ethics: unlawful combatants, national security and healthprofessionals. *Journal of Medical Ethics, 3*: 143–145.

H.R.3734—Personal Responsibility and Work Opportunity Reconciliation Act of 1996. (1996).

H.R.4449—Patient Self Determination Act of 1990. (1990).

Institute of Medicine. (2002). *Unequal Treatment: Confronting Racial and Ethnic Disparities in Health Care.* Washington, DC: National Academies Press.

Kachingwe, A.F., and Huff, R.M. (2007). The ethics of health promotion intervention in culturally diverse populations. In: *Health Promotion in Multicultural Populations: A Handbook for Practitioners and Students,* pp. 40–56. M.V. Kline and R.M. Huff (Eds.). Thousand Oaks, CA: SAGE Publications.

Kleinman, A. (1978). Culture, illness and care: clinical lesson from anthropological and cross-cultural research. *Annals of Internal Medicine, 88*: 251–258.

Kleinman, A. (1988). *The Illness Narratives: Suffering, Healing, and the Human Condition.* New York: Basic Books.

Lee, P.R., Conant, M., Jonsen, A.R., and Heileg, S. (2006). Participation in torture and interrogation: an inexcuseable breach of medical ethics. *Cambridge Quarterly in Healthcare Ethics, 15*: 202–203.

Miles, S.H. (2004). Abu Ghraib: its legacy for military medicine. *The Lancet, 364*(9435): 725–729.

Miles, S.H. (2008). Torture: the bioethics perspective. In:, *From Birth to Death and Bench to Clinical: The Hastings Center Bioethics Briefing Book for Journalists, Policymakers, and Campaigns,* pp. 169–172. M. Crowley (Ed.). Garrison, NY: The Hastings Center.

Miles, S.H. (2011). The new military medical ethics: Legacies of the gulf wars and the war on terror. *Bioethics, 25*: 1-7.

Miller, F.G. and Wertheimer, A. (2007). Facing up to paternalism in research ethics. *Hastings Report.* May/June. Retrieved from http://www.thehastingscenter.org/Publications/HCR/Default.aspx/.

Mitty, E. (2007). Advanced directives: protecting patient's rights. In: *Geriatric Nursing Protocols for Best Practice.* E. Capezuti, D. Zwicker, M. Mezey, D.Gray-Miceli and T. Fulmer (Eds.). New York: Springer Publishing Company.

National Commission for the Protection of Human Subjects of Biomedical and Behavioral Research. (1974). National Research Service Award Act of 1974.

Nuremberg Code (1947). Retrieved from http://ohsr.od.nih.gov/guidelines/nuremberg.html.

Nyamathi, A., Koniak-Griffin, D., and Greengold, B.A. (2007). Development of Nursing Theory and Science in Vulnerable Populations. In: *Annual Review of Nursing Research: Vulnerable Populations,* Vol. 25, pp. 3–26. J.J. Fitzpatrick (Ed.). New York: Springer.

Nyamathi, A., and Koniak-Griffin, D. (2007). In: *Annual Review in Nursing Research: Vulnerable Populations,* Vol. 25, pp. xiii–xv. J.J. Fitzpatrick (Ed.). New York: Springer.

Schulz, A.J. and Mullings, L. (2006). *Gender, Race, Class, and Health : Intersectional Approaches* (1st ed.). San Francisco, CA: Jossey-Bass.

Shi, L., and Stevens, G.D. (2010). *Vulnerable Populations in the United States.* San Francisco: Jossey-Bass.

Susser, I., and Patterson, T.C. (2001). *Cultural Diversity in the United States: A Critical Reader.* Oxford, UK ; Malden, Mass.: Blackwell Publishers.

Taylor, M.D.M. (2010). *Guide to the Code of Ethics for Nurses.* Silver Spring, Maryland: American Nurses Association.

The National Commission for the Protection of Human Subjects of Biomedical and Behavioral Research. (1979). *The Belmont Report: Ethical Principles and Guidelines for the protection of human subjects of research.*

The Hartford Institute for Geriatric Nursing. Retrieved from www.hartfordign.org

The National Commission for the Protection for the Protection of Human Subjects Research. (1974). *Report and recommendations: Research involving prisoners.*

Trossman, S. (2011) Ensuring standards are standard behind bars: Nurses work to review ANA document, promote corrections nursing practice. *The American Nurse,* November/December 2011, pp. 12–13.

Truman, B.I., Tinker, T., Vaughan, E., Kapella, B.K., Brenden, M., Woznica, C.V., et al. (2009). Pandemic influenza preparedness and response among immigrants and refugees. *Am. J. Public Health, 99*(S2): S278–286.

Tunzi, M. (2001). Can the patient decide? Evaluating patient capacity in practice. *American Family Physician, 64*(2): 299–306.

Turner, L. (2005). Is local cultural sensitivity sometimes insensitive? *Canadian Family Medicine, 51*: 478–479.

Urbina, I. (2006). *Panel suggests using inmates in drug trials.* New York Times, pp. 1.1.

U.S. Census (2010). Retrieved from http://www.census/gov/cps.

Wong, J.G., Clare, I.C., Gunn, M.J., and Holland, A.J. (1999). Capacity to make health care decisions: its importance in clinical practice. *Psychological Medicine, 29*(2): 437–446.

World Health Organization. What is the Value-Added of Human Rights in Public Health. Retrieved from http://www.who.int/hhr//hhr_activities_eng.pdf

Yeo, M., Moorehouse, A., Khan, P., and Rodney, P. (Eds.). (2010). *Concepts and Cases in Nursing Ethics* (Third ed.). Ontario, Cananda: Broadview Press.

CHAPTER 5

Ethical Considerations of Care and Research in Mental Health

PAMELA BJORKLUND

In principle, ethics is only meaningful where people—or groups of people—are self-governing and have the opportunity to make choices free from any coercion. Rarely is this the case in the mental health field. (Barker, 2011, p. 3)

5.1. INTRODUCTION

Respect for the autonomy of the human being is a cherished principle of biomedical ethics (Beauchamp and Childress, 2008). The principle derives from Enlightenment liberal traditions where the capacity for self-governance defines personhood and establishes human dignity, and is therefore of supreme value (Radden, 2003). Autonomy assumes the inherent equality and dignity of human beings who are endowed with reason, conscience, free will, and social circumstances free from duress and coercion (United Nations, 1948). The principle of autonomy undergirds the concept of informed consent in health care ethics, practice, and research where fully informed and autonomous decision-making has been a cherished if not fully inviolable right since the *Nuremberg Code*, which established in 1947 the essential right of human beings to voluntary participation in research:

> *This means that the person involved should have legal capacity to give consent; should be so situated as to be able to exercise free power of choice, without the intervention of any element of force, fraud, deceit, duress, overreaching, or other ulterior form of constraint or coercion; and should have sufficient knowledge and comprehension of the elements of the subject matter involved as to enable him to make an understanding and enlightened decision (Nuremberg Code in Shuster, 1997, p. 1436).*

In mental health care, however, some mentally ill persons are coerced into treatment without full and informed consent. Mentally ill persons may lack the capacity for fully autonomous, well-reasoned decisions and thus may be subject to the controlling judgments of disproportionately more powerful persons who act 'in their best interests' and 'for the good of the community.' Such people are not free from any element of force, duress, constraint, or coercion; nor do the connections between their reasons and their decisions insure enlightened choice. This reality defines the core vulnerability of persons with mental illness as well as one of the problems with an impartial, principles- or rights-based ethical framework for mental health practice. Where the mentally ill are concerned, autonomy is neither full nor individual. Often, it is diminished and relational—nested inside a contextual web of care-giving relationships, in particular the therapeutic relationship with the primary mental health care provider.

This chapter explores the unique vulnerability of persons with mental illness; situates an ethical framework for mental health care and research inside the domain of applied, professional ethics; and identifies and describes important ethical issues in mental health care and research. In addition, this chapter locates the source of these ethical issues for psychiatric-mental health nurses in their common, everyday practice routines; identifies the ethical approaches that are most useful to achieving moral understandings in mental health care and research; and provides case studies to illustrate and enlighten the preceding discussions. In all cases, permission was obtained to use ethical narratives and case studies.

5.2. PLACING PSYCHIATRIC-MENTAL HEALTH ETHICS IN CONTEXT

5.2.1. Ethics

Ethics is the scholarly study of morality (Lindemann, 2006). Morality is the subject matter of ethics and is commonly thought of as the right or good way to live, work, treat others, organize social life, and so forth. Ethics sets out to understand, justify, criticize, and correct, if necessary, moral beliefs and the ways of life in which those beliefs are practiced (Lindemann, 2006). Thus, ethics is not so much a 'subject matter' as a 'verb'—a mode of *doing* in thought and action that serves to understand, justify, criticize, correct, and re-establish moral equilibrium in social practices like mental health care and research (Lindemann, 2006; Walker, 2007). Ethics that pertain to the medical specialty of psychiatry/mental health might be termed *psychiatric ethics*. Given the nursing profession's commitment to holism, health promotion, and disease prevention—and because psychiatric disorders and mental health problems are not necessarily one and the same—the term *psychiatric-mental health ethics* is preferred here.

Three recognized branches of ethics include metaethics, normative ethics, and practical ethics (Lindemann, 2006). Metaethics is the study of what constitutes morality and where it originates. Normative ethics is the study of moral theories and concepts. It examines the norms, or standards, that are used to guide and evaluate actions. It proposes to explain what is *right*, what we *ought* to do, and how we *know* what we ought to do. Practical ethics is the study of ethical considerations that arise within specific social practices—for example, business, biomedicine, healthcare research, or advanced practice psychiatric-mental health nursing (Lindemann, 2006).

5.2.2. Professional Ethics

The term *professional ethics* refers to the practical or applied ethics attached to particular professions. Professions have some common characteristics, including specialized bodies of knowledge; responsibility for developing, disseminating, and using that knowledge; a practice orientation that is used for the good of the population served; and the ability to autonomously set educational and behavioral standards for the profession in order to monitor, regulate, and discipline the conduct of its members (Grace, 2009). In contemporary society, a profession's educational institutions, professional associations, and regulatory (licensing and certifying) bodies all play important roles in educating, monitoring, and regulating its members. Contemporary professions, including medicine and nursing, all formulate explicit codes of conduct that represent the discipline's promises to society (Grace, 2009)—for example, the American Psychiatric Association's (APA) Code of Ethics (APA, 2010) and the American Nursing Association's (ANA) Code of Ethics (ANA, 2001), with which all practitioners of psychiatric-mental health care and research should be familiar.

Boxes 5.1 and 5.2 summarize the essential elements of the APA and ANA professional codes. A profession has the autonomy to periodically revise its own standards, scope, and code of conduct to reflect changes in the profession's goals and society's needs as evidenced, for example, by the ever-changing constitution of the *Diagnostic and Statistical Manual of Mental Disorders* (*DSM*), which is scheduled to emerge in 2013 as *DSM-V*; by the routine updating of codes; or by the supplanting of one code by another, e.g., the replacement of the *Declaration of Hawaii* (1977) with the *Declaration of Madrid* (1996).

Box 5.1 - Summary of APA Code of Ethics

Section 1: A psychiatrist shall:

- Not exploit the patient to gratify own needs
- Not violate the boundaries of the doctor-patient relationship
- Not discriminate on the basis of ethnic origin, race, sex, creed, age, socioeconomic status, or sexual orientation
- Not make public appeals based solely upon emotion or utilize patient testimonials
- Not participate in legally authorized execution

Section 2: A psychiatrist shall:

- Conduct himself/herself with propriety in both professional and personal life
- Avoid sexual contact with current or former patients
- Guard against using the inherent inequality of the treatment relationship to influence patients in ways not directly relevant to treatment goals
- Avoid practicing outside his or her area of professional competence
- Intercede with other psychiatrists who jeopardize patient welfare and their own reputations and practices because of mental illness
- Explicitly establish binding contractual arrangements with patients
- Not charge for missed appointments except when this falls within the terms of the explicit contractual arrangement with the patient
- Not split fees, i.e., provide supervision or administration to other physicians or nonmedical persons for a percentage of their fees or gross income

Section 3: A psychiatrist shall:

- Respect the law
- Not engage in illegal activities that bear upon his or her practice
- May protest social injustice without behaving unethically
- May practice acupuncture if allowed by law and if professionally competent to do so

Section 4: A psychiatrist shall:

- Protect the confidentiality of psychiatric records, including the identification of persons as patients
- Release confidential information only with the authorization of the patient or under proper legal compulsion
- Adequately disguise clinical material used in teaching and writing
- Maintain patient confidentiality in consultations where the patient may not have been present and the consultee was not a physician
- Disclose only relevant information and avoid speculation as fact
- Fully describe to examinees the nature, purpose, and lack of confidentiality of examinations performed for security purposes or to determine legal competence or employment suitability

(continued)

Box 5.1 (continued) - Summary of APA Code of Ethics

Section 4 (continued): A psychiatrist shall:

- Assure minors of appropriate confidentiality while including parents and guardians in the treatment, when appropriate
- Reveal confidential information disclosed by a patient only when clinical judgment determines a high risk of danger to patient or others
- May present a patient to a scientific gathering if the patient has provided full and informed consent and the attendees accept the confidentiality of the presentation
- May dissent within the framework of the law if ordered by a court to reveal patient confidences
- May present a current or former patient to a public gathering or news media only if the patient is competent and offers full and informed consent in writing to the enduring loss of confidentiality
- Advise research participants of the investigation's funding sources
- Not evaluate persons charged with criminal acts prior to access to, or availability of, legal counsel
- Avoid sexual involvement with students, trainees, or supervisees

Section 5: A psychiatrist shall:

- Obtain continuing education
- Make referrals only to competent and qualified members of other professional disciplines
- Spend sufficient time to insure that supervisees or collaborating professionals are providing appropriate care
- Never delegate to nonmedical personnel anything that requires the exercise of professional medical judgment
- Agree to the request of a patient for consultation or to such a request from the family of an incompetent or minor patient

Section 6: A psychiatrist shall:

- Hold the therapeutic relationship with the patient above all other considerations in treatment
- Refuse to provide psychiatric treatment to a person who cannot be diagnosed as having a mental illness amenable to treatment

Section 7: A psychiatrist shall:

- Foster the cooperation of those legitimately concerned with the medical, psychological, social, and legal aspects of mental health and illness
- Serve society by advising and consulting with the executive, legislative, and judiciary branches of government
- Clarify his or her status as individual or representative of an organization
- Avoid cloaking public statements with the authority of the profession (e.g., "Psychiatrists know that . . .")

(continued)

Box 5.1 (continued) - Summary of APA Code of Ethics

Section 7 (continued): A psychiatrist shall:

- Never offer a professional opinion on a case unless he or she has conducted an examination and has been granted proper authorization for such a statement
- Permit his or her certification to be used for the involuntary treatment of a person only following his or her personal examination of that person, and only following the finding that the person cannot form a judgment as to what is in his/her own best interests and is likely to harm self or others without such treatment
- Never participate in torture

Section 8: A psychiatrist shall:

- Regard responsibility to the patient as paramount

Section 9: A psychiatrist shall:

- Support access to medical care for all people

APA. (2010). *The principles of medical ethics with annotations especially applicable to psychiatry.* American Psychiatric Association.

Box 5.2 - Summary of ANA Code of Ethics

The nurse:

1. Practices with compassion and respect for the inherent dignity, worth, and uniqueness of every individual
2. Has a primary commitment to the patient, whether an individual, family, group, or community
3. Promotes, advocates for, and strives to protect the health, safety, and rights of the patient
4. Is responsible and accountable for individual nursing practice and delegation of tasks consistent with the nurse's obligation to provide optimum patient care
5. Owes the same duties to self as to others, including the responsibility to preserve integrity and safety, to maintain competence, and to continue personal and professional growth
6. Participates in establishing, maintaining, and improving health care environments and conditions of employment conducive to the provision of quality health care and consistent with the values of the profession
7. Participates in the advancement of the profession through contributions to practice, education, administration, and knowledge development
8. Collaborates with other health professionals and the public in promoting community, national, and international efforts to meet health needs
9. Is a member of a profession that is responsible for articulating nursing values, for maintaining the integrity of the profession and its practice, and for shaping social policy

Source: ANA. (2001). *Code of ethics for nurses with interpretive statements.* Silver Springs, MD: American Nurses Association.

Box 5.3 identifies the historical bedrock for the APA (2010) and ANA (2001) codes. Of particular importance for psychiatric-mental health ethics and mental health practitioners is the *Declaration of Madrid*, which establishes the specific standards for psychiatric-mental health care and research that have been adopted by all 130 societies of the World Psychiatric Association (WPA) (Tasman and Mohr, 2011; WPA, 1996). Boxes 5.4 and 5.5 summarize the essential elements of the *Declaration of Madrid.*

Box 5.3 - Historic Ethical Codes in Mental Health Care and Research

Nuremberg Code (1947)

- Established 10 principles for permissible medical research with human participants, especially voluntary informed consent (Roberts & Roberts, 1999)
- Emphasized protection of human participants from undue harms/ risks and unnecessary pain/ suffering
- Most important document in the history of the ethics of medical research (Shuster, 1997)

Declaration of Geneva (1948, amended 1968)

- An oath that abjures the physician from using medical knowledge "contrary to the laws of humanity"
- A response to atrocities committed by physicians in Nazi Germany (World Medical Association, 1948)

Declaration of Helsinki (1964, amended 1975, 1983, 1989, 1996, 2000, 2002, 2004, 2008)

- Distinguished between therapeutic and nontherapeutic research: All study participants must be assured of the best proven diagnostic and therapeutic method of care (Roberts & Roberts, 1999)
  —Therapeutic research (clinical research that combines biomedical research with professional care)
  —Non-therapeutic research (non-clinical biomedical research involving human tissues or data) (World Medical Organization, 1996)

Declaration of Hawaii (1977, amended 1983)

- Functioned to provide ethical guidance specific to the profession
- Laid down 10 general ethical guidelines for psychiatrists world-wide
- Emphasized the aim of psychiatry to promote health, personal autonomy, and growth (World Psychiatric Association, 1978)

(continued)

Box 5.3 (continued) - Historic Ethical Codes in Mental Health Care and Research

Belmont Report (1979)

- Provided ethical foundations for current federal regulations including Subpart A (Common Rule) and Subparts B, C, and D for "vulnerable populations"
- Specifies three ethical principles that govern research with human participants
  - —Respect for persons
    - * Treat participants as autonomous agents; insure full and informed consent
    - * Protect those with diminished autonomy
  - —Beneficence
    - * Insure favorable balance of risks and benefits
  - —Justice
    - * Insure fair procedures and outcomes in the selection of research participants (National Commission for the Protection of Human Subjects of Biomedical and Behavioral Research, 1979)

Declaration of Madrid (1996, amended 1999, 2002, 2005)

- Declared specific standards for psychiatric practice world-wide
- Adopted by all 130 societies of the World Psychiatric Association as prerequisite for membership

Box 5.4 - Summary of Declaration of Madrid

A psychiatrist must:

- Offer best evidence-based treatment available consistent with ethical principles
- Utilize least freedom-restrictive treatment available
- Seek advice and expertise of others when needed
- Advocate for equitable distribution of healthcare resources
- Keep up with scientific developments in the specialty
- Partner with patients to allow free and informed decisions within relationships of mutual trust and respect
- Safeguard human dignity and legal rights in cases of grave disability or incompetence
- Provide no treatment against the patient's will except in cases of danger to life (patient or third party)
- Uphold the 'best interests' of the patient as paramount in treatment

(continued)

Box 5.4 (continued) - Summary of Declaration of Madrid

A psychiatrist must:

- Assess and treat patients only with their full and informed consent, especially in third-party situations (e.g., consultations, court-ordered evaluations)
- Maintain patient confidentiality and breach only for danger to third party
- Engage in research with psychiatric patients only when:
  —Research is reviewed by ethics committee and is scientifically valid
  —Researcher is properly trained for research
  —Participants are competent to consent
  —Autonomy and physical/mental integrity of participants are safeguarded

Source: World Psychiatric Association (WPA). (1996). *Madrid declaration on ethical standards for psychiatric practice.* WPA, General Assembly, Madrid.

Box 5.5 - Special Situations in Declaration of Madrid

- Euthanasia
  —Duty is to protect life
  —Mental illness may distort patient decisions
- Torture
  —No participation even when under duress
- Death penalty
  —No participation in competency evaluations for execution
- Selection of sex
  —No participation in decisions to terminate pregnancy for purposes of sex selection
- Organ transplantation
  —Role is to insure informed consent and patient self-determination
  —No use of psychotherapeutic skills to influence patient decisions
- Psychiatrists addressing the media
  —Represent the profession with dignity
  —Uphold the dignity of persons with mental illness
  —Make no pronouncements on presumed psychopathology of any person
  —Present research findings accurately and with awareness of their impact
- Discrimination on ethnic or cultural grounds is never permitted

(continued)

Box 5.5 (continued) - Special Situations in Declaration of Madrid

- Genetic research and counseling
  - —Duty to insure full and informed consent of participants
  - —Adequate protection of genetic information against misuse
  - —Referral for genetic testing only to facilities with quality assurance and accessible genetic counseling
  - —Genetic counseling for family planning must respect patients' value systems
- Ethics of psychotherapy in medicine
  - —Practitioners of psychotherapy must have proper training
  - —Approach should be scientific and culturally/ethnically sensitive
  - —Full and informed consent of the patient is required
  - —Power differential in the therapeutic relationship must be recognized
  - —Boundaries must be respected
  - —Confidentiality must be maintained except where mandatory reporting is required (child abuse, elder abuse, danger to third party)
- Conflict of interest in relationship with industry
  - —Avoid accepting gifts
  - —Disclose financial and contractual relationships
- Conflicts arising with third party payers
  - —Principles of good psychiatric practice can conflict with organizational imperatives to maximize profits/minimize costs
  - —Maintain professional independence to apply best practice guidelines
  - —Oppose limits on benefits, parity, or limited access to needed medication
- Boundary violations
  - —Sexual relationships with patients are never permitted
- Protection of the rights of psychiatrists
  - —To live up to the obligations of their profession
  - —To practice at the highest level of excellence
  - —To practice free from abuse by totalitarian regimes or profit-driven economic systems
  - —To practice free from discrimination and the stigma of mental illness
  - —To advocate for patients without media ridicule or professional persecution
- Disclosing the diagnosis of Alzheimer's
  - —Patients have the right to know or not to know
  - —Patients and families should be told as early as possible
  - —Exceptions to disclosure in cases of severe dementia, phobia, severe depression

(continued)

Box 5.5 (continued) - Special Situations in Declaration of Madrid

- Dual responsibilities
  —May arise for insurance or employment purposes or as part of legal proceedings to judge competency, fitness to stand trial, criminal responsibility, or dangerousness to self or others
  —Duty is to disclose to the patient the nature of the assessment as non-therapeutic or potentially damaging
  —Must advocate for separation of records to limit exposure of information only to that which is essential for third-party purposes

Source: World Psychiatric Association (WPA). (1996). *Madrid declaration on ethical standards for psychiatric practice.* WPA, General Assembly, Madrid.

5.2.3. Nursing Ethics

Nursing ethics is a form of practical, professional, or applied ethics. It is in that sense that the terms *nursing ethics* and *professional responsibility* can be considered equivalent concepts (Grace, 2009). However, the term *nursing ethics* is controversial in that some scholars believe nursing ethics is a unique field with considerations that cannot be fully understood by adapting biomedical ethics—that is, the professional ethics of physicians (Veatch and Fry, 2006). Others insist there is nothing morally unique to nursing: Nursing ethics is just a subcategory of bioethics; the same moral issues emerge in health care settings across professions and the same ethical principles apply to those issues whether one is a physician, nurse, patient, or administrator (Veatch and Fry, 2006). Similarly, even though different professions do have unique characteristics, some argue that claims for a unique ethics for each profession are unnecessary: different or specialized ethical demands in the mental health context can be met with a broader sense of what it means to be ethically sensitive in health care (Crowden, 2003). Others argue that impartial principles and broad understandings of healthcare professional ethics cannot account for the unique ethical demands placed on the psychiatric provider; for example, to use the 'personal self' as one's principal therapeutic tool (Radden, 2004; Sadler, 2007). Nor do they recognize the autonomy of the psychiatric patient as relational and the nature of psychiatric treatment as a relationship—more often, as a *web* of relationships wherein influence is inherent; treatment decisions are continuous, not dichotomous; and the subjectivity of the clinician, who is a fundamental component of the situation as a *person*, is inescapable (Olsen, 2003).

Here, nursing ethics is differentiated from healthcare ethics broadly to emphasize the roots of nursing ethics in everyday nursing practice as opposed to a transcendent realm of universal, impartial ethical principles. Thus, the term *nursing ethics* refers not merely to the professional ethics of the nursing discipline. More specifically, it refers to the study of nurses' moral concerns, nurses' moral knowledge, and nurses' moral judgments as they arise, are experienced, and are acted upon in the everyday, routinized, but nevertheless unique context of psychiatric-mental health nursing practice at multiple levels across multiple sites (J. Liaschenko, personal communication, September, 2006).

5.3. ETHICAL CONSIDERATIONS IN MENTAL HEALTH CARE

5.3.1. Vulnerability in Mental Illness

5.3.1.1. Diminished Autonomy/Forced Treatment

The mentally ill are vulnerable on several counts, not least of which is their frequently diminished autonomy and decisional capacity. Mental illness is one of the few forms of illness that is commonly treated by force against the person's expressed wishes (Barker, 2011), including such treatment as seclusion, restraint, involuntary medication, involuntary commitment, and restriction of a patient's rights to such things as visitors, phone calls, personal possessions, and taken-for-granted 'privileges' like the right to leave one's room, watch television, eat in a dining room, or associate with others. Clearly, the model of the autonomous patient or research participant is problematic, if not also unrealistic with respect to patients whose self-control, judgment, insight, reasoning ability, and capacity to effectively recognize and communicate needs and concerns waxes and wanes.

Even psychiatric patients who clearly lack adequate decisional capacity may nevertheless retain their moral agency and can still make self-interested choices which, although irrational, are not necessarily harmful to self or others. Autonomy or the capacity to self-govern is predicated upon agency, that is, one's status as a moral agent—a person with inherent dignity and worth who acts in the world for reasons of his or her own. Respecting the autonomy of psychiatric patients entails upholding their moral agency: "To be 'cured' against one's will and cured of states which we may not regard as disease is to be put on a level with those who have not yet reached the age of reason or those who never will; to be classed with infants, imbeciles, and domestic animals" (C.S. Lewis in Barker, 2011, p. 45).

Thus, a major challenge in mental health care and research is to establish whether or to what extent psychiatric patients possess decisional capacity and are capable of giving or withholding informed consent for either treatment or participation in research. In some cases, competence to give or withhold consent must be formally evaluated and documented, usually by a physician, as specified by law. Judgments of competency are typically made in the context of treatment refusals whereupon risks, benefits, and interests must be weighed in the matter of paternalistic interventions like involuntary commitment, forced medication, or any other serious restriction of patient rights. Such paternalistic interventions require not only that the patient lacks decisional capacity but also that the forced treatment or restrictions are in the patient's 'best interests' (Szmukler and Appelbaum, 2008). While the person's best interests may be difficult to determine, considerations include:

- The past and present wishes and feelings of the person concerned, to the degree they can be ascertained, along with the factors the person would consider if able to do so;
- The need to permit and encourage the person to participate as fully as possible in any decisions made for him or her;
- The views of others in the person's relational network with whom it would be appropriate to consult about the person's wishes, feelings, and best interests; and
- Whether the purpose for which any decision is required can be as effectively achieved in a less restrictive manner (Szmukler and Appelbaum, 2008, p. 241).

While 'the protection of others' may be invoked to rationalize forced treatment or restrictions of rights, a potential for dangerousness to others should not be confused with the person's 'best (health) interests,' which can justify involuntary treatment where decisional capacity is lacking. As an ethical and legal consideration, 'protection of others' may justify involuntary detention and treatment, depending on the credibility, seriousness, and magnitude of the risk to others; but it does not hinge on the individual's lack of decisional capacity. The potential for dangerousness to others may be high while the health interest may be minor, and the individual may be fully competent to make treatment decisions despite community safety concerns (Szmukler and Appelbaum, 2008). In sum, the legal justification for involuntary psychiatric treatment in all 50 U.S. states requires the presence of mental illness, which presumes impaired decisional capacity, along with either the potential for dangerousness to oneself or others or grave disability, which is an extension of the potential for danger to self by means of inability to care for oneself sufficiently to meet basic conditions necessary for life (Olsen, 2003).

5.3.1.2. Treatment Pressures/Therapeutic Relationships

Psychiatric-mental health patients are also vulnerable because they receive mental health care and treatment in the context of a therapeutic relationship in which influence is inherent and unavoidable. The character, or person of the clinician, including his or her virtues, is ethically significant for patient outcomes. The clinician's skills at building, maintaining, and repairing ruptures in the therapeutic relationship are more significant for therapeutic outcome than the clinician's theoretical orientation or therapy-specific training (Olsen, 2003; Radden and Sadler, 2008; Safran and Muran, 2003). This emotionally charged interpersonal process may be the key to treatment outcome; over the course of approximately 50 years of psychotherapy research, the quality of the therapeutic relationship has turned out to be the most robust indicator of treatment success (Muran and Barber, 2010; Safran and Muran, 2003).

The influence inherent in the therapeutic relationship exists on a spectrum of coercion, or treatment pressures that range from (a) persuasion, suggestions, and recommendations to (b) interpersonal leverage; (c) inducements, incentives, or offers; (d) threats; and (e) involuntary, or 'forced' treatment (Szmukler and Appelbaum, 2008). Persuasion appeals to the patient's reason, respects the patient's autonomy, and is least problematic. Suggestions and recommendations lie at the boundary between persuasion and interpersonal leverage, which uses the patient's less powerful position and sometimes emotionally dependent relationship with the clinician to exert pressure in a particular direction (Szmukler and Appelbaum, 2008). Inducements present the patient with goods, services, monetary rewards, or other incentives for cooperation with recommended treatment. Although more extreme and problematic, threats approximate inducements in that both involve conditional propositions: If the patient accepts treatment, then the clinician will do X. If the patient does *not* accept treatment, then the clinician will be 'forced' to do Y. At this point, the term *coercion* rather than *treatment pressure* is clearly appropriate (Szmukler and Appelbaum, 2008). Forced treatment, of course, lies at the extreme end of the spectrum and deprives the patient of all autonomy. While inducements, incentives, and threats are ethically questionable if not morally repugnant, they nevertheless are commonly used in the U.S. to leverage psychiatric treatment (Monahan *et al.*, 2005; Robbins, Petrila, LeMelle, and Monahan, 2006; Szmukler and Appelbaum, 2008).

5.3.1.3. Exploitation/Boundaries

Due to such factors as impaired reality-testing, limited insight, poor judgment, and other aspects of their diminished autonomy, the mentally ill are especially vulnerable to exploitation, dependence, abuses of power, and the inherent influence and inequality of the treatment relationship. According to the APA Code of Ethics, the therapeutic relationship is "such a vital factor in effective treatment" that preservation of optimal conditions for development and maintenance of a strong therapeutic alliance takes "precedence over all other [ethical and technical] considerations" (APA, 2010, p. 9; Radden, 2002a). Because each individual clinician has a unique and powerful potential to help or harm the patient, extra care must be taken by the mental health provider to observe the boundaries of the treatment relationship, especially because of the "private, highly personal, and sometimes intensely emotional" nature of the relationship (APA, 2010, p. 3; Radden, 2002a). The intensity of the therapeutic relationship can activate needs and fantasies in both patient and provider "while weakening the objectivity necessary for control" (APA, 2010, p. 4; Radden 2002a). Such interventions as advice-giving, self-disclosure, and other deliberate or inadvertent boundary crossings exploit the power differential in the therapeutic relationship and further weaken the patient's autonomy if they are not accompanied by a clinically sound, contextually appropriate, and well-documented therapeutic rationale.

So important is the issue of boundaries that much of psychiatric-mental health ethics could be considered discourse on boundary violations. All human relationships have boundaries (Jorgenson, Hirsch, and Wahl, 1997). In personal relationships, boundaries tend to evolve over time as a relationship develops or the parties to it grow and change: "For example, the parent and child renegotiate boundaries as the child moves toward adulthood, and the boundaries in an intimate relationship shift as trust between the parties grows" (Jorgenson *et al.*, 1997, p. 50). Boundaries in professional relationships are more rigid; once set, they typically are not crossed or violated without justification. Boundaries flow from the fiduciary nature of the professional relationship, which exists because the professional possesses knowledge and/or skills that the patient lacks and thus seeks. In accepting the trust and confidence of the patient, the fiduciary, or trustee, agrees to act only in the patient's 'best interests' as collaboratively defined (Jorgenson *et al.*, 1997).

Gutheil and Gabbard (1993) have distinguished between benign boundary crossings and harmful boundary violations in mental health care with respect to time, place and space, money, gifts, physical contact, language, self-disclosure, and patient and therapist roles. They have suggested that boundary crossings are benign, therapeutic variants that advance the treatment in a productive way and do not harm the patient. Some of these boundary crossings could be completely appropriate human responses to unusual events that involved physical contact. For example, "[a] patient stumbled as she was leaving the office and fell to the floor. The therapist helped the patient up and made sure that she was all right" (Gutheil and Gabbard, 1998, p. 410); or, "[a] patient entered her therapist's office and announced that she had just received news that her son had died. The patient reached out to embrace the therapist, and the therapist accepted the embrace as the patient sobbed" (Gutheil and Gabbard, 1998, p. 410). Failing to respond humanely at such times might have a negative impact on the patient, perhaps leading to premature termination of treatment, which would be more harmful to the patient than the inadvertent boundary crossing.

A boundary violation, on the other hand, is obviously harmful, constitutes exploitation of the patient, and is likely to destroy the treatment over time. Unlike a boundary crossing, the therapeutic rationale for a boundary violation is usually not identified, discussed, or documented and may be part of an unexamined, repetitive practice (Gutheil and Gabbard, 1998). The harm may range from wasting the patient's time and money to inflicting severe trauma including the following examples: the therapist who hugs the patient at the end of each session, the therapist who asks the patient to run errands for him, the therapist who conducts sessions outside the office or discloses his or her own personal problems in a way that burdens the patient, and the therapist who makes overt sexual contact with the patient (Gutheil and Gabbard, 1998).

The "edge of appropriate behavior" that defines a boundary is not always clear in mental health care due to the diversity of psychotherapeutic approaches, the need to individualize treatment with targeted strategies for a wide range of variously functioning people in unique situations, and professional norms which change with historical and social conditions (Gutheil and Gabbard, 1998, p. 410). Freud, for example, analyzed his own daughter, Anna; similarly, he analyzed his friend, Sandor Ferenzi, while walking through the countryside during vacations (Gutheil and Gabbard, 1993). Today, mental health treatment of family, friends, and/or self—outside the office, no less—constitutes a boundary violation for which investigation by the appropriate regulatory agency would be required along with professional sanctions.

The purpose of clear boundaries is to create a safe and predictable environment for both patient *and* provider, in which the therapeutic alliance can flourish and external boundaries create the possibility of productively crossing psychological boundaries through potentially therapeutic mechanisms including empathy, interpretation of transference and countertransference, and identification with the therapist (Gutheil and Gabbard, 1998). Boundary crossings have both patient care and risk management dimensions. A boundary crossing has the potential to either enhance or compromise patient care, while knowledge of boundaries is important to effective risk management (Gutheil and Gabbard, 1993). Court decisions suggest a trend toward findings of liability for boundary violations even in the absence of gross therapist misconduct; and fact finders—civil or criminal juries, judges, ethics committees of professional organizations, or state licensing boards—often believe that the presence of even minor boundary crossings is presumptive evidence of, or corroborates allegations of, gross therapist misconduct including sexual misconduct, which usually begins with relatively minor boundary crossings (Gutheil and Gabbard, 1993).

Crossing boundaries for therapeutic purposes is an advanced psychotherapeutic skill, and mental health practitioners should practice within both their professional and personal scope. A boundary crossing may be important for a patient's growth and development, but it is not always easy to know how or when to do this. New practitioners typically find it awkward, unnecessarily rigid, inauthentic, or lacking in empathy to strictly and consistently maintain the boundaries of time, place, money, gifts, physical contact, self-disclosure, and role (Gutheil and Gabbard, 1993). It takes sensitivity, knowledge, experience, technical skill, and risk tolerance to know when crossing a boundary is clinically indicated. However, basic risk management requires clear documentation in the patient record of the indications and clinical rationale for deliberate boundary crossings.

Most clinicians make unintentional self-disclosures. For example, they decorate their offices in ways that reflect who they are. Their manner of speech and dress, their style of greeting patients, and all other verbal and nonverbal communications reveal information to the patient. A clinician self-discloses anytime he or she chooses to comment on any particular aspect of the patient's dialogue. The clinician is telling the patient something about what he or she thinks is important. Patients are generally quite expert at noticing and picking up on these inadvertent self-disclosures, which are not the same as deliberate, conscious choices to reveal something personal about oneself as a therapeutic technique, although deliberate *and* inadvertent self-disclosures both require discussion with the patient. "The boundary issue is not whether self-disclosure occurs or does not occur. Rather, the key issue is *what* the therapist self-discloses and whether the therapist burdens the patient with personal problems in a manner that reverses the roles in the dyad" (Gutheil and Gabbard, 1998, p. 412).

The vulnerability of the psychiatric patient to harmful boundary crossings imposes a special burden on the provider. With greater opportunity to exploit and dominate, the provider must adhere to stricter standards of good conduct, or virtuous behavior (Radden, 2002b). Virtue ethics, a character-focused approach to ethics, is a helpful, perhaps necessary, if not entirely sufficient model for understanding ethical concerns in mental health care and research (Radden and Sadler, 2008; Sadler, 2007). Virtues are defined as the personal qualities attributed to a person's character and are identifiable through outward action as well as through more subtle manifestations of the person's inner, mental life (Radden and Sadler, 2008). Virtue is evidenced in practice and requires rehearsal, planning, focus, effort, and discipline. Virtue may be acquired through habituation, taught through educational processes, and utilized in the practitioner's capacity for practical reasoning and practical judgment in resolving ethical conflicts (Radden and Sadler, 2008). Because virtue ethics emphasizes everyday conduct, which is laden with ethical significance (Radden and Sadler, 2008), and everyday practice gives rise to the ethical concerns most salient to nurses (Chambliss, 1996), the virtues are important to nurse professionals. Indeed, the virtuous character traits of integrity, compassion, courage, honesty, and humility, to name a few, are explicitly identified in the ANA Code of Ethics as essential to nursing practice (ANA, 2001; Crigger and Godfrey, 2011; Grace, 2009).

5.3.1.4. 'Personal Self'/Stigma

The ethical significance of the 'personal self' of both the patient and the mental health provider cannot be overstated. The personal self of the clinician is an important instrument in effective treatment (Sadler, 2007). The 'self' is a complex amalgam of knowledge, skills, values, ideals, experiences, affects, character traits, self-representations, and outward behavior. It is the practitioner's most salient and valuable therapeutic tool, essential to the therapeutic alliance, which in turn is *the* most important factor for successful mental health outcomes. The personal self, a commonsense concept with ethical and psychiatric significance, is characterized by *agency*, the ability to act in the world for reasons of one's own; *identity*, which distinguishes the self from all else; *trajectory*, movement along a course that stretches forward into the future; *history*, awareness of a past belonging uniquely to oneself; and *perspective*, a standpoint from which to view and experience the world (Sadler, 2007). The personal self is owned; it is 'mine.' However, treatment requires the patient not only to share intimate aspects of the personal self but to reform and reconstruct it in a therapeutic project that is unmatched in our culture with the exception, perhaps, of childrearing (Radden, 2002a). It is an endeavor that heightens both the patient's vulnerability and the responsibilities imposed on the practitioner.

For the patient and others, the boundary between self and mental illness is not always clear. What the clinician considers signs and symptoms of illness may be, for the patient, "prized aspects of the personal self" (Sadler, 2007, p. 116). What Sadler (2007) terms *self-illness ambiguity*, or more descriptively, the "invasion of the personal space by mental illness," contributes to the vulnerability of psychiatric patients (p. 118). They can feel offended, harassed, and intruded upon by the presumptions and ministrations of well-meaning others who may not themselves fully recognize or appreciate the difference between, for example, the 'person with schizophrenia' and 'the schizophrenic' who has become the illness (Sadler, 2007). Distrustful of their own experience, such patients may question their very identity: "Is this me or is this my illness?" Successful treatment depends in part on "making the self-illness ambiguity less ambiguous" as more aspects of the personal self become visible, comprehensible, and manageable (Sadler, 2007, p. 117).

The conflation or fusion of the patient's personal self with his or her mental illness contributes to social stigma, which compounds the vulnerability of psychiatric patients in presenting them with yet another burden to manage. Not only must they struggle with the mental illness, but they must also contend with the shame, humiliation, and mistreatment that attends social stigma (Sadler, 2007). Stigma occurs as a function of attaching a negative, misunderstood, and exaggerated attribute to a social group that results in global devaluation of group members (Goffman, 1963; Halter, 2008). People with the undesirable attribute may be considered to have brought it upon themselves as a matter of moral failure, poor self-control, or lack of willpower (Halter, 2008). In cases of the mentally ill, the special vulnerability of psychiatric patients extends to the societal reaction to mental illness, which feeds back into conceptions of the personal self (Sadler, 2007). As a function of stigma, their psychic pain is often less recognizable than physical pain no matter how debilitating the mental illness may be. Others in society may still find the pain of mental illness unpersuasive, if they see it at all (Sadler, 2007).

The confusion of personal self with mental illness manifests not only in the patient's distrust of personal experience but also in society's pervasive distrust of the psychiatric patient's psychological integrity, capacity for self-control, responsibility for personal conduct, and ability to safely and cooperatively live in community with others (Sadler, 2007). Radden (2002b) best articulated the problem:

> *[S]cience may eventually allow us to identify and explain states of mental disorder with reference to specific biological markers and underlying causes, thus eliminating much of the negativity, mystery and fear presently surrounding them. Yet some of the systemic prejudice and stigma attaching to such states seem likely to remain as long as our cultural values are unchanged, values which include autonomy, rationality, self-control, personal identity and psychological integrity. With roots deep in the Greek origins of Western culture, these values are entrenched, long lived and antithetical to the ravages wrought by mental disorder. Nothing less than the elimination of these states through prevention and cure . . . could entirely end the negativity attaching to them (Radden, 2002b, p. 411).*

The stigma of mental illness may abate as science advances, but the state of psychiatric science to date has certainly not yet made this possible.

5.3.1.5. Dual Relationships/'Dirty Hands'

Dual relationships are constituted by the necessity of providers working for the benefit of parties other than, or in addition to, the patient. Dual agency exacerbates the vulnerability of the psychiatric patient and creates ethical problems for the mental health practitioner, whose allegiance might be divided between a patient who needs a certain level or kind of care and an agency that needs to cut costs. Gutheil and Simon (2003) recommend that providers follow the conclusions of the Hastings Center (1978) with respect to issues of double agency: separate functions should reside in different roles, and patients should be fully informed not only of treatment objectives but also of any conflicts within the provider's priorities or between different professionals' agendas. Tasman and Mohr (2011) advise clinicians to completely avoid treatment situations that place them in a conflict between therapeutic responsibility to patients and third parties. Examples of dual relationships include clinicians treating their own relatives and friends, the same therapist employing concurrent family and individual therapy with a given patient, and clinicians testifying as forensic witnesses for current psychotherapy patients.

A major area for ethical concern in mental health care has been generated by the ways in which health care is financed and access to care and its associated costs are controlled. Managed care may achieve its financial goals with practices that promote dual relationships. Managed care organizations may place strains on confidentiality, privacy, trust, and other aspects of the therapeutic relationship (Radden, 2002b) by their need to control costs and access to care. Mental health practitioners may find it necessary to act as gate keepers, limiting and rationing health care to insure the viability and/or profitability of the organization (Radden, 2002b). Specific issues of concern include restrictions on the number of clinicians listed on provider panels for a given community, increasing numbers of MCO personnel with access to confidential treatment records, transfer of authority for treatment decisions from providers to less knowledgeable treatment reviewers, refusal to pay for integrated treatment, and insistence on split treatment models in which the patient obtains psychotherapy from a social worker or psychologist and only brief, infrequent medication management visits with a psychiatrist or psychiatric nurse practitioner (Tasman and Mohr, 2011). Such restrictive practices fragment patient care, limit the capacity of medical providers to insure high quality care, and create an ethical bind in which "medical responsibility is not accompanied by a commensurate degree of authority to direct the treatment process" (Tasman and Mohr, 2011, p. 66).

In the world of managed care, the ethical principle of beneficence tends to give way to an ethic of utility. As a consequence, it is increasingly likely that nurses may be forced to act in ways that may be incompatible with ethical practice. The phenomenon of 'dirty hands' is a moral dilemma marked by the experience of being morally compromised and suffering moral distress by doing what is required (Mohr and Mahon, 1996). In mental health care environments that are increasingly driven by market forces, practitioners may find themselves in circumstances where they must adhere to prescribed clinical decisions that may not be in the best interest of the patient (Mohr and Mahon, 1996). There are inherent difficulties and contradictions in a system that treats health care as a market commodity and not as a social good. The fundamental nature of mental health care is relationship, not market transaction.

5.3.1.6. Diagnosis/Explanatory Models

Managed care's approach to containing costs and controlling access to care rests upon a technical, instrumental view of both human beings and mental health care (Phillips, 2002). The challenge of explaining mental illness may be a result of this approach (Brendel, 2002). Explanatory models in mental health care and research have ethical significance because they demonstrate how human existence is construed and what is of value in making human behavior intelligible. Explanatory models lead the practitioner to treat the human suffering of mental illness in particular ways (Brendel, 2002; 2003). Often, the person with mental illness is reduced only to that which can be observed and identified from the outside (Phillips, 2002). The complexity of an individual life is distilled to a cluster of observable, behavioral signs and symptoms organized around a DSM category set to which a treatment algorithm or protocol can then be applied. The bio-psycho-social-ethno-cultural uniqueness of the particular person situated in his or her unique historical context is missing (Phillips, 2002).

Adopted from contemporary biological psychiatry, managed care's construal of human existence relies heavily on technical reason, derived from Aristotle's distinction between techne (technical reasoning) and *phronesis* (practical reasoning) (Phillips, 2002). From the standpoint of technical rationality, a particular problem is always an instance of a general type (Phillips, 2002). Technical reason uses systematized knowledge of the general type, along with specific rules for knowledge application, to address particular problems as if they actually were the general type—that is, without the variability created by individual patients' lives and histories and/or individual providers' varying levels of skill, training, artistry, and experience (Phillips, 2002). Psychotherapies with instruction manuals, treatment algorithms, and other formulaic solutions derive from this kind of reasoning. Such approaches are helpful but insufficient, given human complexity and the limits of the scientific evidence base. They rely *solely* on the science of the practice, leaving out the practical wisdom of the experienced practitioner (Phillips, 2002).

Brendel (2002) asserts that science and ethics are equal partners in any project to explain mental illness and that the scope of psychiatric-mental health ethics includes focus on the values and norms that guide explanatory models. Explanatory models for mental health care and research are deeply value-laden because they must involve the best interests of patients and participants who are people who generally want to be accurately understood and treated as persons, not as disorders or disease entities reduced to diagnostic labels (Brendel, 2002). Pragmatic philosophers such as William James and John Dewey believed that the essential aim of science ought to be favorable practical outcomes for people in their everyday lives and that any explanatory model of mental illness could only be 'true' to the extent it actually promoted beneficial, real-world results for people with mental illness (Brendel, 2003). Consistent with pragmatism of this type, an explanatory model of mental illness that also promotes ethical patient care is more widely applicable within clinical science, where explanations are coherent and plausible only insofar as they are useful and empirically testable in clinical settings (Brendel, 2002; 2003). An explanatory model of mental illness must not only be evidence-based but must promote the beneficial, practical, ethical outcomes of easing mentally ill patients' pain and suffering while achieving more adaptive real-world functioning consistent with their best interests (Brendel, 2002; 2003).

Brendel (2003) has identified three pragmatic, empirical-ethical principles that can guide the mental health clinician to a more widely applicable, outcomes-oriented approach to clinical explanation and treatment. The first pragmatic principle is methodological pluralism. An explanatory model of mental illness based solely on neuroscience ignores the mounting evidence of complex etiological interactions between genetic predispositions and psychosocial stressors and of the treatment utility of combining psychopharmacological and psychotherapeutic approaches (Brendel, 2002; 2003). Mental health clinicians and researchers are ethically and scientifically disadvantaged if limited to a single, reductive, either biological or psychological model of mental illness that cannot account for the indeterminate, open-ended, corrigible nature of both psychiatric diagnosis and etiologies of psychiatric disorder (Brendel, 2002; 2003).

The second pragmatic principle is full participation of the patient in treatment planning in order to achieve optimum results in achieving a mutually acceptable, positive outcome. From a pragmatic view, truth is "the outcome of a deliberative social process aimed at identifying what works in a given situation" (Brendel, 2003, p. 571). In mental health care, the explanation for the patient's difficulties develops over time as the patient, provider, family, and others collaborate and deliberate about the complex, changing dynamics of the clinical situation (Brendel, 2003).

The third pragmatic principle central to mental health practice is the provisional nature of psychiatric explanation (Brendel, 2003). To provide patients with ethical care, practitioners must formulate cases based on the current evidence-base and do so with an awareness of the pluralistic and provisional nature of psychiatric explanation. In mental health care and research, current explanatory models and concepts are never adequate or final (Brendel, 2003).

5.3.1.7. Confidentiality/Privileged Communication

The sensitive nature of the patient's communications in mental health care heightens the stakes for potential breaches of confidentiality. *Confidentiality* refers to the therapist's responsibility to not release information obtained in the course of treatment to third parties. This is essential for the development of a safe, trusting, therapeutic relationship (Sadock and Sadock, 2007). *Privilege* refers to the patient's right to prevent disclosure of treatment information in judicial hearings; mental health clinicians must treat their patients' communications as privileged as determined by state statute (Sadock and Sadock, 2007; Tasman and Mohr, 2011). Privileged communication is provided by statute in each state in the U.S.; however, not all states extend the privilege to nurses, psychologists, or other non-physician mental health professionals (Tasman and Mohr, 2011).

Although courts uphold the duty of confidentiality between patient and therapist, which endures after a patient's death, they recognize a higher duty to protect the public safety. This means breaches of confidentiality may be required by law in cases of child abuse, threats of suicide, threats of harm to a third party, and allegations of sexual misconduct made against a therapist (Tasman and Mohr, 2011). Other exceptions to confidentiality include patient requests for release of records to third parties, the duty to warn potential victims of a patient's threats to harm them, emergencies, court-ordered psychiatric evaluations, and malpractice litigation initiated by a patient (Tasman and Mohr, 2011). Members of a treatment team may share information with each other without specific permission from a patient; however, team membership should be clarified.

Means of preserving confidentiality may include having all employees of mental health facilities sign confidentiality agreements and/or attend regularly scheduled, continuing education events; obtaining signed authorization from patients before releasing information; explaining the need for confidentiality to parents of children and adolescents; obtaining confidentiality agreements from all participants in family and group psychotherapy; avoiding gossip or stray communications with relatives of patients or employees not directly involved in the care of patients; properly disguising case presentations; and, as a clinician, refusing to discuss privileged information with one's own family, friends, students, or co-workers (Tasman and Mohr, 2011).

5.4. ETHICAL CONSIDERATIONS IN MENTAL HEALTH RESEARCH

Clinical care and research are both areas for practice, broadly speaking; the ethical considerations of mental health care for people with the particular vulnerabilities identified above are also relevant for mental health research with this subset of policy-designated 'vulnerable participants.' The same historic codes and declarations which form the basis for research ethics policies have guided clinical care and professional practice ethics. Conversely, research ethics principles and policies have derived in part from practice ethics, which is appropriate given that research informs effective practice and in part derives its justification from that supporting role (Spetie and Arnold, 2007).

Contemporary research ethics policies began with the *Nuremberg Code* as a result of reflection and judgment on the atrocities perpetrated upon concentration camp inmates by Nazi physicians (Rhodes, 2010). Since then, the protection of human participants in biomedical research has been the focus of research ethics policy. Informed consent, based on both the principle of autonomy as an *ideal* of pure self-determination as well as the principle of respect for the *actual* autonomy of the real human participant, resides at the core of research protections and constitutes the centerpiece of regulatory attention (Rhodes, 2010). The focus on protection of the participants of human research is justified by the lessons of history, by the results of research in experimental psychology that point to a number of pernicious human tendencies across a wide range of societies (Nussbaum, 2010), and by the fact that research inherently involves relationships of asymmetrical power. Relationships with asymmetrical power roles are common in society. (Juritzen, Grimen, and Heggen, 2011; Foucault, 1980). Research ethics is based on a concept of the asymmetry of power. It views the researcher as powerful and potentially harmful, the participant as less knowledgeable and therefore disadvantaged and potentially disempowered within this unequal relationship, and review boards as necessary to protect the participant by striking a better balance of power (Juritzen *et al.*, 2011).

Few ethicists dispute the necessity of protecting those who are least able to protect themselves. Long after the Nuremberg judgments and the widespread revelation of Nazi research practices, history has documented the necessity of such protections (Juritzen *et al.*, 2011). Existing codes of research ethics did not prevent the research abuses and questionable research practices illustrated by (a) the 1963 revelation of investigators injecting uninformed elderly patients with live cancer cells at the Jewish Chronic Disease Hospital; (b) Henry Beecher's 1966 publication in *The New England Journal of Medicine* of 22 examples of unethical or questionably ethical U.S. research studies; (c) the 1971 debate in *The Lancet* of the ethics of feeding live hepatitis virus to mentally disabled children at Willowbrook State School from 1955–1970; (d) the 1972 *Associated Press* exposé of the 40-year Tuskegee syphilis study that was still running 25 years after a reliable treatment for syphilis had been developed; (e) the 1975 U.S. Army acknowledgment of experiments with hallucinogenic drugs on unaware civilians; or (f) the 1999 death of 18-year old Jesse Gelsinger in a University of Pennsylvania/ Schering-Plough gene therapy trial (Beecher, 1966; Edsall, 1971; Goldby, 1971; Krugman and Shapiro, 1971; Pappworth, 1971; Rhodes, 2010; Stolberg, 1999; Weiss and Weiss, 1999).

Social science research also points to the necessity of protecting those who are least able to protect themselves. Replicated findings in social and experimental psychology show that people cannot be relied upon to do what they know is right under certain social conditions—for example, when they can defer to authority and not be held personally accountable, or when group pressure induces them to violate the clear evidence of their own senses where they are the sole voice of dissent (Nussbaum, 2010; Zimbardo, 2007). Numerous examples from experimental psychology show that reliable, apparently decent citizens can be induced by social situations to dehumanize, stigmatize, inflict pain on other human beings, or otherwise violate conventional norms of moral behavior (Nussbaum, 2010; Zimbardo, 2007). Research investigators are not themselves immune to such social pressures; thus, ongoing vigilance in the area of protection of human participants in research is warranted. People with mental illness may be at risk of further psychological distress and exacerbation of their symptoms when enrolled in a research study, and they may be at risk for exploitation and coercion by researchers, clinicians, and even family members in the manner by which informed consent is obtained (McCauley-Elsom, Gurvich, Lee, Elsom, O'Connor, and Kulkarni, 2009). However, many mental health problems and illnesses are episodic in nature or have a fluctuating course, meaning that people's mental state—and thus, their capacity to comprehend information and offer informed consent—vary over time (McCauley-Elsom *et al.*, 2009). Autonomy and decisional capacity vary for some of those with mental illness. A subset of people with a wide range of mental health problems may never experience a loss of decisional capacity or ability to give full and informed consent for research participation, which can lead to claims that the classification of all mental health services users as 'vulnerable' is itself disempowering (Allbutt and Masters, 2010). *The Belmont Report* supports the notion that people with mental illness should have fair access to opportunities to reap the benefits of research. As a social good, research should extend in fair ways to those whose immense and costly suffering is of concern to society as a whole (National Commission for the Protection of Human Subjects of Biomedical and Behavioral Research, 1979).

Weiss and Weiss (1999) reviewed the history of evolving ethics guidelines for the conduct of psychiatric research, including the 1998 report of the National Bioethics Advisory Commission (NBAC), which took an overall stance of protectiveness and placed emphasis on the role of government regulation in safeguarding those with mental illness against exploitation in psychiatric research. The NBAC (1998) report offered 21 specific recommendations across six categories, including the following highlights: (a) With respect to informed consent and decisional capacity in individuals diagnosed with mental disorders, those who are capable of consent should be allowed to consent or refuse research participation without the involvement of others and without coercion. With or without decisional capacity, all conscious people with mental illness have the right to refuse research participation, and decisional capacity should be formally and independently assessed in potential study participants when the research protocol presents greater than minimal risk (Weiss and Weiss, 1999). (b) Psychiatric research must be classified according to risk including "minimal risk," "greater than minimal risk with the prospect of direct medical benefit to subjects," and "greater than minimal risk that does not offer the prospect of direct medical benefit to subjects." Within each of these classifications, there are stringent directives about IRB review and personal and surrogate informed consent (Weiss and Weiss, 1999). (c) Surrogate decision makers have specific duties and must identify and act on the wishes of the study participant; a 'best interest' standard is insufficient for consent to participate in psychiatric research (Weiss and Weiss, 1999).

According to Weiss and Weiss (1999), the NBAC report, which recommended a moratorium on research with participants with impaired decisional capacity, had significant drawbacks that derived from five principal problems including: (a) insufficient awareness of the subtle, widely varying, and fluctuating clinical features of psychiatric disorders; (b) insufficient recognition of the immense societal impact of mental illness and the pressing need for research to address it; (c) insufficient respect for the autonomy and personhood of people with mental illness; (d) insufficient awareness of the practical dimensions of the scientific context; and (e) insufficient integration of existing ethics data on psychiatric research (Weiss and Weiss, 1999).

Overall, people with mental illness are capable of informed consent but have greater difficulties with consent processes compared to medically ill and healthy populations because the symptoms of mental illness can adversely affect the information-based, cognitive aspects of consent (Weiss and Weiss, 1999). Subjective factors such as attitudes, values, motivations, and context may affect research enrollment decisions (Weiss and Weiss, 1999). Beyond the issue of informed consent, little is known about the effectiveness of ethical safeguards in protecting human research participants. In mental health research, much more education about ethics is needed in the areas of regulatory requirements, the role of the IRB in psychiatric research, differences between clinical care and clinical research, scientific conduct and misconduct, scientific merit and ethical issues in study design, participant recruitment and selection, symptom-provoking studies, medication-free research, placebo-controlled clinical trials, genetics studies, better protection of participants during research participation, relationships between patient volunteers and members of the research team, conflicts of interest in industry-sponsored research, and psychiatric research with children and pregnant women (Rosenstein, Miller, and Rubinow, 2001).

Much of the current controversy surrounding psychiatric research focuses on the ethical problems of: (a) employing placebo controls instead of comparing new drugs to existing treatments; (b) discontinuing medications for clinical trials, which provokes symptoms and can complicate a patient's recovery; (c) the predominance of industry-sponsored clinical trials and the push to find new uses—that is, new patients with different psychiatric diagnoses—for 'old' psychotropic drugs that are going off patent protection; (d) protecting privacy and confidentiality in genetics research; and (e) conducting psychopharmacology research with children (Angell, 2005; Kolch, Ludolph, Plener, Fangerau, Vitiello, and Fegert, 2010; Rosenstein *et al.*, 2001; Spetie and Arnold, 2007).

The latter is a particularly charged issue. Children and adolescents with psychiatric disorders are doubly vulnerable by virtue of both their mental disorder and the fact of being children with a developmental status that entails normal dependency and limited decisional capacity. Along with the historical reluctance of researchers to expose children and adolescents to unnecessary risk during research trials, their protected status as 'vulnerable' has led to a paucity of data on the effectiveness, safety, and pharmacokinetics of psychotropic drugs in children (Spetie and Arnold, 2007). As a result, and with the rationale of not wanting to keep potentially helpful treatments away from children and adolescents who suffer from severe psychiatric symptoms, clinicians may treat pediatric patients by prescribing psychotropic medications 'off-label'—that is, without an FDA-approved indication and without the benefit of any evidence base. This is disturbing for many reasons. At these young ages, the boundary is often obscure between normal and abnormal behavior, which is better understood in adolescents and adults. At younger ages, it is sometimes normal to see such developmental phenomena as separation anxiety, negativism, hyperactivity, tantrums, imaginary playmates, unmodulated aggression, and heightened reactivity to environmental change (Spetie and Arnold, 2007).

Kolch *et al.* (2010) reviewed and integrated the findings of 138 publications on the ethical and legal issues entailed by psychopharmacological research in children. The need for research with this population is clear; off-label medication use in minors is soaring. The strict paradigm of excluding mentally ill children from research is changing as society recognizes the need to balance the protection of emotionally disturbed children from research against the widespread use of unsafe, ineffective medication. Clinical trials with children may increase; however, legal, ethical, and practical hurdles exist including legislative barriers, conflicts of interest, problems with assent and consent, problems with study design and small samples, problems insuring minimal risks and burdens, and problems with global justice; e.g., with respect to limited supplies of extremely expensive pharmacogenetic therapies (Koch *et al.*, 2010). Practitioners must guard against the pressures of both direct-to-consumer pharmaceutical advertising and large monetary incentives to enroll pediatric clients in clinical trials. They must also remember that, in the case of research, children and adolescents are never able to provide consent until they come of age. Parental involvement and consent, even if ethically problematic, is required. As legally guaranteed, minors do have the right to information about the research project and to decline to assent to participate. If a child declines participation, his or her competence to refuse should be formally evaluated.

5.5. ETHICAL SIGNIFICANCE OF EVERYDAY LIFE IN MENTAL HEALTH CARE

The richness and moral complexity of everyday life in mental health care and research cannot be overestimated. When nurses at any level of practice are asked about their ethical concerns, the responses are typically about their everyday, work lives. Stories are typically the format because narrative and analogy are the forms that moral reasoning takes (Walker, 2007). Nurses spend their professional lives as boundary workers, practicing in the interstitial spaces between multiple professions with their multiple competing interests (Chambliss, 1996). In the health care organization, for example, nurses work at the boundaries of medicine, nursing administration, occupational therapy, respiratory care, radiology, housekeeping, dietary, admissions, volunteer services, health information management, pharmacy, and many other departments (Chambliss, 1996). In all practice contexts—inpatient or outpatient, basic or advanced, independent or group practice—nurses may find themselves case managing patient care in order to negotiate the goals and tasks of treatment and to mediate agreement between patients, families, referral sources, physicians, and all other team members. This reality shapes their ethical concerns.

A multi-year ethnographic inquiry observed and described how emergency department nurses in several mid- to large-size American medical centers conceptualized and responded to the ethical problems they encountered in their everyday work (Chambliss, 1996). Nurses' moral concerns were not abstract; they were not the bioethics issues that interest many physicians—stem cell research, human enhancement, physician-assisted suicide, and medical futility—except as those issues affected the particular persons subject to their care. While the participants were not psychiatric-mental health nurses, this classic work in medical sociology demonstrated that nurses' conceptions of ethical problems were the result of a complex process of socially negotiating the everyday demands of their "in-between" spatial location. Moreover, Chambliss found that responsibility to meet one's ethical obligations was not an individual attribute enacted within the relatively narrow boundaries of the nurse-patient relationship. Rather, it was created and constrained by the larger social context.

In other words, nurses' understanding of what was responsible for them to do was fundamentally shaped by their social location vis-à-vis patients and by their position as subordinates in healthcare systems (Chambliss, 1996). To illustrate the former, by virtue of their proximity to patients, their location in the 'in-between zone,' and their own sense of professional responsibility to advocate for patients, nurses often pick up the slack when things fall through the cracks and other departments or professions default on responsibilities for important (but often unseen) elements of patient care or agency housekeeping. Nurses may also be deeply constrained by the limits of their professional autonomy to follow hospital or agency policies as well as physician directives (Chambliss, 1996).

Every day, nurses juggle the demands of this in-between spatiality, including the orders or directives of health care providers (both physicians and advanced practice registered nurses), the needs of patients, the demands of families, the rules of the law, the boundaries of their legal scope of practice, the bureaucracy of the workplace, the defaulted responsibilities of other departments or agencies, the dictates of administrators, their expectations for professional autonomy, and their own physical and emotional limits (Chambliss, 1996). These conflicts are some of the ethical problems of nursing and explain why nurses' patient care concerns so often involve systems issues and/or conflicts with physicians or administrators—and are construed (or even trivialized) as something 'other' than ethical problems because they do not meet the threshold for the traditional ethical *dilemma* of biomedical ethics. The higher nurses advance in the healthcare system, the more intense these kinds of conflicts become (Chambliss, 1996).

For example, as nurses'—especially advanced practice nurses'—status, power, authority, knowledge, competence, and skills have grown, their responsibilities have changed, which challenges medical hegemony and/or dominance in health care organizations. Nurses at all levels of practice, but especially at the higher levels, have come to feel that they must—and have a right to—define and answer ethical questions for themselves. In part, 'professionalization' describes a shift from a technical to a moral orientation to one's work (Chambliss, 1996). As power goes up, so do responsibilities—and so do ethical conflicts with those who have competing responsibilities and interests. As the organization of health care work changes, so too do the ethical conflicts, as in the case of the surgical nurse who creates a new protocol that changes the work flow of physicians on the surgical team: "The resulting quarrels are seen as moral conflicts, framed in the formal terms of a moral debate. Such debates . . . only arise when there are speakers to deliver them, and with a voice strong and clear enough to be heard" (Chambliss, 1996, p. 99). This is where advanced practice nurses have a critical role to play in educating, informing, supporting, and facilitating the verbal and behavioral expression of nurses' moral knowledge at basic levels of practice as well.

5.6. MORAL FRAMEWORKS FOR MENTAL HEALTH CARE AND RESEARCH

The profession of nursing applies moral theories and frameworks from moral philosophy to understand nursing practice, including utilitarianism or consequentialism, deontological or principles-based ethics, and virtue ethics. Enlightenment moral philosophy, Kantian ethics in particular, produced the moral theories used most often by bioethics and consequently by nursing. American nursing's code of ethics (ANA, 2001) is based on both a Kantian, deontological ethics of duty and an ethics of virtue, outlining both the duties and moral obligations of nurses and the virtues that make for excellence in nursing practice.

5.6.1. Ethics of Responsibility

A useful, alternative model for healthcare ethics essentially encapsulates and describes the narrative, socially negotiated, interpersonal process observed in practice. Walker's (2007) alternative model of moral inquiry has given rise to an ethics of responsibility which maintains that morality consists of a system's *actual* social practices and not moral theories. In an ethics of responsibility, the practices characteristic of morality are the practices that implement commonly shared understandings about how responsibilities are to be divided or deflected within a social system (Walker, 2007). These practices of responsibility are commonly shared understandings about who is obligated to do what for whom and who will get to avoid or even remain unaware of certain kinds of obligations. Our various responsibilities, and what it takes to meet them, so often remain invisible to others. An ethics of responsibility tries to shed light on them so that members of a social system can see more clearly how they are all in it *together* (Walker, 2007). Thus, in this model, a system's practices of responsibility are identified and examined to get at the content of the organization's shared morality so that members can achieve new moral understandings in a continuous process of revising and recreating the present moral order. So how might an ethics of responsibility work in real life?

The social organization of healthcare systems creates and shapes the ethical problems of its members. When power relationships are stable and unchallenged, few ethical crises emerge (Chambliss, 1996). When professional groups such as nursing develop new levels of practice that may challenge the existing social order, then moral agendas tend to come into conflict. Practices of responsibility that flow from particular divisions of labor show us these sorts of problems very clearly. For example, a DNP-prepared APRN working in an emergency department had concerns about the hospital's practice of assigning to nursing the responsibility of ratifying current patient medication regimens with hospital admission orders. A form required that providers, both APRNs and physicians, verify home medication regimens with admission and new medication orders. The APRNs ratified their own orders while the physicians simply initialed a form prepared by RNs. The signed or initialed form constituted medication orders for admission. The ratification process was extremely time-consuming for the nurses. Moreover, when quality control reports revealed a deficiency in compliance, it was seen as a *nursing* failure; and the nurses at all levels were asked to be more careful in drawing the attention of physician providers to these requirements.

Whose responsibility is it to wrestle with this problem and find a solution? Do benefits and burdens of current practices of responsibility fall proportionately on those to whom the responsibility belongs? This seems to be a systemic problem that falls by default to nursing for unexamined reasons. Is that where it belongs? If not, where or with whom? Where would a more ethical system of care place this kind of responsibility? These are the sorts of questions an ethics of responsibility might ask.

5.7. CONCLUSION

5.7.1. Ethical Significance of Proximity/Empathy in Mental Health Care

Moral knowledge is inextricable from social knowledge and from one's social location in the larger community, especially with respect to one's responsibilities to and for other human beings (Walker, 2007). Moral knowledge comes from one's proximity to, connections with, and empathy for other people. This informs conscience, or the 'still, small voice within.' Proximity, or closeness to others, shapes and sustains the responsibilities moral agents understand themselves to have. It tends to shape what we think we owe each other (Walker, 2007). For example, a mother tends to feel the weight of her moral responsibility to her child—to whom she is very close—to a different degree than the stranger's child. A nurse tends to feel the weight of her moral responsibility to the long-term patient—for whom she has cared for many weeks or years—to a different degree than the newly arrived referral. In order to comprehend a clinical situation and respond morally to one's child, the stranger, the long-term patient, or the newly referred patient, one must exercise the capacity for empathy—the capacity to understand what it must be like to stand in another's shoes.

Empathy is an important source of ethical knowledge. It may be the mental health clinician's most valuable asset. Mutual empathic responsiveness stimulates moral imagination, moral intuition, moral sensitivity, and the capacity for moral distress. One cannot respond morally to others unless one can also see, struggle with, feel with, and ultimately comprehend what is suffered, experienced, and endured by other sentient beings. Morality is anchored in powerful feelings such as love and fear, and it relies on our ability to read each other's emotions and intentions.

Enlightenment philosophers believed that the exercise of reason brings human beings to moral knowledge. Religious leaders believe that moral knowledge derives from divine law or the exercise of faith (Taylor, 1985). What guides a person to moral response is conditioned by empathy, which cannot develop and grow in the human organism without human connection, attachment, proximity, and opportunities for reciprocal recognition and response to the subtleties of human expression. Faith and reason do not fully inform moral judgments in either the child or the mentally ill person who may have no strong attachment to a faith tradition and may not yet have the capacity for formal operations or abstract reasoning. The gaps in their systems of logic can be wide. They may understand what parents and the larger community hold to be right and wrong; however, the child, like the person with a serious mental illness, is not yet what philosophers would call 'the fully formed, autonomous moral agent.' Yet, both are capable of moral behavior, and mental health providers have a responsibility to facilitate it.

5.8. WEBSITES FOR FURTHER INFORMATION

Box 5.6 - Websites for Further Information

American Psychiatric Association: Principles of Medical Ethics with Annotations Especially Applicable to Psychiatry
http://www.psych.org/mainmenu/psychiatricpractice/ethics.aspx

American Psychiatric Nurses Association: Position Papers (ECT, Seclusion and Restraint, Workplace Violence, Roles of Psychiatric Mental Health Nurses in Managed Care)
http://www.apna.org/i4a/pages/index.cfm?pageid=3335

American Psychological Association: Ethical Principles of Psychologists and Code of Conduct
http://www.apa.org/ethics/

Geriatric Mental Health Ethics: A Casebook
http://www.springerpub.com/samples/9780826103192_chapter.pdf

Psychiatry Online: Case Studies in Ethics
http://focus.psychiatryonline.org/Mobile/article.aspx?articleid=114955&RelatedWidgetArticles=true

World Psychiatric Association: Declarations on Ethical Standards
http://www.wpanet.org/detail.php?section_id=5&category_id=9&content_id=31

5.9. CASE STUDIES

5.9.1. Case Study #1

The patient was an elderly woman with all mental capabilities intact. She was admitted for a hip replacement. A newly certified nurse anesthetist was told by the patient in the pre-op patient interview that she desired a spinal anesthetic instead of a general anesthetic. There were no contraindications to a spinal, so this was the plan decided by both patient and CRNA.

The anesthesiologist assigned to the case (the chair of the department) also interviewed the patient, and he decided that general anesthesia would be used. The CRNA informed him that the patient desired a spinal anesthetic. The MD replied, "Just give her some Versed; she'll never remember." The CRNA felt very uneasy about this and knew that it was wrong, but was intimidated and didn't want to rock the boat. The CRNA went along with the anesthesiologist's plan and did as was instructed.

Over the subsequent nine years, the CRNA never forgot this patient and her inability to be a patient advocate for fear of retribution. She states that now she has grown in confidence and would not let this happen again without some valid reason to override a patient's wishes.

Questions for Discussion:

1. To whom did the CRNA owe her fidelity? Is the principle of fidelity sufficient to understand the CRNA's ethical conflict? What else requires ethical consideration?
2. Does analysis of this case from a feminist ethics perspective lead to a different ethical outcome? Could the concept of 'gender' be operating in this scenario? How? Where?

5.9.2. Case Study #2

A female in her late 50's was admitted for evaluation because she was not seeking the necessary treatment for her infected leg ulcers. She was a hoarder living in a house that has been condemned. She had been able to obtain groceries and keep herself fed with a roof over her head, despite the deplorable condition of the building. The Department of Public Health had cleaned out the house several times in order to get rid of cat urine, feces, and strange collections of things like her hair, which lay in bowls all over the house. She underwent outpatient commitment, is now in assisted living, and is very unhappy about not being in her own home. The patient is often medication non-adherent, but when she faces revocation of her provisional discharge, she begins to takes them again. At what point does she have a right to live in a 'bizarre' way and be left alone, versus having treatment forced on her? Her health was in jeopardy, as her leg ulcers were infected and she was facing amputations if she continued to refuse treatment. She is now miserable because she is not able to live on her own.

Questions for Discussion:

1. Is there any point in a patient's care when treatment should/must be forced?
2. What are this patient's 'best interests,' and how should they be determined?
3. What actions might support the 'diminished autonomy' of this patient?

5.9.3. Case Study #3

An ACT team specializes in the care and treatment of young adults aged 18–24 with serious and persistent mental illness (SPMI). The teams are composed of social workers from the county health department, the mental health center, and the state; nurses from the mental health center; a psychiatrist; and an advanced practice registered nurse. The teams are funded from the Department of Human Services and do not have adequate funds for supplies or patient needs. The primary goal of the team is to assist patients in goals related to rehabilitation of their mental illness in order to avoid hospitalization and keep them living in the community. Specific goals include maintaining stable housing, learning to stick to a budget, medication and treatment adherence, effective parenting, sobriety, socialization, better physical health, staying out of jail, and staying out of the hospital.

The ACT team has found that money can be effective in getting patients to complete tasks. For example, they sometimes pay non-compliant patients $2/day to take their medications in front of the staff, or the patients are given gift cards to Subway or Target after a week of medication compliance. The team has also given money ($10–$20) for patients to get necessary lab work they would not otherwise do and also have given a patient with extreme hand contractures $20 for each visit to the physical therapist.

Birth control options are discussed with all female patients. Many already have children and have declined birth control options in the past for various reasons. A young woman with schizophrenia came into the office and said she had run out of money. She asked to borrow $50 from the team's flex fund. She had borrowed money in the past and not paid it back. The case managers and the nurse decided not to loan the money to the patient, but instead offered her $50 to get a Depo Provera injection that day plus an additional incentive of $50 every three months for subsequent injections. She agreed to get the injection in exchange for the money even though she had refused birth control in the past.

Questions for Discussion:

1. Is it ethical to pay a patient to receive birth control? For any reason?
2. Do these scenarios describe inducement or coercion? What is the difference? Informed consent?

5.9.4. Case Study #4

A clinical nurse specialist (CNS) in an outpatient psychiatric clinic evaluated a patient who presented with several psychiatric complaints and an extensive history of major medical problems, including many surgeries and chronic pain. The patient had previously been receiving treatment from another provider and was also being treated at the pain clinic in the same building.

A patient service assistant (PSA) who worked in the psychiatric clinic happened to be passing by the pain clinic one day and saw the patient and recognized her from the psychiatric clinic. She asked a pain clinic staff person why the patient was receiving treatment there and learned that the patient had chronic pain. The patient was in a wheelchair, which shocked the PSA because she had seen the patient outside the clinic, coaching a youth sports team, clearly not in a wheelchair and not apparently in pain. At a subsequent sports event, the PSA took a video of the patient to prove that the patient was not using a wheelchair, and she brought the video to the pain clinic as evidence. The patient was also observed going to her vehicle, standing up from the wheelchair, and effortlessly putting the wheelchair into her vehicle.

Because of the patient's extensive medical history and unsolicited information relayed by the PSA, the CNS diagnosed the patient with Factitious Disorder and met with the collaborating psychiatrist to discuss treatment options. The psychiatrist concurred with the diagnosis. The PSA's information influenced the providers' diagnosis of the patient; however, the CNS believed that she had a duty to perform the most comprehensive assessment possible, including collateral information from others, to arrive at the best diagnosis and treatment plan for the patient. This breach of confidentiality had the potential to benefit the patient if the diagnosis was accurate and treatment was successful.

Questions for Discussion:

1. Do therapeutic ends ever justify unethical means? Do they justify the ends in this case?
2. Where, when, how was patient confidentiality breached? Was it? Would it be different if the pain clinic was in a different building?
3. Is it legal/ethical to film someone without their permission?
4. Should the patient be told about the breach?

5.9.5. Case Study #5

Many psychiatric medications have not been approved by the FDA for use in children and adolescents. Most of these medications have not gone through clinical trials with children and adolescents.

An adolescent was admitted for a first psychotic episode. At that time, this unit had only one child/adolescent psychiatrist, who was from a foreign country and was a new graduate He was not yet board certified, and there was a language barrier between him, the patients, the parents, and the staff on the unit. An antipsychotic medication was tried for this adolescent with no significant clearing of the psychosis. The psychiatrist met with the patient for two to three minutes each day, leaving the nursing staff to assess the patient's current condition. The psychiatrist did not meet face to face with the family; all his communications occurred via telephone. After two weeks of this medication trial and no clearing of the psychosis, the psychiatrist decided to perform electroconvulsive therapy (ECT) and communicated this to the family. The psychiatrist did not seek a second opinion with another psychiatrist and did not offer a second medication trial. The psychiatrist left the signing of the informed consent and explanation of the procedure to the nursing staff. When the family arrived, they did not know any details of the procedure or the risks. They agreed to the procedure based on the recommendation of the psychiatrist.

The ECT occurred over the course of a few weeks concurrently with a second medication trial that the psychiatrist decided to begin with the ECT. To complicate matters , the adolescent later admitted that he had been 'huffing' and using 'mushrooms' prior to his hospital admission, which the parents did not know. The patient got better over time, but it is unknown whether the psychosis cleared in response to the ECT, the new medication, or the time away from street drugs.

When asked about the rationale for ECT, the psychiatrist later reported that he felt pressured by the insurance company to get the patient discharged quickly. In addition, the language and cultural differences of the physician, the lack of informed consent obtained by the physician, the lack of a second opinion (which is required for ECT), and only one medication trial before ECT was obtained all present issues.

Questions for Discussion:

1. Although it commonly occurs, is it ethical to give psychotropic medications to children and adolescents that are not FDA-approved for use with children?
2. What could or should a nurse have done with ethical concerns about the practices of the psychiatrist and the care of this adolescent?
3. As a subordinate in the healthcare hierarchy, and constrained by 'doctor's orders', what are the boundaries of a nurse's role and responsibilities in this scenario?

Identify the psychiatric-mental health ethics issues that are illustrated by this case.

5.9.6. Case Study #6

A psych/mental health department was downsized. Over 50% of the staff was cut. As part of this process, case managers also had to shrink their caseloads. From nearly 600 patients, more than 300 patients were cut. The decisions about which patients would no longer receive services were delegated to two nurse practitioners still remaining on the service. All of the patients had a primary physician and a geriatric nurse practitioner (GNP) assigned to them. The decision of the two NPs was to not make the cuts themselves. Instead, they spent many days on the phone calling all the assigned GNPs to discuss each patient—all 600 of them. The GNPs determined which patients they were comfortable managing on their own and which ones they were not. When the calls were completed, a caseload fewer than 300 patients remained.

Questions for Discussion:

1. Were responsibilities and roles appropriately matched in this scenario? Should the moral distress of cutting a large caseload in half have been shared by anyone else? Who? Why?

2. Have the 300 patients who lost case management services been treated fairly and justly?
3. What ethical issues, or legal ones, arise from making medical decisions based on finances?

5.10. REFERENCES

Angell, M. (2005). *The Truth About the Drug Companies: How They Deceive Us and What To Do About It.* New York: Random House.

Allbutt, H., and Masters, H. (2010) Ethnography and the ethics of undertaking research in different mental healthcare settings. *Journal of Psychiatric and Mental Health Nursing, 17*: 210–215.

American Nurses Association. (2001). *Code of Ethics for Nurses with Interpretive Statements.* Silver Springs, MD: American Nurses Association.

American Psychiatric Association. (2012). *The Principles of Medical Ethics With Annotations Especially Applicable to Psychiatry.* Arlington, VA: American Psychiatric Association.

Barker, P. (2011). *Mental Health Ethics: The Human Context.* London: Routledge.

Beauchamp, T. L. and Childress, J. F. (2008). Principles of Biomedical Ethics, 6th Edition. New York: Oxford University Press.

Beecher, H. K. (1966). Ethics and clinical research. *The New England Journal of Medicine, 274*(24): 1354–1360.

Brendel, D. H. (2002). The ethics of diagnostic and therapeutic paradigm choice in psychiatry. *Harvard Review of Psychiatry, 20*: 47–50.

Brendel, D. H. (2003). Reductionism, eclecticism, and pragmatism in psychiatry: The dialectic of clinical explanation. *Journal of Medicine and Philosophy, 28*(5–6): 563–580.

Chambliss, D. (1996). *Beyond Caring: Hospitals, Nurses, and the Social Organization of Ethics.* University of Chicago Press.

Crigger, N. and Godfrey, N. (2011). *The Making of Nurse Professionals: A Transformational, Ethical Approach.* Sudbury, MA: Jones and Bartlett.

Crowden, A. (2003). Ethically sensitive mental health care: Is there a need for a unique ethics for psychiatry? *Australian and New Zealand Journal of Psychiatry, 37*: 143–149.

Edsall, G. (1971). Experiments at Willowbrook. *The Lancet 298*(7715): p. 95.

Foucault, M. (1980). *Power/Knowledge: Selected Interviews and Other Writings 1972–1977.* New York: Pantheon Books.

Fry, S. T. and Veatch, R. M. (2006). *Case Studies in Nursing Ethics, 3rd ed.* Sudbury, MA: Jones and Bartlett Publishers.

Gallup Organization. (2010, December 3). *Nurses Top Honesty and Ethics List for 11th Year.* Available: http://www.gallup.com/poll/145043/nurses-top-honesty-ethics-list-11-year.aspx

Goffman, E. (1963). *Stigma: Notes on the Management of Spoiled Identity.* Englewood Cliffs, NJ: Prentice-Hall.

Goldby, S. (1971). Experiments at the Willowbrook State School. *The Lancet, 297*(7702): 749.

Grace, P. J. (2009). *Nursing Ethics and Professional Responsibility in Advanced Practice.* Boston: Jones and Bartlett Publishers.

Gutheil, T.G. and Gabbard, G.O. (1993). The concept of boundaries in clinical practice: Theoretical and risk management dimensions. *American Journal of Psychiatry, 150*(2): 188–196.

Gutheil, T.G. and Gabbard, G.O. (1998). Misuses and misunderstandings of boundary theory in clinical and regulatory settings. *American Journal of Psychiatry, 155*(3): 409–414.

Gutheil, T.G. and Simon, R.I. (2003). Abandonment of patients in split treatment. *Harvard Review of Psychiatry, 11*: 175–179.

Halter, M.J. (2008). Perceived characteristics of psychiatric nurses: Stigma by association. *Archives of Psychiatric Nursing, 22*(1): 20–26.

Hastings Center. (1978). In the service of the state: The psychiatrist as double agent. *Hasting Center Report, 8*(2): 1–23.

Jorgenson, L.M., Hirsch, A.B., and Wahl, K.M. (1997). Fiduciary duty and boundaries: Acting in the client's best interest. *Behavioral Sciences and the Law, 15*: 49–62.

Juritzen, T.I., Grimen, H., and Heggen, K. (2011). Protecting vulnerable research participants: A Foucault-inspired analysis of ethics committees. *Nursing Ethics, 18*(5): 640–650.

Kolch, M., Ludolph, A.G., Plener, P.L., Fangerau, H. Vitiello, B., and Fegert, J.M. (2010). Safeguarding children's rights in psychopharmacological research: Ethical and legal issues. *Current Pharmaceutical Design, 16*: 2398–2406.

Krugman, S. and Shapiro, S. (1971). Experiments at the Willowbrook State School. *The Lancet 297*(7706): 966.

Lindeman, H. (2006). *An Invitation to Feminist Ethics.* Boston: McGraw-Hill.

McCauley-Elsom, K., Gurvich, C., Lee, S., Elsom, S., O'Connor, M., and Kulkarni, J. (2009). Vulnerable populations and multicentered research. *International Journal of Mental Health Nursing, 18*: 108–115.

Mohr, W.K., and Mahon, M.M. (1996). Dirty hands: The underside of marketplace health care. *Advances in Nursing Science, 19*(1): 28–37.

Monahan, J., Redlich, A.D., Swanson, J., Robbins, P.D., Appelbaum, P.S., Petrila, J., McNiel, D.E. (2005). Use of leverage to improve adherence to psychiatric treatment in the community. *Psychiatric Services, 56*: 37–44.

Muran, J. C., and Barber, J. P. (2010). *The Therapeutic Alliance: An Evidence-Based Treatment Guide to Practice.* New York: The Guilford Press.

National Bioethics Advisory Commission. (1998). Research involving persons with mental disorders that may affect decision making capacity, Volume 1. *Report and Recommendations of the National Bioethics Advisory Commission.* Rockville, MD: National Bioethics Advisory Commission.

National Commission for the Protection of Human Subjects of Biomedical and Behavioral Research. (1979). *The Belmont Report: Ethical Principles and Guidelines for the Protection of Human Subjects of Research.* Washington, DC: U.S. Government Printing Office.

Nussbaum, M.C. (2010). *Not For Profit: Why Democracy Needs the Humanities.* Princeton, NJ: Princeton University Press.

Olsen, D.P. (2003). Influence and coercion: Relational and rights-based ethical approaches to forced psychiatric treatment. *Journal of Psychiatric and Mental Health Nursing, 10*: 705–712.

Pappworth, M.H. (1971). The Willowbrook experiments. *The Lancet 297*(7710): 1181.

Peter, E. and Liaschenko, J. (2004). The perils of proximity: A spatiotemporal analysis of moral distress and moral ambiguity. *Nursing Inquiry, 11*(4): 218–225.

Phillips, J. (2002). Managed care's reconstruction of human existence: The triumph of technical reason. *Theoretical Medicine, 23*: 339–358.

Radden, J. (2002a). Notes towards a professional ethics for psychiatry. *Australian and New Zealand Journal of Psychiatry, 36*: 52–59.

Radden, J. (2002b). Psychiatric ethics. *Bioethics, 16*(5): 397–411.

Radden, J. (2003). Forced medication, patients' rights and values conflicts. *Psychiatry, Psychology, and Law, 10*(1): 1–11.

Radden, J. (2004). The debate continues: Unique ethics for psychiatry. *Australian and New Zealand Journal of Psychiatry, 38*: 115–118.

Radden, J., and Sadler, J.Z. (2008). Character virtues in psychiatric practice. *Harvard Review of Psychiatry, 16*(6): 373–380.

Rhodes, R. (2010). Rethinking research ethics. *The American Journal of Bioethics, 10*(10): 19–36.

Robbins, P.C., Petrila, J., LeMelle, S., and Monahan, J. (2006). The use of housing as leverage to increase adherence to psychiatric treatment in the community. *Administration and Policy in Mental Health Services, 75*: 49–59.

Roberts, L.W., and Roberts, B. (1999). Psychiatric research ethics: An overview of evolving guidelines and current ethical dilemmas in the study of mental illness. *Biological Psychiatry, 46*: 1025–1038.

Rosenstein, D.L., Miller, F.G., and Rubinow, D.R. (2001). A curriculum for teaching psychiatric research ethics. *Biological Psychiatry, 50*: 802–808.

Sadler, J. Z. (2007). The psychiatric significance of the personal self. *Psychiatry, 70*(2): 113–129.

Sadock, B.J., and Sadock, V.A. (2007). *Kaplan and Sadock's Synopsis of Psychiatry: Behavioral Sciences/Clinical Psychiatry, 10th edition.* Philadelphia: Wolters Kluwer/Lippincott Williams and Wilkins.

Safran, J.D. and Muran, J.C. (2003). *Negotiating the Therapeutic Alliance: A Relational Treatment Guide.* New York: The Guilford Press.

Shuster, E. (1997). Fifty years later: The significance of the Nuremberg Code. *New England Journal of Medicine, 337*(20): 1436–1440.

Smith, D.E. (1990). The statistics on women and mental illness: The relations of ruling they conceal. In: *The Conceptual Practices of Power: A Feminist Sociology of Knowledge,* pp. 108–138. D.E. Smith (Ed.). Boston: Northeastern University Press.

Spetie, L., and Arnold, L.E. (2007). Ethical issues in child psychopharmacology research and practice: Emphasis on preschoolers. *Psychopharmacology, 191*: 15–26.

Stolberg, S.G. (1999, November 28). The biotech death of Jesse Gelsinger. *The New York Times Magazine,* 9136–9150.

Szmukler, G., and Appelbaum, P.S. (2008). Treatment pressures, leverage, coercion, and compulsion in mental health care. *Journal of Mental Health, 17*(3): 233–244.

Tasman, A., and Mohr, W.K. (2011). *Fundamentals of Psychiatry.* Wiley-Blackwell.

Taylor, R. (1985). Ethics, Faith,and Reason. Englewood Cliffs, NJ: Prentice-Hall, Inc.

United Nations General Assembly. (1948, December 10). *Universal Declaration of Human Rights.* Available: http://www.ohchr.org/en/udhr/pages/language.aspx?langid=eng

Walker, M.U. (2007). *Moral Understandings: A Feminist Study in Ethics, 2nd Edition.* New York: Oxford University Press.

Widiger, T.A. (1998). Invited essay: Sex biases in the diagnosis of personality disorders. *Journal of Personality Disorders, 12*(2): 95–118.

World Medication Association (WMA). (1948). *Declaration of Geneva.* Geneva: WMA, General Assembly. Available: http://www.cirp.org/library/ethics/geneva/

World Medical Organization. (1996). Declaration of Helsinki. *British Medical Journal, 313*(7070), 1448–1449. Available: http://www.cirp.org/library/ethics/helsinki/

World Psychiatric Association (WPA). (1978). Declaration of Hawaii. *Journal of Medical Ethics, 4*: 71–73. Available: http://www.ncbi.nlm.nih.gov/pmc/articles/PMC1154636/pdf/jmedeth00167-0017.pdf

World Psychiatric Association (WPA). (1996). *Madrid Declaration on Ethical Standards for Psychiatric Practice.* Madrid: WPA, General Assembly. Available: http://www.wpanet.org/detail.php?section_id=5andcontent_id=48

Zimbardo, P. (2007). *The Lucifer Effect: How Good People Turn Evil.* London: Rider.

CHAPTER 6

Ethical Considerations in the Care of Pediatric Patients

RITA MARIE JOHN

6.1. OVERVIEW

There is a broad range of ethical issues for Advanced Practice Nurses (APNs) who practice in pediatrics, ranging from limiting care for the very premature newborn to reproductive health issues in adolescents. There are no simple answers to ethical problems that arise in clinical practice. The APN faces ethical problems in practice whether she works on an inpatient unit and faces distress due to end of life issues and treatment refusal; works in a NICU with critically ill newborns or in ambulatory care with abusive parents, or works with parents who refuse vaccines for their children. Competence in ethics is essential in clinical practice. There are challenges that the APN must identify, analyze, and manage. It can be difficult to manage the therapeutic alliance with families, to protect patient privacy and confidentiality, and to use professional authority in an appropriate manner. This chapter serves as an introduction to the problems of pediatric ethical issues. It will review pediatric health care decision-making, practice issues, and role conflict unique to pediatrics. In addition, it will discuss the special problems unique to newborn, infant, child, and adolescent healthcare, followed by a brief discussion of pediatric subjects in a research study. The chapter will conclude with several case studies for further discussion.

6.2. HEALTH CARE DECISION MAKING

Pediatric ethical dilemmas are significantly different than adult ethical dilemmas. With an adult, the provider presents all the options to the competent adult who then decides on the course of action based on his/her best interests. The ethical principle of autonomy allows a person to make decisions freely, without interference. Respect for autonomy is a core concept in modern ethics (Cummings and Mercurio, 2010; Ross, 1998). The competent adult has the right to control any actions affecting his or her body and providers cannot override that decision. The adult consent must be voluntary, informed and competent (Ross, 1998).

In addition, autonomy allows the patient the right to refuse treatment and dictates that the APN must respect that decision. A surgeon who performs a procedure without the consent of the competent adult patient commits assault. Thus, an adult's refusal of treatment is accepted. Adult autonomy is based on the adult having adequate capacity to make the decision, but does not allow the adult to demand treatment that is not medically necessary (Cummings and Mercurio, 2010). In pediatrics, the degree of autonomy in decision-making depends on the child's age, maturity, and intellectual capacity. Children cannot be truly autonomous. Thus, with babies, toddlers, and preschool children, their surrogates make decisions for them; with older children and adolescents, they have some decision making capacity.

The principle of beneficence requires that the APN act in the best interest of the patient, including preventing harm, helping those in danger, and protecting others. This means that the APN will act in the best interest of the child At times, autonomy is in conflict with beneficence. This occurs when the APN feels that a particular treatment would be in the best interest of the child, but the patient and the family refuse the treatment. Autonomy usually overrides beneficence.

Nonmaleficence assures that the APN will protect the patient and do no harm. This principle is associated with the expression "above all, first do no harm" (Beauchamp and Childress, 2001). For APNs, this requires that the care rendered be performed with skill, knowledge, and diligence. Nonmaleficence asks for the obtaining of a consultation when there is doubt. Undoubtedly, this principle comes into play during end of life issues, when sustaining life may not be the best alternative. Lack of training to counsel and inform patients about end of life care choices, genetic counseling, and/or devastating diagnosis may be an area where APNs and others should defer to other professionals in order to protect patients and avoid harm (Okun, 2010). The American Association of Pediatrics (AAP) Committee on Bioethics (1997) states, "All children are entitled to medical treatment that is likely to prevent serious harm, or suffering, or death".

APNs should present all benefits, risks, and alternatives to surrogate pediatric decision-makers. APNs have a moral obligation to make sure that their own biases do not interfere with presenting all possible treatment options. At times, providers may not present alternative treatments to parents due to the provider's biases; as providers, they may not believe that certain alternatives are reasonable (Ross and Frader, 2009). The APN must consider all alternatives and be aware of bias before approaching patients with treatment plans. Withholding information about reasonable options is not acceptable for the APN as it could lead to an exercise of power that is unacceptable in this diverse society (Ross and Frader, 2009). APNs must not substitute their personal beliefs without information about treatment options. In pediatrics, it is critically important that providers educate parents in order to foster fully informed decision making with a process that allows the risks, benefits and alternative interventions to be fully explored so that parents can act in the best interest of the child.

The Internet has changed the way that families interact with providers as eight out of ten patients now use online resources to explore health issues (Eckler, Worsowicz and Dowley, 2009). Morahan-Martin (2004) reported that Internet searches affected patients' decisions about treatment for a health problem (44%), enabled them to ask more questions or obtain a second opinion (38%), gave them new ideas about how to handle a health problem (34%), helped them discover the relationship between diet, stress and exercise (30%), gave them new ideas about how to cope with a chronic disease (25%), and affected a decision about whether or not to seek health care (17%). Thus, information that providers give to parents must be clear and reflect current research to avoid the informed parent deducing that the provider was not up to date or even misled them. Coulter and Ellins (2007) reported that effective health care communications between patients and professionals are most effective when enhanced by health education materials, self-management action plans, and other technologies used to educate patients. The paternalistic model of healthcare is no longer acceptable in clinical practice, since the Internet has made patients informed consumers.

Even if the APN feels strongly about an issue, she must ensure that she fully informs the parent of all options to assure the parent or guardian can fulfill their moral duties (Mears, 2010; Ross and Frader, 2009). There are several reasons for parental refusal, including: lack of understanding, cultural beliefs, religious beliefs, denial of the health problem, fear of the treatment, lack of resources, fear regarding side effects, and the belief that alternative treatments may have no side effects (Ross, 2011). Thus, the parent needs continued, ongoing conversation before understanding why a particular treatment has been recommended.

The principle of justice is involved in the decision-making process, as it provides that each person should be treated equally. Nondisclosure of critical information for a surrogate is considered a breach of the principle of justice. It also requires that the APN treats each person equally and not on the basis of the race, socioeconomic class, age, sex, or social class. This is an area of concern for practitioners in neonatology, where the neonate may be at risk for receiving less care than an older child (Janvier, Bauer, and Lantos, 2007). Health insurance differences may also lead to managed care constraints and may affect how children with the same disease are treated.

6.2.1. Decision Making in Pediatrics

Young children do not participate in decision-making as they lack the capacity to decide on treatment plans. In adolescents, the principle of autonomy is less clear. The reason for children's lack of autonomy is based on their age, developmental disability, or mental illness, whether temporary or permanent. The role of surrogates in pediatrics is held to a much higher standard in the decision making process, especially if the surrogate is not related (Ross, 2009).

In pediatrics, a surrogate decision-maker is usually designated for the child. This surrogate is typically the parent, as it is felt that the parent will act in the child's best interest. This Best Interest Standard is the guiding principle used by decision makers who must make choices for minors or others who lack the ability to make decisions (Kopelman and Kopelman, 2007). This principle is an umbrella concept as it is used to make good, or at the very least acceptable, choices for those who cannot make their own (Kopelman and Kopelman, 2007). It is the principle to which parents and guardians are held when making decisions. However, the Best Interests Standard has been criticized as being vague, or unobtainable (Kopelman, 2007).

Parental authority and the Best Interest Standard go hand in hand. Parental authority allows a parent to speak for a child who does not have decision-making capacity. It is based on several beliefs: that parents know what is best for their child; parents must live with decisions that are made about their child's medical care; parents have the ultimate responsibility for bringing up their child; and that bonds between family members make the parent most likely to make decisions based on the best interest of the child (Cummings and Mercurio, 2010). Parents' decision-making capacity is more limited than patient autonomy. While an adult decides about their own treatment course, parents must base their decisions on what is in the child's best interest and in the family's best interest. Surrogate decision-making must be made in the best interest of the child. If the decision is not made in the best interest, parents can be charged with abuse and neglect. As a result, the court will likely overturn the parents' decision if it is determined that it is not in the best interest of the child.

Neonates, infants, toddlers, and preschoolers lack the ability to make decisions about health care. On the other hand, school age children and adolescents should be included in the decision making process to the degree to which they have the capacity to assent to treatment (Committee on Bioethics, 1995). This is particularly true as the child matures into adolescence, a period where there is increasing autonomy and the adolescent is more active in decision-making regarding treatment decisions. By asking for a child's participation in the process, a child's dignity is recognized. However, there may be limitations depending on age, psychological status, developmental status, and medical condition.

The child's role in the final decision is less clear. An understanding of children's cognitive level helps to clarify why children may not be fully competent to make a decision (Ross, 1998). Piaget described children between two and seven years of age as preoperational. In this stage of development, the child is not able to consider the whole picture and can only see one aspect of an event at a time. The child is egocentric and is unable to generalize from one experience to a similar one. By the time the child reaches seven, he is less egocentric and has some logic at a concrete operational stage. Around age 11, the child is able to begin to think abstractly and to consider long- and short-term consequences of their decisions. This does not mean that the decision-making capacity is fully developed. New research indicates that their ventromedial prefrontal cortexes are developing through early adulthood (Hazen, Schlozman and Beresin, 2008). This area of the brain is responsible for improvements in memory and emotional stability, as well as the ability to have long-range plans (Hazen, Schlozman and Beresin, 2008). Complicating this new information about brain physiological maturation is fact that ill children tend to regress to earlier stages of development.

The issues around decision-making for pediatric patients are complex. The APN must consider the ethical principles of autonomy, beneficence, nonmaleficence, justice, parental authority, and the Best Interest Standard. The child's surrogate must consider the greater good for the whole family unit. All of this must be viewed within a cultural context (Turner, 2010). The concept of shared decision making is a key part of the decision making with families (Mercurio, Adams *et al.*, 2008). This is a very Western view of childhood assent and may not be accepted by all cultural groups. Some cultural groups view elders as key decision-makers (Mercurio, Adams *et al.*, 2008).

6.2.1.1. Decision Scenarios

Decision-making is easier when both the surrogate and the child agree with the APN on the course of treatment. Childhood assent requires four key elements:

1. The child should be assisted in understanding his or her condition.
2. The child should be told what will happen during proposed treatment.
3. An assessment must be conducted determining what the child understands and what factors are influencing this understanding.
4. A gathered response from the child regarding the proposed treatment (Mercurio *et al.*, 2008).

Parental/surrogate authority is respected in defining the child's best interest and it is best when an adolescent also agrees with the plan to treat. If the parent and child of less than 18 years agree to treat, then the APN can go ahead with the treatment plan. When there is an agreement to treat, and that agreement is what the APN believes is correct, there is no problem in the decision making process. These scenarios are not problematic since both the parent and the adolescent agree on the course of treatment.

If the parents' preference is to treat, but the child refuses treatment, then the child's wishes will generally be overturned by the parent's as the child does not have full understanding of the need for treatment. The child's ability to agree to a treatment plan is largely determined by the child's age and maturity (Spencer, 2000) and determined by his/her competency. Depending on the age of the child, the refusal of the child may need to be considered. This may put the APN in conflict with the parents and other providers. However, the key lies in the child's cognitive ability to carefully weigh all the options. If the APN asks a 4 year old if he wants his booster shots, he is likely to reject this treatment option. Cognitively, he is unable to weigh the pros and cons of missing vaccines. However, in adolescence, nontreatment decisions should be considered. If the parents' preference is to treat, but the adolescent refuses, the competency of the adolescent must be fully assessed. In this scenario, the APN should try to educate the adolescent about the need for treatment. Working with families is key to a successful outcome. It is always better to reach a compromise rather than allow the case to go to court. In general, the younger the child, the more likely the child's refusal will not affect outcome of the case.

In a different scenario, the parent or surrogate may disagree with a treatment plan and refuse treatment for a child who is not competent. In this case, the state can intervene if the parent's decision is deemed to be either abusive or neglectful. The APN must consider the efficacy of the proposed treatment before seeking a court order to override the parent's refusal. Thus, with a young child, if the parents, as the surrogate decision makers, go against a life-saving treatment for the child, the APN and other health care providers can seek court intervention. However, if a treatment option's benefit is not as clear, the APN must weigh the pros and cons of overriding the caretakers' wishes.

When there is a clearly life-saving intervention for a school age child or younger which is refused by the parents, the parent's authority as decision makers usually will be overturned by the court, particularly if the objection is religious (Ross, 2008). The United States Supreme Court has ruled that religion is not a valid legal defense when it is used to harm the child (Mercurio *et al.*, 2008). The AAP does not believe that a religious defense should be used as a reason to deny treatment of a child when there are highly effective treatments available (Committee on Bioethics, 1997). However, as the child grows, it is possible that if both the parents and the adolescent object to the treatment on a religious basis, the court may uphold the refusal. This was the case in November 2007, when Dennis Lindberg, a Jehovah's Witness with leukemia, refused a blood transfusion and was supported by his guardian, who was also a Jehovah's witness. The Washington State Court upheld the refusal. Within 12 hours, the child died (Black, 2007).

There is a recent trend of supporting adolescent refusal, particularly if the parents are also refusing treatment (Ross, 2008). A "mature minor" is an adolescent who has not yet reached the age of adulthood (18 in the United States), but who is being treated as an adult. This may be difficult for APNs when they do not believe that the parent is acting in the child's best interest. These are cases where the APN may feel the need to take the parent to court. Conversely, if the minor's preference is treatment and that minor is an adolescent , the APN may need to go to court in order to treat the child if the APN believes that the parent is not acting in the child's best interest. Consultation with other team members along with an ethics team consultation should be considered prior to reporting the case to child protective services. Child protective services will initiate court proceedings, so the individual practitioner does not have to pay for a lawyer. Again, the main consideration is the efficacy of the treatment. When the treatment is highly efficacious, it is more likely that the court will rule in favor of the APN. However, when the treatment is not as effective, the APN must carefully consider the best action. Certainly, the best option with a less efficacious treatment is for the APN to work with the parents or guardian and the adolescent minor in deciding on the treatment plan.

There are, of course, examples in which an adolescent patient adamantly refuses treatment even when it is advised by both his parents and the APN. The adolescent may refuse treatment and ask for legal counsel to help them receive no further treatment or may even run away. This happened in the case of 16-year-old Billy Best in 1994, when he refused further chemotherapy for Hodgkin's disease after five treatment rounds. He decided to run away and his parents asked him to come back home. In their plea, they promised Billy that he would not have to resume chemotherapy if he came home. Keeping their promise, the family then refused further treatment and the medical team reported them to Child Protective Services. However, the Massachusetts Court ultimately dismissed the case and the family pursued alternative treatment. Billy is still alive today, and is now publishing a book about his life. His doctors believe that the five treatment courses that he received adequately treated his cancer, but the family believes that their alternative treatment is the reason he is alive today (Ross, 2009).

In a similar case, 16-year-old Abraham Cherrix, also diagnosed with Hodgkin's disease, refused a second round of chemotherapy after the disease reappeared in 2006. The child refused treatment and his family traveled to Mexico for an alternative treatment. When they returned, the parents were charged with neglect and an additional treatment of radiation therapy with a complementary and alternative treatment (CAM) was instituted (Simpson, 2007).

The APN, faced with parental and mature adolescent refusal of treatment, must be aware of current trends which allow families with mature minors to refuse treatment. In February 2007, the State of Virginia passed a law that allowed families with adolescents 14 and over the right to refuse treatment (Simpson, 2007). Decisional authority was previously clearly in the hands of parents; however, recent trends in decision-making with mature adolescents have changed the way these cases are being decided in court. In cases of refusal where the risk of harm is such that it would constitute medical neglect and place the child at risk for harm, reporting to child protective services and going to court may be the only option. It is important to recognize that going to court to allow for a particular treatment to occur is usually fatal to the APN-family relationship (Ladd and Forman, 2010). It is critical to work with these families so that the best possible outcomes can occur. The APN should consider not terminating care, but to educate and negotiate with the family so the medical care can continue. In some cases, seeking the state's help may be needed.

The APN may ensure better outcomes if mutually acceptable treatment plans using shared decision making are utilized. If the APN and the family cannot come to an acceptable decision, care may be transferred to another provider, but the APN cannot abandon the patient.

6.3. PRACTICE ISSUES

6.3.1. Access to Care Issues

6.3.1.1. Insurance Issues

Insurance and managed care constraints may be an area of conflict for the APN (Butz *et al.*, 1998). Institutions may only accept one kind of insurance, and at times, the best care for a rare problem may be in a hospital in a neighboring state where a family on a state-funded Medicaid program will require approval to go out of network. Different insurance providers may require different information and knowing what this information is can be difficult (Okun, 2010). It may take considerable effort on the part of the primary care provider to get a nonparticipating provider covered by the insurance provider. In addition, if the APN is employed by a particular institution, she may feel an obligation to refer to a provider within the institution even though the APN believes another provider may be more knowledgeable in a specific area. An example of this is a child with a rare liver disorder. In this case, the participating gastroenterologist does accept the child's insurance, but there is no hepatologist that accepts this child's insurance. The APN must discuss the issue with the medical director of the insurance company in order to get the child taken care of by the appropriate specialist. This usually takes extra time on the part of the APN. Meanwhile, this has delayed treatment and is an access to care delay due to managed care constraints. This can lead to moral distress as the APN cannot provide the same level of care to all the patients she sees. The APN needs to get involved in policy through involvement with state and national organizations.

6.3.1.2. Unavailable Treatment

APNs have reported unavailability of treatments that APNs felt were necessary because of lack of insurance coverage (Butz *et al.*, 1998). In some cases, a pediatric advanced practice nurse may find that there are no providers in a particular subspecialty on an insurance panel. For example, there may be no pediatric neurosurgeon on the insurance panel but the child has a bony tumor of the head. In order to obtain these services, the APN must contact the insurance company and must generate a request with the rationale for the need for a pediatric neurosurgeon. The APN who is pressed for time needs to decide when she will do the forms needed for the referral while providing care to patients and balancing her own family demands. This is another area of moral distress for the APN.

6.3.1.3. Prescription Conflicts

It is not uncommon to find that a particular drug is not covered by insurance and the available alternatives do not have the same action and will not work as effectively. To get this medication for the family, the APN must fill out appeal paperwork, taking it to the next level after the insurance has refused the medication. This is a time consuming process and takes time away from patient care or from the family. Balancing resources can be difficult for the APN provider who may have several medically fragile children in her practice. However, without insurance to cover the cost of the medication, there will be an additional financial burden for the family which may lead to lack of compliance with the ideal treatment regime.

In addition, recent legislation in over sixteen states has limited Medicaid services to the poor including restriction on the number of prescriptions per month. Illinois limits the number of prescriptions that a Medicaid recipient can receive to four per month (Galewitz, 2012). This kind of limitation may cause families to restrict medical care to children, and APNs may find that they balance the ideal care with the best possible care given the insurance restrictions. Rationing of resources limits each person's right to equal care. Providers do not see patients in isolation, but within a larger community, and they should consider the larger community needs as they prescribe. The right of equal treatment requires that careful consideration be given to the treatment plan so that community resources are not distributed disproportionately to a few individuals (Camosy, 2011). This can lead to moral distress for the practitioner as she makes treatment decisions.

There are other areas in prescription writing that may cause conflict for the APN. Families may request a specific antibiotic for treatment of a common pediatric entity such as acute otitis media. While evidence-based guidelines call for the first-line drug to be high dose Amoxicillin, the family may prefer a third generation cephalosporin which comes at a higher cost for both the insurance company and the family. It also may not be the best first line agent. From a public health standpoint, using the stronger medication when it is not needed can lead to bacterial resistance. It is important to spend the time educating families rather than being pressured to do something that is against good medical practice. A family of a young infant may demand medication for the baby's upper respiratory tract infection. As new warnings about the risk of stroke have been issued by the CDC which warn against the use of this medication in young children, the practitioner must follow the ethical dictum of nonmaleficence: "First do no harm." The family must be educated about the proper use of such medications. The APN must prescribe treatments that provide the evidence based care and not give in to parental demands. This is another situation leading to moral distress for the APN.

Families may ask providers to write for a variety of medications just in case they get sick before their insurance coverage is terminated. Documenting the reasons for these prescriptions may present an ethical dilemma for the APN. Families want to make sure they have enough medication, but prescribing medications for conditions that are not present is against the law and therefore neither ethically nor legally sound practice. The APN cannot write for medications for conditions that the patient does not have just because the insurance will cover it for one condition, but not for another.

In some instances, one child in a family may be covered under the insurance, but another child may not. Providers may be asked to write prescriptions for an uninsured child in the insured child's name and to forge diagnoses that the insured child does not have. Although it is difficult to turn needy families down, providers cannot commit fraud and violate the Health Care Fraud Act. The APN must offer the parent alternative means of getting the prescription filled (John, 2009). While the APN must follow the ethical principle of beneficence, the APN must always follow the law first.

6.3.1.4. Preferential Treatment

Some practices may ask APNs to give preferential treatment to patients with private insurance by seeing them out of order, putting the private insurance patient or self-pay before the patient with state insurance. This may lead to moral distress for the APN because the practice is making it difficult to do the right thing. This leads to longer waits for patients with state insurance. Preferential appointment times may be given to families with private insurance or they may be allowed to walk in without appointments, whereas patients with state Medicaid are required to make appointments.

6.3.1.5. Diagnostics

Insurance companies may designate certain practices as premium practices if they practice more cost effective healthcare. In cost-sharing systems in some managed care companies, a practice's remuneration is inherent on the ability to limit health care costs. There is an incentive to reduce health care expenditures. Practices will be specially designated by the companies if they are deemed more cost effective, and they will be reimbursed for their services at a higher rate. This is a dubious ethical practice (Okun, 2010). The APN should provide care based on evidence rather than on whether or not the reimbursement to the practice will be higher. These are conflicts that are clearly professional constraints on practice. Section 6.5 contains case examples of ethical conflicts described in this chapter.

6.3.2. Conflicts of Pediatric Advanced Practice Nurses

6.3.2.1. Patient Management

One of the major ethical conflicts for pediatric advanced practice nurses stems around autonomy and the disagreements that arise about patient management. An example of this is when the APN believes that a patient requires inpatient care and a pediatrician or family practitioner colleague disagrees. Some of the moral distress associated with this conflict might be resolved by having the APN's practice agreement include the involvement of a third party if there is disagreement between the APN and the medical consult. When these instances occur, the practice agreement would allow for resolution without conflict between the disagreeing members of the health team. Ideally, a discussion about the best course of action for the patient should be a joint decision that includes all providers and the family.

6.3.2.2. Billing Issues

Most insurers today cover APN services at 85% of the insurer fee-for-service schedule (physician rate). To avoid getting a reduced rate, a physician may decide to bill under his name and bill at 100% of the usual fee. This is an ethical dilemma for the APN, but it is also illegal to bill for services under another's name. APNs must clearly state in writing in her practice agreement that her employer may only bill at the legal rate.

6.3.3. Institutional Problems

6.3.3.1. Practice Conflicts

Practices may offer providers a bonus if they increase their patient population or shorten the time that they spend with patients. While time is not the only measure of effective care, it is one of many things that enters into the health care encounter. The APN may wish to see as many patients as possible to increase billable visits, but may experience moral conflict by not providing the length of visit necessary to adequately care for her patients. This can also be a professional and legal issue.

6.3.4. Family and Pediatric Advanced Practice Nurse Relationships

The issues in this area center around maintaining appropriate boundaries with families, caring for children of friends and family members, accepting gifts, romantic relationships with adolescent patients, being intimate with families and children, and nonmonetary payment for services (Ladd and Forman, 2010). It is important to maintain professional relationships and avoid becoming over involved with families.

6.3.5. Using Professional Authority Appropriately

APNs may be asked by families to write letters to outside agencies to request further services. In some cases, this may require that the APN document something that is not true or is not clear from the medical record. Examples of this include writing letters for utilities to get reduced rates or better housing, to confirm parental competence, or about conditions for social security long-term disabilities (Moon *et al.*, 2009). It can be quite difficult for the APN not to sympathize with the family. The need to recognize sympathy for the family must be balanced against the need to avoid being unethical and using the APN's authority inappropriately. The principle of justice must prevail and the APN must be truthful. While it is important to advocate for the child and the family, the principle of justice demands fairness from the APN.

6.4. SPECIFIC AGE GROUPS

6.4.1. Neonates and Preterm Infants

Today, the treatment of premature newborns is usually based on the patient's Best Interest Standard and recognition of parental authority. However, there is no specific gestational age threshold that enables the APN to withhold intensive care. In some cases, resuscitation is done but when it is clear that the prognosis is poor, treatment is withdrawn. The AAP (2007) has stated there is no difference between the initiation of treatment of newborns and the withdrawal of treatment once it has been instituted. Some providers may find it difficult to withdraw treatment once it has been started. A 2005 survey study of 781 clinicians including physicians, house officers, and nurses used several statements and asked clinicians for their agreement and disagreement with them. They reported that only 14% of critical care physicians agreed with the false statement that 'there is an agreement among ethicists that withdrawal of treatment is different from withholding it'. However, among other doctors and nurses, there was a 40 to 47% agreement with this false statement. This lack of knowledge about starting or withholding treatment was confirmed when the question was asked in reverse. When the question was restated, 'There is no ethical difference between not starting a life support measure and stopping it once it has been started', 50 to 60% of nurses and other physicians disagreed with the statement (Solomon *et al.*, 2005). This points to a lack of knowledge among pediatric intensive care providers about ethics.

6.4.1.1. History

To understand the present ethical dilemmas in neonatal care, it is important to review some cases that have shaped the landscape of ethical issues in neonatology. In 1963, a neonate was born with Down syndrome and duodenal atresia. The family did not want life-saving surgery done as caring for the child in the future would have posed undue financial stress on the rest of the family. After two weeks, the infant died secondary to lack of ability to absorb nutrition. In 1973, in an essay in the New England Journal of Medicine, Duff and Campbell supported the non-treatment decision, saying that the decision to treat neonates belonged in the hands of families.

Subsequent to this case, there was a profoundly compromised newborn in Maine that the family and physician decided not to treat. Other physicians objected and the case went to the Maine Supreme Court who found that human life took precedence and that the child should have all medical procedures done if this could save his life. The infant died after the court-ordered surgery (Paris *et al.*, 2007).

In contrast, in the Stinson case (1983), an 800 gram newborn with a survival rate of less than 5% was kept alive after he was transferred from a community hospital (where the family had requested no resuscitation) to Children's Hospital of Philadelphia (CHOP). At CHOP, the family was told that the baby would be kept alive at all costs unless he was brain dead. The child was kept alive through several illnesses including a brain hemorrhage. Finally, the baby extubated himself and was allowed to die.

In 1982, in Indiana, Baby Doe was born with Down syndrome and tracheoesophageal fistula. The baby was allowed to die without surgical treatment at the request of the obstetrician and the family (Paris, Schreiber and Moreland, 2007; Pless, 1983). The Indiana Supreme Court upheld the parent's decision, but the federal government felt that physicians are obliged to treat every child. The following year, in New York, an infant was born with a meningomyelocele and multiple congenital defects. The family elected no treatment, but a Vermont lawyer, Lawrence Washburn, brought suit against New York for non-treatment of the child. The Department of Health and Human Services was notified about non-treatment and the case was referred to the New York State Child Protective Service, who did not feel that the case involved child neglect. The child died, but the Surgeon General at the time, C. Everett Koop, informed Congress of the need for treatment for these children (Chambers, 1983).

As a result, Congress passed the Baby Doe Amendment or Baby Doe Law in 1984, effective June 1, 1985. It was an addition to the child abuse law, which stated that withholding food, fluid, and medically indicated treatment from disabled children was a form of child abuse. A 1983 editorial in the *New England Journal of Medicine* critiqued the law, stating it "was based on the premise that all life, no matter how miserable, should be maintained if technically possible" (Angell, p. 659). The law was challenged in Federal court and ultimately the United States Supreme Court struck down the amendment in 1986 (Paris, 2005). Out of this act, the "Best Interest Standards" were formed and became the ethical basis for deciding treatment decisions for pediatric patients that could not talk for themselves.

By the late 1980s, one third of neonatologists admitted that they provided medical interventions for sick neonates even when they disagreed with the benefit of the treatment (Kopelman, Irons and Kopelman, 1988). The case of Sammy Linares (1989) and baby boy Messenger

(1996) furthered the rights of parents to make decisions regarding their children. In both cases, the fathers removed their infant sons from ventilators and were charged with their murders. Both fathers were set free. In the Linares case, the grand jury never returned a homicide indictment (Paris, 2005). Foregoing medical treatment of critically ill newborns by health care professionals and parents is fairly common and such cases have not been successfully prosecuted (Sklansky, 2001).

Research completed around this same period showed that there was disagreement among practitioners about treatments for newborns with genetic problems and medical issues. Shaw, Randolph and Manard (1977) surveyed 457 pediatricians and pediatric surgeons about whether they would let parents decide whether to operate on a newborn with biliary atresia and Down syndrome. In their study, 51.7% of the pediatricians would let the parents decide, and 38.4% of pediatric surgeons would let the parents decide. In the same study, 16.5% of the pediatricians and 27.9% of the surgeons would try to persuade the parents to let them operate on the child but would not bring them to court if they would not. Todres, Krane, Howell and Shannon (1977) reported on a survey of 230 pediatricians regarding the same issue. Their study reported that 40.2% of physicians would pursue a court order, and 54.2% would not bring the parents to court. In this study, religious beliefs and affiliations of the physicians significantly affected whether they would pursue a court order.

6.4.1.2. Decisions to Treat the Preterm Infant

The benefit/burden assessment in assessing the viability of the sick neonate considers survival rates along with neurodevelopmental status including anencephaly (Paris, 2005). When there is a risk of mortality greater than 50% and an associated high risk of morbidity, there is a grey area as to whether to continue treatment. Often, extremely premature infants are treated in a "wait and see" approach when there is uncertainty about the outcome (Paris *et al.*, 2007). In a highly publicized 2003 case in Texas, a 23-week gestation, 615 gram newborn was treated against the parent's wishes. The administrator of the hospital insisted on treatment because the child was more than 500 grams. The parents initially won 60 million dollars in punitive damages, as the child now requires 24-hour care. The Texas Supreme Court overturned the jury verdict because they believed that if the physician is unsure, treatment should be initiated over parental objections (Paris *et al.*, 2007).

In the 2007 AAP guidelines on non-intervention or withdrawal of intensive care for the high-risk infant, critical elements in the decision-making are outlined (AAP, 2007). These elements include communicating in a direct, open manner with parents; involving the active decision-makers in the care of the child; continuation of comfort care; and making sure that treatment decisions are centered on the Best Interest Standard. Parents may have difficulty making decisions based on the Best Interest standard and may consider their own interest over that of the baby (Hentschel, Lindner, Krueger, and Reiter-Theil, 2006). In Hentschel *et al.* (2006), a small observational study of 40 neonates in a German NICU (single institution) found that restriction of ongoing intensive care was decided in 32 neonates, but in 9 cases, the team had no knowledge of the parent's wishes. In a different study done in the Netherlands, 79% of the parents were involved in decision making (van der Haide *et al.*, 1997). While the ideal is comprehensive informed consent, parents may feel overwhelmed by details and may ask a provider to help them and share some responsibility in the decision making process. A major weakness of both studies is that parents were not interviewed—only the medical team. A parent's decision is frequently made with the information that they receive about the infant's prognosis from the healthcare team. It is critically important that this information be clear and based on current statistics of morbidity and mortality, as neonatal medicine has made significant advances over the past twenty years. In order for parents to make a decision, the benefits and burden of treatment must be completely discussed. The APN involved must be sure that the information is complete in order to assure that parental authority is based on what would be in the best interest of the child (Mercurio, 2010).

Good ethics begins with good data (Mercurio, 2010; Townsend, 2012). Patient outcome estimators are available at the NICHD website: http://www.nichd.nih.gov/about/org/cdbpm/pp/prog_epbo/epbo_case.cfm. At this website, the provider must put in the infant's gestational age, birth weight, sex, and whether antenatal steroids were given within 7 days of delivery along with whether it was a singleton birth. For example, a female, singleton birth at 24-weeks' gestation weighing 700 grams and receiving antenatal steroids has a 72% survival rate, with 59% of those infants having no profound neurodevelopmental impairments, but 44% of the 72% having moderate or severe impairments. There is a 59% risk of death or moderate to severe developmental impairment based on this website's patient outcome estimator. An APN must consider that these statistics will not reflect whether an extremely premature baby received maximum treatment and therefore the rates of death and impairment may be statistically lower. The AAP concluded that treatment decisions for high-risk neonates should consider the physiologic maturity of the infant, the seriousness of the neonate's medical conditions including birth defects, and the probability of death and disability.

In a study by Kempf *et al.* (2009), 95 high risk mothers were counseled about fetal risk in advance of delivering their child. The study results demonstrated that palliative comfort care only was desired by 100% of parents when the child was delivered at 22 weeks; but by 24 weeks, only 38% desired palliative comfort care only; and by 26 weeks, none of the parents wanted palliative comfort care only. The results of counseling about morbidity and mortality outcomes of premature infants less than 26 weeks resulted in a substantial proportion of parents desiring comfort care. The importance of discussing outcomes of extremely premature infants prior to delivery in high-risk mothers helped families make difficult decisions.

The AAP divides the types of decision making with premature or high-risk neonates into three categories (AAP, 2007). The first decision-making scenario occurs when death is likely and if the infant lives, there will be an unacceptably high rate of morbidity. In this case, intensive treatment is not indicated (AAP, 2007; Mercurio, Maxwell *et al.*, 2008). Therefore, it is acceptable to withdraw or withhold treatment because it is not in the best interest of the newborn. It is important to work with families who want to continue treatment even if there is no medical reason to hope for recovery. If continued treatment is not in the best interest of the child, the APN should obtain an ethics consult if the family continues to want to treat (Mercurio, 2010). This is consistent with the AAP policy, which states that "medical professionals should seek to override family wishes only when those views clearly conflict with the interests of the child" (AAP, 2008).

In the second type of decision-making, the infant has a high chance of survival with an excellent prognosis in terms of long-term neurodevelopmental outcome. In this case, intensive treatment in an NICU makes sense. The APN must place the interest of the patient over the parents or their own interest and provide life-sustaining treatment. The APN has an ethical responsibility to the infant and must provide care. In this case, parental requests to not provide treatment should be questioned.

The third decision-making scenario is more problematic, as the prognosis is uncertain and the outcome of intervention is less clear. In these cases, parental authority determines the treatment course. The infant should always receive full supportive and comfort care. There is a controversy regarding whether to initiate treatment of very premature infants less than 23 weeks who present vigorously at birth.

6.4.1.3. Allocation of Resources

Some ethicists feel that preterm infants do not receive full treatment because there is less value put on the life of a newborn (Janvier *et al.*, 2007). The argument here is that people would fully treat a 2 month old with sepsis, but would let a 24-week gestation newborn die because he only had a 50% chance of survival without sequelae. The question around newborn resuscitation and care is that fetuses are not viewed as living by some and therefore in the initial minutes following birth, may be seen as less of person (Janvier, Bauer and Lantos, 2007). According to Janvier *et al.* (2007), the newborn is placed in a special moral category, resulting from the transition from fetus to person. Decisions to treat newborns differently from other age persons suggest that newborn's lives are less valued (Javier, Bauer and Lantos, 2007), or that the law makes definitive cut off dates. NICU treatment for preterm and critically ill newborn infants is scrutinized more than adult intensive care units. Many associations believe that resuscitation under 24 weeks should not be done due to a poor prognosis (Javier *et al.*, 2007). Ross (2007) writes, ". . . what is best for a child is complex, evolving, and situationally-dependent. Clinicians and families must work together and regularly assess the benefit/burden calculation" (p. 351).

Kipnis (2007) also defends the importance of parental decision making in cases where the prognosis is not as clear, but points out that there are blurred boundaries in which high risk infants might benefit from treatment intervention. There is a group of newborns who will benefit from NICU care, but in some cases, it is unclear at the time of the decision making whether or not a specific infant would be harmed or helped from treatment. Some neonatologists initiate treatment, waiting to see what the course of the newborn will be. However, once they treat and the baby has a bad outcome, the baby may not die when life support is withdrawn. While treatment may offer a good outcome, there are situations in which the outcome is less clear and parents should be involved in the final decision (Kipnis, 2007).

6.4.1.4. Maternal-Fetal Conflict

When a mother is pregnant, she has full power of decision-making regarding her obstetrical treatment at the time of delivery, which may be at odds with the best choices for the baby. The principles of respect for patient autonomy, beneficence, nonmaleficence, and justice guide decisions, whereas feminist theory and the ethics of care help frame the answer. A woman who refuses to have a cesarean delivery when faced with a large fetus with heart rate abnormalities should be educated about the consequences of such a decision, but the autonomous pregnant woman has the right to refuse treatment. The American College of Obstetrics and Gynecology states that with regard to maternal decision making capacities, they would not support going to court to force a cesarean section to protect the fetus (American College of Obstetricians and Gynecologists, 2005; Townsend, 2012). Guidelines should be in place within hospitals and birthing centers to resolve conflicts, and shared decision-making should be used when there is a conflict. The APN/nurse midwife may be involved in the care of the infant and may be called on to educate the mother about the care of these infants and the possible outcomes. Open communication is the key to ethical decision-making, with intervention by the courts rarely needed.

6.4.1.5. Newborn Screening

In the early 1960s, phenylketonuria (PKU) testing of infants was introduced and by 1967, the test was mandatory in 37 states (Paul, 2008). The expansion of newborn screening to congenital hypothyroidism took place in 1973, and by the mid-1980s, several other metabolic conditions were added to newborn screening panels. In the late 1980s, it became clear that early introduction of penicillin prophylaxis prevented death in patients with sickle cell disease. Therefore, screening for sickle cell disease was added to the panel. In the early 1990s, tandem mass spectrometry was developed and its use in newborn screening increased the number of conditions tested. The use of tandem mass spectrometry technology led to expansion of the newborn screening program. These new tests also raised questions about the necessity of screening for conditions that could not be effectively treated (Paul, 2008).

Today, more than 98% of the 4.3 million babies born in the United States undergo newborn screening done at birth (Gonzales, 2011). The guidelines for testing newborns at birth include that the disease tested for should be an important public health problem, that there is an effective treatment, and that the test is acceptable to the population (Wilson and Junger, 1968). Categories of newborn screening include hemoglobin disorders, metabolic disorders, endocrine disorders, and other diseases such as cystic fibrosis (National Newborn Screening and Genetic Resource Center, 2012). In 2005, the Health Resources and Services Administration recommended that 29 core conditions be included in the newborn screen with an additional number of 25 conditions that are second tier recommendations (Gonzales, 2011; Paul, 2008). Different states' newborn screening programs vary, but all screen for the 29 core conditions. New tests continue to be added to the panel based on observational data and expert opinion (Tarini, Burke, Scott and Wilfond, 2008).

Today, the Secretary of Health and Human Services' Advisory Committee on Heritable Disorders and Genetic Diseases in Newborns and Children makes recommendations regarding what tests should be included in the newborn panel. More recently, there is a proposal to screen for severe combined immunodeficiency and for congenital cyanotic heart disease, which would bring the core panel to 31 different screening tests. All states have not yet implemented these two new recommendations.

Advocacy groups have played an important role in the addition of tests to the panel. However, some of these groups are tied to industry and some of the diseases now included in some state panels are not a large public health threat. An example of this is Krabbe's disease, which was added to the New York State newborn screening panel despite the fact that the condition only affects 40 infants per year nationwide. In addition, the treatment of Krabbe's disease is controversial (Paul, 2008). Conversely, screening for congenital hypothyroidism has prevented developmental disabilities as newborn screening allows this disease to be picked up before there are any physical manifestations of hypothyroidism. If parents refuse newborn screening, they may opt out of early identification of diseases like PKU and hypothyroidism that can be effectively treated in the newborn period. Early treatment of these diseases reduces mortality and morbidity as the diagnosis of the disease before the development of symptoms is critical. Some recommendations of the newborn screening panel are problematic as there are no effective treatments to date.

Newborns are now screened for both cystic fibrosis (CF) and sickle cell disease (SCD). As a result, there is an increase in the number of patients identified as of carrier of the disease. While genetic testing of children is not recommended in order to protect the child's privacy and autonomy, newborn screening is an exception to this rule. There has been considerable debate about the potential benefits and harm. Table 6.1 outlines the pros and cons of carrier state identification. It could be argued that disclosure of sickle cell carrier state is important because of the increased risk of heat stroke associated with the carrier state (Ross and Clayton, 2009). A recent systematic review reported that the issues surrounding SCD carriage identification by newborn screening is underexplored (Hayeems, Bytautas and Miller, 2008). There is no data about cystic fibrosis carriers having increased risk of any disease. The confirmation of CF carriage requires a burdensome confirmatory pro-

TABLE 6.1. Pros and Cons of Carrier State Identification.

Pros	Cons
Awareness about Clinical implications of carrier status	Anxiety or distress from learning of an abnormal test
Awareness of future reproductive choices	Misunderstand of genetic implications
Empowered by knowing genetic information	Potential discrimination and stigmatization on the carrier
	Continued worry about the carrier
	Possibility of non-paternity

cess to distinguish between a false positive and truly positive testing (Hayeems *et al.*, 2008).

While the American Academy of Pediatrics (2001, reaffirmed in 2009) recommends that parents be informed that screening tests are being done and that parental permission should be obtained, most states continue with the newborn screening program as an "opt out" test and therefore no permission is required before the testing is done. In order for parents to opt out, they must know in advance that a test is being performed and then must proactively opt out of the program if they do not want their baby screened in the nursery. The issue is whether or not the broadening of these tests continues to fulfill the criteria for a public health screening program. Parents should be educated about these tests and active consent should be obtained to fully respect parental autonomy (Ross and Clayton, 2009). If the parent refuses newborn screening, the child may be placed at risk for long-term sequelae such as intellectual disability from untreated PKU or hypothyroidism.

In addition, there are pilot programs to screen for lysosomal storage disorders, fragile X, and Duchene's Muscular dystrophy. Since these disorders may not show up until later in life, there are questions as to whether it is ethical to test newborns for diseases that will not be symptomatic until later. Some of the concerns about newborn screening for the infant include psychological harm, stigmatization, and discrimination from being identified as having a costly disease (AAP, 2001, reaffirmed 2009).

The introduction of new tests to the newborn screening panel should be carefully studied for long-term effects. Some ethicists feel that children should have the right to determine whether they want testing for genetic conditions (Ross and Clayton, 2009; Hayeems *et al.*, 2008), while others argue that it is acceptable to waive informed consent for newborn screening research if there is an excellent test and definitive therapy (Tarini *et al.*, 2008). Clearly, there are issues related to parental refusal of newborn screening, as some of these screening tests do screen for very treatable conditions. However, the need for newborn screening and the risk and benefits must be thoroughly explained to the parent.

6.4.1.6. Vaccine Refusal

Refusal of accepted medical treatments such as vaccines is a source of concern for both physicians (Talati, Lang and Ross, 2010) and pediatric nurse practitioners (Butz, Redman, Fry and Kolodner, 1998). Childhood immunizations are still a persistent area of concern for parents and providers.

State laws requiring vaccines stem from a 1905 landmark case in which the United States Supreme Court endorsed school immunization requirements and gave states the right to reinforce these laws (Omer *et al.*, Salmon, Orenstein, deHart and Halsey, 2009). In 1922, the Supreme Court found that school immunization requirements were constitutional (Omer *et al.*, 2009). Recently, the trends in immunization policies and ethics have made universal vaccination more difficult (Feudtner and Marcuse, 2001). Due to changes in molecular immunology, there are an increasing number of vaccines available. In addition, cost-effectiveness analyses are changing policy decisions around immunizations.

Early in the 1900s, vaccination was mandatory and required to protect the public health. Today, the ethical issues around universal vaccination revolve around securing the greatest good for the greatest number of people versus protecting the rights of individuals. In the United States, a parent cannot be forced to vaccinate a child.

If there was a national mandatory requirement for vaccination of all children despite parental objections, society would minimize the effects of deleterious disease consequences, promote societies' duty to protect children, and maximize equal distribution of health programs and their prudent use. If the vaccination of children was an elective decision, it would promote the personal liberty to refuse or choose, and would minimize any adverse vaccine events. Today, vaccines are recommended and are not mandatory in the hopes that the Best Interest Standard will prevail, and families will want to protect their children against vaccine preventable diseases.

There are three reasons that parents can elect to exempt their children. There are exemptions for children who have valid medical reasons for not taking the vaccine such as allergies, exemptions for parents whose religious beliefs oppose immunizations, and exemptions for parents who have philosophical beliefs that can be cited when they refuse to immunize their child (Omer *et al.*, 2009). All states allow medical exemptions and all but two states, Mississippi and West Virginia, allow religious exemptions, but only 40% of states allow philosophical exemptions (National Conference of State Legislators, 2012). States where philosophical reasons for exemptions are allowed have a higher rate of immunization refusal (Omer *et al.*, 2009). In general, recent parental concerns due to perceived vaccine safety issues have led to increasing numbers of parents refusing or delaying vaccines.

Halperin (2000) categorized vaccine hesitant parents into five groups and these are seen in Table 6.2. The first three groups are easier to work with and the last two are the most difficult to convince. It is possible with targeted education to overcome vaccine resistance. The ethical issues for a provider are centered on how to deal with the resistance. A recent study showed that 4.8% of pediatricians would always refuse to continue as the child's medical provider and 18.1% would sometimes tell the parent that they would not continue as the child's medical provider if the parent refused to vaccinate their children (American Academy of Pediatrics, 2001). The position of the American Academy of Pediatrics is that providers should continue to work with families.

The APN must be aware of parents' need for correct information about vaccines. The results of a recent study reported that new mothers wanted to be provided with vaccine information in advance of the two month health supervision visit (Vanice *et al.*, 2011). While the information ahead of the visit did not change the immunization rate in a study of 272 mothers, it did change their attitude about vaccines. Another study showed that parents who refuse vaccines are not all the same

TABLE 6.2. Five Groups of Vaccine Hesitant Parent.

Pros	Cons
Uninformed but educable	Seeks information to counter an anti-vaccination message
Misinformed but correctable	Are not aware of the benefits
Well read and open minded	Explored the pro-vaccine and vaccine hesitancy message and want to discuss the vaccine
Convinced and contented	Strongly vaccine hesitant but want to demonstrate their willingness to listen to the other side of the argument
Committed and missionary	Want to convince provider to agree with them about being against vaccines

Adapted from Halperin.

and have different reasons for refusing vaccines (Gust *et al.*, 2008). The largest portion of parents who changed their minds did so because of information from health care providers (Gust *et al.*, 2008). Another study reviewed United States newspaper print information from 1995 to 2005 and found that 37% of the articles gave negative information about immunizations (Hussain *et al.*, 2011). Thus, APNs must be aware of the importance of providing appropriate evidence-based resources for vaccine information.

A study of vaccine attitudes, concerns and information sources showed that parents of young children felt the most important resource of information about vaccines was the child's doctor or nurse (Kennedy, Basket, and Sheedy, 2011). Due to the dissemination of unreliable information to parents, parents may refuse and want to space out vaccines (Pineda and Myers, 2011). A list of reliable websites and books are found in Box 6.1. If the family refuses to immunize their child, the APN should ask the family to sign a release from liability to a malpractice suit if the child was infected with the vaccine preventable disease and had a bad outcome. This is available from the following website--http://www.aap.org/immunization/pediatricians/pdf/refusaltovaccinate.pdf

The American Academy of Pediatrics has endorsed continued involvement with families who refuse vaccines (Diekema and the Committee on Bioethics, 2005). Ohio has a free one-hour training program for providers to help them overcome barriers to immunizations [http://www.ohioaap.org/program-initiatives/maximizing-office-based-immunization-(mobi)].

From an ethical standpoint, the APN must assess the level of information that the parent has and explore the beliefs of the parent. The APN then can educate and give appropriate information including websites and books (See Table 6.3) (Pineda and Myers, 2011). Parents must have misinformation corrected and the correct information communicated in an effective forum so that informed decisions can be made in the best interest of their children (Boom and Healy, 2011).

Some of the reasons that providers give to validate their reasons for terminating patient relationships include philosophical differences, and the risks of exposing immunized patients to non-immunized patients with diseases that are vaccine preventable. For example, a child with cough whose parent has refused immunization against pertussis may be present in the waiting room along with infants who have not yet been fully protected against vaccine. It has been shown that children with nonmedical exemptions of vaccines are at increased risk of acquiring or transmitting vaccine-preventable diseases (Salmon *et al.*, 2000; Feikin *et al.*, 2000). One study showed that children who did not get immu-

TABLE 6.3. Websites and Books with Reliable Information about Vaccines.

Websites with Reliable Information about Vaccines
• www.medlineplus.gov—National Library of Medicine • www.cdc.gov—Centers for Disease Control • www.nih.gov/icd—National Institute of Health • www.who.int—World Health Organization • www.aap.org—American Academy of Pediatrics • www.childandfamily.info—Tufts University Child and Family Web Guide • www.immunizationinfo.org—National Network for Immunization Information • www.vaccine.chop.edu—Vaccine Education Center at Children's Hospital of Philadelphia website • www.immunize.org—Immunization Action Coalition Website • www.vaccinateyourbaby.org—Put out by two websites • http://immunize.cpha.ca/en/default.aspx—The Canadian website encouraging immunizations. • www.caringforkids.cpc.ca—Canadian Pediatric society • www.iom.org—Institute of Medicine • www.meningitis-angels.org • www.hispanichealth.org • www.nfid.org—National foundation for infectious disease • www3.niaid.nih.gov/dmid/vaccine • www.nmaus.org—National Meningitis Association • www.immunizationinfo.org—National Network for Immunization Information • www.pkids.org—Parents of Kids with Infectious Disease • www.vaccine.texaschildrens.org—Center For Vaccine Awareness and Research, Texas Children Hospital
Books with Reliable Information about Vaccines
• Offit, P.A. and Bell, L.M. (1999) Vaccines: What Every Parent Should Know. New York, NY: IDG Books. • Humiston, S.G. and Good, C. (2000) Vaccinating Your Child: Questions and Answers for the Concerned Parent. Atlanta, GA: Peachtree Publishers. • Fisher, M.C. (2005) Immunizations and Infectious Diseases: An Informed Parent's Guide. Elk Grove Village, IL: American Academy of Pediatrics. • Myers, M.G. and Pineda, D. (2008) Do Vaccines Cause That? A Guide for Evaluating Vaccine Safety Concerns. Immunizations for Public Health. • Your Child's Best Shot from the Canadian Pediatric Society

nized for measles have 22 times greater risk of measles (Feikin *et al.*, 2000). In 2012, Washington State declared a pertussis epidemic. Non-medical exemption from vaccination has ranged from a low of 0.2% in Rhode Island to a high of 5.7% in Washington State (Stokley *et al.*, 2011). If the rates of immunizations are higher at school entry, there is a lower incidence of measles and mumps (Orenstein and Hinman, 1999). There is a relationship between vaccination rates and rates of infectious disease that could be prevented by vaccines. Some providers feel that parents should vaccinate their children for the child's and community greater good and feel that if they do not want vaccines, they will discharge the patient. This is not the position of the AAP, which encourages continued involvement with the family (Diekema and the Committee on Bioethics, 2005). However, if the APN wants to terminate the relationship, she must transfer the care of the patient to another provider before she terminates the relationship. She cannot abandon the patient and refuse to care for the child (Gilmour *et al.*, 2011).

6.4.2. Child and Adolescent

6.4.2.1. Predictive Genetic Testing

Genetic advances have developed rapidly over the last twenty years and tools for genomic analysis were developed to help map genes. While these advances may help improve the lives of Americans, they also lead to new ethical dilemmas. Personalized information about modifiable risk factors may provide children and adolescents with the information they need to modify their lifestyle in order to avoid disease. However, this generation is the first group of children and adolescents that have the ability to get this information, but how this will affect them is not yet known. In addition, decision-making ability in adolescents is controversial and it also may be influenced by peers (Gardner and Steinberg, 2005).

Predictive genetic testing can be divided into categories of diseases that manifest in adults, diseases that manifest in childhood, and testing that identifies carrier information. There is universal consensus in the AAP that predictive testing in children for adult onset disease and testing for carrier status should be delayed. A mature adult must make decisions about genetic testing (American Society of Human Genetics (ASHG)/American College of Medical Genetics (ACMG), 1995; American Academy of Pediatrics, 2001). The kind of genetic condition and the possibility of preventive treatment determines whether geneticists will provide genetic testing (Borry *et al.*, 2008). Borry *et al.* (2008)

surveyed 600 geneticists. He reported that if there was a medical treatment for a genetic disease such as with Familial adenomatous polyposis or multiple endocrine neoplasia, then the geneticist might be willing to test children at 6 years and at 16 years. However, with diseases with no known cure such as Alzheimer's, and Huntington's, the geneticists would not test a child (Borry *et al.*, 2008).

There are psychosocial, clinical, and reproductive implications to these tests and there is not yet enough research as to the long-term effects of knowing this information. Table 6.4 outlines the important points to consider before doing genetic testing of children (ASHG/ACMG, 1995). There are harms of knowing a genetic diagnosis for the child and adolescent that may increase anxiety for the parent and child, increase guilt for the parents, problems with employment and insurance, detection of paternity, changes in how the child is viewed by the parents, and alteration of self-image for the child. For example, in a family with history of retinoblastoma, knowledge of whether a child has the gene for retinoblastoma can allow for surveillance and early detection of the disease, thereby preventing loss of vision. However, if the family refuses the genetic test, the question may be asked: "Are they acting in the child's best interest?" In the case of muscular dystrophy, a child may appear unaffected at birth, but by early childhood is symptomatic. If the family does not know their proclivity for the disease, they may not be able to plan their future family appropriately. If the parents know predictive information, they will have the information they need for family planning (Ross, 2008).

In the case of Fragile X syndrome, the number of trinucleotide repeats is often associated with the severity of the disease, so knowing the genetic make-up of the child can determine the prognosis. In terms of reproductive issues, parents may avoid having further children in order to prevent having another child with the disease and may make family planning decisions based on the knowledge of their disease (Borry *et al.*, 2009). Genetic testing can also allow families to make life decisions about retirement based on the information.

Knowledge that a child has a genetic disorder may affect family relationships and the child may be rejected, overindulged, or scapegoated. Vulnerable child syndrome (Green and Solnit, 1964) may result, causing the parents to treat the child as though something is going to happen to the child, and restrict his activity. Unaffected children may be treated differently as a result of the identification of a problem with their sibling.

Ethical issues regarding genetic testing also center on privacy and confidentiality as well as the right to know and the right to not know.

TABLE 6.4. Important Issues in Genetic Testing in Children and Adolescents.

Potential Benefits and Harms of testing	• Medical benefits is the main reason to test a child or adolescent • Psychosocial benefit to an adolescent • If the disease is adult onset, delay genetic testing • If the risk or benefit is not clear, the parent and adolescent must make the decision after the potential benefits and harms completely reviewed • Testing should be discouraged if the potential harm outweighs the benefits to a child or adolescent
Family and Decision Making	• The child and parent should receive education and counseling based on their ability and maturity • The provider must obtain parental permission along with adolescent's or child's voluntary assent • The competent adolescent's request for the results should outweigh the refusal of the parent to give the adolescent the information • If the provider feels the test is not in the best interest of a child, the provider needs to advocate on the behalf of the child
Research	• Research must focus on the genetic test's proposed benefits to the child as well as the psychosocial impact of the results of the genetic test

A family member who has knowledge of his genetic disease may not choose to disclose the disease if is not likely to result in serious harm to another family member.

Testing for certain diseases may be supported by the APN if there is clear benefit to the child. For example, in hypertrophic cardiomyopathy, drug therapy may be of benefit to the child to prevent sudden death (ASHG/ACMG, 1995). If the APN is in doubt, she should refer the patient to the geneticist. If the APN believes that the genetic test may cause more harm than benefit to the child, the APN must act as an advocate for the child. They can refuse to do the testing as it does not benefit the child.

As genetic testing becomes available via public websites such as 23andMe.com, it is possible that a child's saliva can be tested by parents without their permission. These public websites provide a report about risks of over 200 diseases and are given without a healthcare provider's counseling. While the site states that the testing of children requires a special kit and additional charge, it would be possible for parents to collect saliva of their adolescent without permission.

6.4.2.2. Special Needs Children

Families who care for children with special health care needs (CSHCN) have multiple demands on them that are different from families raising well children. The enormity of the obligations can change the family dynamics—limiting attention to other children, changing employment status of a parent, limiting recreational activities, and making day-to-day decisions. The family is responsible for carrying out complex regimes with little support from outside agencies. This may lead to lack of adherence and trigger a referral to child protective services for medical neglect. The APN must develop a plan using shared decision-making that meets the needs of the family and the CSHCN. For the seriously ill CSHCN, the APN should raise the issue about advanced care plans and palliative care before the child is actually dying. Discussion around what should be done for a child with a terminal condition must be discussed before an acute event occurs (Okun, 2010).

For providers, one of the issues with special needs children is the extra time required in caring for these children versus caring for a well-child, often without appropriate reimbursement (Okun, 2010). While a sense of duty and obligation to patients is part of clinical practice, providers must be compensated for the time spent caring for these patients as they do take away time for other patients. There is additional paperwork for insurance companies to approve equipment and medication and this additional time is also not compensated.

The APN must develop expertise in counseling and informing patients about issues around death, sexuality, genetic risk, and prognosis. Discussion around harm versus benefit for a variety of procedures and surgical options must be held to promote beneficence. Families who want treatments that are not proven may be refused by providers if there is no clear benefit to the child (Okun, 2010). This may lead to difficult communications with families regarding refusal to give unproven treatment. However, good ethics demand refusal of unproven treatments.

6.4.2.3. Nondisclosure of a Diagnosis to a Child or Adolescent

While patient autonomy may be clearer in adult ethical situations, pediatric patients require a significantly different approach due to the importance of family and their necessity to act in the best interest of their child. Over the past 30 years, the decision to disclose or not disclose a diagnosis of HIV to a child or adolescent has become a new ethical dilemma in pediatrics. There have always been religious and cultural beliefs that might prevent disclosure of a diagnosis to a child and their family members against the wishes of their parents (Kulkarni *et al.*, 2001; Wells and John, 2002). Disclosure of a disease may carry the burden of stigmatization and discrimination along with cultural and religious concerns for families (Kulkarni *et al.*, 2001).

While the AAP recommends disclosure of HIV status to a child, the AAP also recommends that clinical status, social situation, age, and psychosocial maturity be considered (Committee on AIDS, 1999). However, culture clearly needs to be considered in disclosures (Betancourt, Green, and Carrillo, 2011). Outside Western cultures, communication by innuendo rather than direct communication is the norm. Telling a patient a diagnosis directly may be seen as disrespectful and can disrupt family relationships (Kuldarni *et al.*, 2001). In certain cultures, family autonomy is far more important that individual autonomy and reflects the fact that different cultures handle ethical considerations in different ways (Swota and Hester, 2011). Therefore, when discussing disclosure with families, the APN must consider the entire life of the patient, including an understanding of the family, community, and culture (Swota and Hester, 2011).

Ethical issues about nondisclosure center on basic concepts in pediatric ethics such as child autonomy, truth telling, beneficent deception, nonmaleficence, confidentiality, cross cultural considerations, and family autonomy. The APN may meet families who request nondisclosure of any diagnosis to the child due to religious or cultural reasons. Family autonomy must be considered in cross-cultural ways. In Western society, moral dilemmas may require consideration of family autonomy. Most professionals prefer to be truthful with their pediatric patients. Truth telling is closely aligned with the ethical duty of respecting the autonomy of others (Kuldarni *et al.*, 2001).

The military's previous policy of "Don't ask, don't tell" regarding sexual orientation and passed by Congress in 1996 reflects the concept of beneficent deception (Kuldarni *et al.*, 2001). The concept of avoiding telling the truth, if truth can do more harm than good, has lost popularity. In cases where parents do not want an older child or adolescent told of a diagnosis, the diagnosis must be considered. For example, in an adolescent, where HIV is often a sexually transmitted diagnosis, the responsibility to protect the rest of society must be considered. While it can be argued that the strongest argument for nondisclosure is the wishes of the parents, consideration of the public's health also must be considered in a sexually active adolescent. Legal concerns may overshadow these decisions, and in cases where there is a risk to the rest of society, the APN can get a court injunction based on the principle of beneficence and the Best Interest Standard.

The patient may also feel a loss of trust and significant anger toward the members of the healthcare team who failed to disclose the diagnosis. The APN may experience guilt, fear, empathy, liability, and anger about failing to be honest with the patient. Nondisclosure may lead to frustration, as the APN may not be able to talk directly to the patient and get his/her input into medical treatment decisions. Some of the reasons for nondisclosure cited by the parent may be the child's age, the lack of symptoms, and the reduction in self-esteem if the child knew about his disease.

Medical decision-making is problematic when the interests of the child and the interest of the parents are not in concert. The child or adolescent who does not know the diagnosis cannot weigh in on treatment options. In an adolescent who is able to consider treatment options, the nondisclosure takes this right away from the child. A pragmatic right-based justification seems appropriate in the adolescent who is able to make decisions (Kulkarni *et al.*, 2001). In these cases, an ethics consult may be helpful to the APN and the health care team.

6.4.2.4. Caring for Abused Children

According to legal mandates, the APN is required to report suspected child abuse. Child abuse may take the form of physical abuse, psychological abuse, sexual abuse, or neglect (Centers for Disease Control, 2012). At times, questioning parents lead the APN to suspect that the child is being exposed to excessive violence, which also needs to be reported even if the APN is concerned about the therapeutic relationship with the parent. It is important to remember that the APN must act in the best interest of the child no matter what the relationship is with the guardian or parent—protecting the child is the focus of the APN's care.

There are several different ethical situations around child abuse in which the APN may experience moral distress. Parents may suffer from mental illness, substance abuse, or domestic violence leading to child abuse. A child should ideally be raised in an environment that will foster his growth and development. While this may mean the removal of the child from the natural guardians, all efforts should be made to keep the family together with supports and ongoing treatment. Placement in a foster care may result in multiple homes, multiple school placements, loss of parental and family support and the termination of foster care at 18, leaving the child without adequate life skills for adult life (Fisher,

2011). Placement with foster care may not be the best option for the child in the long run, so it should be used only if the parent's situation is unable to be remediated (Fisher, 2011). The APN who cares for foster children must monitor their progress and report concerns to child protective services.

APNs may be involved in child abuse cases in which the child experiences a severe injury as a result of abuse. This can occur in the ED, PICU, or in long term care facilities. In these cases, lifesaving medical treatment may be needed. In some of these children, the perpetrator is not clear and the parent—perhaps one of the perpetrators—may be involved in making decisions. If it is determined that the child is suffering, will not recover, and the quality and extent of life will not be restored, consideration of termination of lifesaving support should be raised with the parents. In cases where the parents might be charged with a crime if the child's life support is terminated, the parent may be more concerned about what is best for them instead of the child (Gladsjo *et al.*, 2004). In these cases, the court will appoint a guardian ad litem, who is an attorney who advocates for the best interests of the child. These attorneys explore the situation based on interviews with the healthcare team, including the APN and the parents. They issue a report to the judge about the child's situation in order to help the court make a decision. Discontinuing life-sustaining interventions may cause disagreements between the health care provider and families (Fisher, 2011; Gladsjo *et al.*, 2004). Parents may not be able to consider the best interest of child when there is a potential conflict of interest, an insufficient understanding of their child's condition, or parental refusal to acknowledge the seriousness of the child's condition. Difficult decision-making can be helped by a referral to an ethics team to review the decision making process and improve the parent's understanding. This may also help avoid court involvement in these cases.

Covert surveillance is another issue in cases of Factitious Disorder by Proxy, also known as Münchausen syndrome. This disorder occurs when a well-child is subjected to multiple medical procedures to find out what is wrong with the child when, in truth, the parent or guardian is making up a child's symptoms for medical attention. About 10% of the children die as a result of their parent's attempt to falsify their symptoms. Most perpetrators are careful about their deceitful activities and finding them in the act of falsification of symptoms is difficult. This may lead to planting cameras or using hidden mirrors to catch the parent in the act. There are two ethical sides to the use of covert spying. One side believes that the spying will lead to a loss of trust and set up a dishonest relationship between the parent and the provider (Fisher,

2011). The child is used as bait, which some believe is unacceptable and leads to the provider losing sight of their main responsibility of child protection. As the family is unlikely to do this in a hospital setting, this method is difficult to implement. On the other hand, if the parents are confronted openly about the problem and asked to participate in a recovery program, the relationship may be preserved.

APNs may have negative feelings about guardians who have abused their children. It is important to acknowledge those feelings if the APN is going to continue to work with the family. If the APN's feelings cannot be worked through, the care of the family should be transferred.

6.4.2.5. End of Life: Palliative Care

The most fundamental choice in care of the child with a terminal illness is when to discontinue treatment and allow the child to die (Freyer, 2004). One of the goals of palliative care is the relief of pain and suffering. There are clear guidelines for pediatric palliative care by a number of professional societies, including the AAP and the National Hospice Foundation (Friebert and Huff, 2009; Committee on Bioethics and Committee on Hospital Care, 2000). Despite this, the current estimate is that only 10 to 20 percent of dying children receive hospice services (Friebert and Huff, 2009; Committee on Bioethics and Committee on Hospital Care, 2000). There are four values that form the basis of palliative care for children (Mercurio, Forman *et al.*, 2008):

1. Pain and suffering is unacceptable and should be alleviated.
2. Pain and suffering include physical pain but have a psychological, emotional, and spiritual dimension.
3. Each child should be treated with respect.
4. The family of the pediatric patient is the responsibility of the primary care provider.

APNs, similar to other providers, may lack formal training in palliative care and may not have the knowledge base to set up high quality programs. Davies *et al.*'s 2006 study of 117 nurses and 81 physicians examined the barriers to palliative care in an academic children's hospital. The authors listed 26 barriers to primary care and the participants agreed that 12 of them occurred frequently or almost always. The most commonly perceived barrier is uncertain prognosis since in pediatrics there are a wide variety of uncommon diseases. The top five barriers after uncertain prognosis are family's inability to acknowledge incurable condition, language barriers, time constraints, family preference for more treatment, and staff shortages. Nurses pointed to the lack of a palliative care consultation team as a barrier to palliative care more than physicians and physicians felt that cultural differences were more of a barrier than nurses.

The provision of palliative care to children is a new area of pediatrics healthcare and there are many unknowns in caring for these patients. At present, pediatric palliative care teams are not available in every hospital. In a survey of 6 hospital- based palliative care teams done from January to March 2008, there were 515 new referrals made to the service (Feudtner *et al.*, 2010). The predominant conditions were genetic and congenital (40.8%). In contrast to adult palliative care, at the 12-month follow-up, only 30.3% of the cohort died. Those that died within 30 days of cohort entry had cancer or a terminal cardiovascular condition. This study reinforces the fact that pediatric patients referred to palliative care services have a wide variety of conditions with an unclear duration of survival. The APN working in palliative care must be clear with families that there are many unknowns about palliative care including time of death.

Pharmaceutical companies may not provide information about symptom- relieving medications, nor are there suitable formulations for pediatric patients (Committee on Bioethics and Committee on Hospital Care, 2000). Thus the APN must acknowledge that palliative care pain management may not relieve pain in a suitable way initially, but the APN should continue to work with the family to provide optimal treatment. The APN must also acknowledge that caring for a patient with a rare disease may require continued reassessment to provide optimal comfort care.

There are several pediatric palliative care programs available for APNs who wish to improve their care of terminally ill children. Table 6.5 is a list of curricula that are now available for APNs and other members of the healthcare team who want additional training in palliative care.

For the adolescent who is diagnosed with a terminal illness, the issues around decisions are more complex due to determination of decisional capacity. In the case of a dying adolescent who has been through multiple treatment regimes, maturity levels may be remarkable and patients should be granted their preferences on how they want to spend the rest of their life (Frey, 2004). Adolescents may deny their impending death and continue to act as though they will survive. Acceptance of this may take time and the APN must gently communicate the reality of their present illness (Frey, 2004). As with adults, adolescents should be allowed to determine the aspects of palliative care intervention

TABLE 6.5. Palliative Care Training.

Association/Name of Curriculum	Website
American Association of Colleges of Nursing ELNEC Core Curriculum	http://www.aacn.nche.edu/elnec/trainings/national#core
Initiative for Pediatric Palliative Care	http://www.ippcweb.org/curriculum.asp
National Hospice and Palliative Care Organization	http://www.nhpco.org/i4a/pages/index.cfm?pageID=5889
Center to Advance Palliative Care	http://www.capc.org/palliative-care-professional-development/clinical-site-visit-directory
American Academy of Hospice and Palliative Care	http://www.aahpm.org/certification/default/resources.html This is a physician website but it has good resources for learning more about palliative care.

which they desire (Committee on Bioethics and Committee on Hospital Care, 2000; Frey, 2004). The adolescent must understand the risks of all the treatment options, understand the medical information, make a voluntary choice, and comprehend the nature of the decision (King and Cross, 1989; Leikin, 1989). An adolescent's conception of death should be considered in order to allow him to make end of life decisions (Leikin, 1989).

A parent may oppose the disclosure of the adolescent's transition to a terminal illness. To avoid any problems, the provider should initiate a conversation about truthfulness about the diagnosis and prognosis with the family from the beginning. This will help reduce anxiety in the adolescent and foster a trusting relationship. Most parents understand the importance of truthfulness and good ethical practice. At times, the parent may not want the child to be told about the transition to palliative care. The APN must make sure that the parents know that if the child directly asks, the APN will be truthful. In these cases, having the family talk with a spiritual advisor may be helpful. Again, an ethics consult may be needed in difficult cases.

6.4.3. Adolescents

6.4.3.1. Issues in Reproductive Health

Ethical issues are frequent in adolescent healthcare centered on the right to confidential reproductive healthcare. In the past half-century, laws to give adolescent access to reproductive health care without parental consent have enabled adolescents to obtain confidential reproductive health care (Feierman *et al.*, 2002). The reason for expanded adolescent's rights in the past 30 years stems from the knowledge that some teens will not seek health care if their parents are required to be notified. Statutes known as "state minor consent laws" allow adolescents to seek treatment for sexually transmitted diseases, contraception, and reproductive issues without the consent of parents (English, 2007).

6.4.3.1.1. Disclosing Adolescents' Information to Parents/Guardians

Clinics with public funding may give adolescents access to confidential family planning services, contraception, and pregnancy-related care. Depending on the state, these laws also allow adolescents to consent for treatment for mental health and substance abuse treatments. APNs may treat adolescents for these issues without the consent of the parent depending on the state law. However, there are states where parent's rights have been infused into the right of adolescents to seek reproductive health care. In the case of abortion, in 37 states as of August 2012, at least one parent must be notified before an abortion can take place (Guttmacher Institute, 2012a). However, the Supreme Court ruled that parents cannot overturn the adolescent's right to an abortion, and in some states, the laws allow a judge to override parental notification if the adolescent can show maturity in health care decision making process.

Adolescents are allowed to consent to a variety of health care services such as sexual and reproductive health care, mental health care, and substance abuse treatment. Despite the advances in minors' rights, not all states allow adolescents to have access to the above services. Recent parental rights notifications now state that state consent laws apply to minors 12 and over or in some cases, only if they are married, pregnant, or already parents in order to consent (Guttmacher Institute, 2012b). In some states there is no case law and APNs may provide medical care if they feel the minor is mature. For example, 26 states and the district of Columbia allow minors to consent for contraceptive services; only 20 states limit which categories of minors can consent, and only 4 states have no law (Guttmacher Institute, 2012b).

When an adolescent is pregnant, only 37 states allow adolescents to seek health care without parental permission. There are 13 states where there are no explicit policies regarding providing care to adolescents. In

14 states, the APN can notify the parent of the adolescent's pregnancy if the APN feels it is in the best interest of the child (Guttmacher Institute, 2012c). In these 14 states, there is no requirement to notify the parent. Only North Dakota requires parental notification when providing care to adolescents in the second and third trimester of pregnancy. The APN must always consider what is in the best interest of the child. Depending on the state law, once the pregnancy ends, these adolescents may be considered minors again even though they are parents. It is the responsibility of the APN to know state law for adolescents. Some pregnant adolescents seek to become emancipated minors after their pregnancies. An emancipated minor has the right to consent to treatment regardless of the parent's wishes. The adolescent must follow the procedures required to obtain a certificate of emancipation for that state and the APN must actually see the certificate to provide routine medical care. For homeless adolescents, some states allow treatment without documentation.

The Guttmacher Institute website is an excellent current resource of information regarding adolescent healthcare and state laws. The ethical issues concern the importance of adolescent confidentiality. If the law requires reporting, then the APN must tell the patient the reason that they will notify parents.

Finally, in caring for adolescents for reproductive issues, parents may find out about the office or emergency room when they receive an insurance statement either via the Internet or by a paper statement. Adolescents must be informed that this may happen and there is no way of preventing the insurance company from issuing an explanation of benefits.

6.4.3.1.2. Sterilization of Minors with Developmental Disabilities

The issues around sterilization of minors with developmental disabilities are controversial due to the long history of abuse of sterilization of women in the United States (Mercurio, Adam *et al.*, 2008). In 1942, the Supreme Court declared human procreation was a fundamental right (Committee on Bioethics, 1999, reaffirmed 2006). This law made the sterilization of any individual more difficult and by the 1970s, there were several regulations that prevented federal programs from sterilizing individuals with developmental disabilities (Mercurio, Adam *et al.*, 2008). The surgical sterilization of the developmentally disabled remains controversial and there are significantly different laws from state to state (AAP Committee on Bioethics, 1999, reaffirmed 2006). The AAP encourages pediatricians to develop relationships with local agencies and legal resources to understand and sort through the complex information around state and federal law (Committee on Bioethics, 1999).

The argument against sterilization of developmentally disabled minors focuses on respecting the integrity of the body, risks of surgical sterilization, and avoidance of limitations on the child's development and decision-making (Goldman & Quint, 2011). Parents of developmentally disabled children may have hygiene, mood change, pregnancy, and sexual activity concerns. It is argued that sterilization does not change an adolescent's sexual desire and only changes the risk of pregnancy. Parents must understand that sterilization carries risks and the benefit of sterilization must be for clear medical indications. The family with a child with developmental disabilities should consider that sterilization will prevent pregnancy, but it will not prevent sexual abuse or exposure to sexually transmitted diseases. Ethical concerns about sterilization of adolescents with development disabilities focus on the right of the child not to be treated as an object, but as a human being with basic rights (Goldman and Quint, 2011).

The APN caring for these families should start the discussion about sexuality as the child enters puberty, exploring the concerns of the family and discussing contraception options to prevent pregnancy. Aside from the legal issues, there are religious beliefs that may interfere with presenting the pros and cons to parents. In cases where the APN cannot give unbiased care because of religious beliefs, transfer of care to another provider is imperative.

6.4.4. Issues Surrounding Social Media

Social media such as Facebook, Twitter, Linkedin, and internet searches of patients can be way of obtaining information about patients (Jent *et al.*, 2011). Social media is a way of developing and maintaining relationship across distances. However, depending on the privacy setting, significant personal information can be obtained via these sites. A preliminary study of 302 graduate students showed that 27% of providers sought information about their patients via social media sites (SMS) (Lehavot, Barnett and Powers, 2010). By exploring an adolescent's SMS posting, the APN may find herself in a unique dilemma, as the APN must decide what to do with the information that is obtained especially if the patient is posting information about self- or other-directed violence. If the APN fails to act, she may be liable for not acting on the posting information even though she may have believed that the posting was not truthful (Lenhart and Madden, 2012). The adolescent may also believe that an APN's searches are an invasion of privacy and this can disrupt the therapeutic nature of the relationship (Jent *et al.*, 2011).

Jent *et al.* (2011) reported a survey of 109 pediatric medical residents, interns, and medical students in South Florida who used medical vignettes to explain that they had visited the SMS of a patient and presented the subjects with options after reading the patient's personal posts. Both faculty and trainees reported that they felt SMS to be public information. However, the trainees were the only ones who reported going on to SMS for information. Although going onto a patient's website may be an ethical violation, this did not appear to influence health provider's decision-making to do so.

Given the exposure of the younger generation to technology and SMS, the APN must consider ethical guidelines before using SMS in clinical practice and obtain permission before seeking information about patients on their websites. Providers should not seek information about a patient from an Internet or SMS search. Using social media together with an adolescent, and with the parent permission, may be a more acceptable way of exploring information posted on a SMS with a provider.

6.4.5. Pediatric Subjects in a Research Study

The ethical principles of respect for persons, justice, and beneficence are important in pediatric as well as adult research. The application of these principles in pediatric research must be considered against a child's developmental level, family decision-making, and risk to the child. Institutional Review Boards (IRBs) involved in approving pediatric research protocols view children as a vulnerable population and therefore focus on maximizing safety in pediatric research protocols (Boss, 2010). Healthy children usually participate in research studies that involve no more than minimal risk unless it offers direct benefit to the child or it offers only minor increase over minimal risk (Boss, 2010). While the Institute of Medicine has tried to standardize minimal risk, each local IRB will view this differently and there is variability in the risk assessment of each IRB (Boss, 2010).

Informed consent of both the child and parent is important in pediatric research. When there is more than minimal risk, both parents may be required to sign the consent. In the AAP policy statement (1995), in order to obtain pediatric asset, the researcher must make sure that the child has an understanding of health and must have a clear explanation of the tests. The child should agree to the study without any coercion and should understand what participation in the study involves. Pediatric patients can benefit from research but maximizing pediatric safety in studies is important. Pediatric patients pose unique problems in all aspects of healthcare. The APN caring for children must consider their special ethical dilemmas and work with families to promote the best outcomes.

6.5. CASE STUDIES

1. The parents of a 32-week gestation age infant girl do not want intervention for the neonate. The child is otherwise well, but has respiratory problems and needs intervention. What is your approach to this problem?
2. A 39-year-old mother was recently diagnosed with breast cancer. She is BRA-2 gene and wants her 16 year old tested for the gene. The child does not want to be tested. How would you approach this issue? What are the ethical principles in this situation?
3. During a pertussis outbreak, there are five parents in your practice with young infants refusing the DTaP vaccine. What is your approach and why?
4. A mother of an 8 year old brings the child to your office for a well-child visit. The mother has refused vaccines and today tells you that if you want to give vaccines you will need to negotiate with the child. How do you approach this situation? What are the ethical dilemmas with vaccine refusal?
5. A 13 year old discloses that she is sexually active with her boyfriend. She is not using birth control but is using condoms consistently by her report. How do you approach this situation? What are the ethical and legal issues with reproductive healthcare for adolescents?
6. A fifteen-year old boy has a green penile discharge. He appears in the office without his parents. The clinic staff states he cannot be treated. What are the APN's responsibilities? How do you approach this situation? How would you educate the staff?
7. A 15 year old child with muscular dystrophy is developing increasing shortness of breath. He has previously expressed his desire to not have life support. The mother wants the child have a tracheostomy. What is the APN's response? What ethical dilemma does this cause?
8. A mother of a 19 year old who is mildly developmentally delayed is concerned about her daughter's interest in boys. What is the APN's response? Why?

6.6. REFERENCES

American Academy Pediatrics Committee on Bioethics. (1997). Religious objections to medical care. *Pediatrics, 99*: 279–281. doi: 10.1542/peds.99.2.279

American Academy Pediatrics Committee on Bioethics. (2001, reaffirmed in 2009). Ethical issues in genetic testing in pediatrics. *Pediatrics, 107*: 1451–1455. doi: 10.1542/peds.107.6.1451

American Academy of Pediatrics, Division of Health Policy Research. (2001). *Periodic Survey of Fellows No. 48: Immunization Administration Practices.* Elk Grove Village, IL: American Academy of Pediatrics.

American Academy of Pediatrics Committee on Fetus and Newborn. (2007). Non initiation or withdrawal of intensive care for high-risk newborns. *Pediatrics, 119*: 401–403. doi: 10.1542/peds.2006-3180

American College of Obstetricians and Gynecologists. (2005). Maternal decision making, ethics, and the law. Committee Opinion No. 321, Available at http://www.acog.org/~/media/Committee%20Opinions/Committee%20on%20Ethics/co321.pdf?dmc=1&ts=20120722T1602359868. Accessed July17, 2012.

American Society of Human Genetics (ASHG)/American College of Medical Genetics (ACMG). (1995). Points to consider: ethical, legal, and psychosocial implications of genetic testing in children and adolescents. *American Journal of Human Genetics, 57*: 1233–1241 Available at http://www.ncbi.nlm.nih.gov/pmc/articles/PMC1801355/?tool=pubmed retrieved July 12, 2012.

Angell, M.A. (1983). Handicapped children: Baby Doe and Uncle Sam. *New England Journal of Medicine, 309*(11): 659. Available at http://www.nejm.org/toc/nejm/309/11/

Annas, G.J. (1984). The case of Baby Jane Doe: Child abuse or unlawful federal intervention? *American Journal of Public Health, 74*(7): 727–729. doi: 10.2105/AJPH.74.7.727

Beuchamp, T.L. and Childress, J.F. (2001). *Principles of Biomedical Ethics* (5th edition). New York, NY: Oxford Press.

Betancourt, J.R., Green, A.R. and Carrillo, J.E. (2011). Cross-cultural care and communication. In: *UpToDate.* H.N. Sokol (Ed.). Available from http://www.uptodateonline.com.

Black, C. (2007, November 29). Boy dies of leukemia after refusing treatment for religious reasons. *Seattle Post-Intelligencer.* Available at http://seattlepi.nwsource.com/local/341458_leukemia29.html

Boom, J.A., and Healy, C.M. (2012). Standard childhood vaccines: Parental hesitancy or refusal. In: *UpToDate.* M.M. Torchia (Ed.). Available from http://www.uptodateonline.com.

Borry, P., Goffin, T., Nys, H. and Dierickx, K. (2008). Attitudes regarding predictive genetic testing in minors. A survey of the European Clinical Geneticists. *Journal of Medical Genetics, 34*(5): 370–374. doi:10.1136/jme.2007.021717

Borry, P., Evers-Kiebooms, G., Cornel, M.C., Clarke, A. and Dierickx, K. (2009). Genetic testing in asymptomatic minors: background considerations towards ESHG Recommendations. *European Journal of Human Genetics, 17*(6): 711–719. doi: 10.1038/ejhg.2009.25

Boss, R.D. (2010). Ethics for the pediatrician: pediatric research ethics: evolving principles and practices. *Pediatrics in Review, 31*(4): 163–165. doi: 10.1542/pir.31-4-163

Brody, H. (2012). From an ethics of rationing to an ethics of waste avoidance. *New England Journal of Medicine, 366*: 1949–1951. doi: doi:10.1056/NEJMp1203365

Butz, A.M., Redman, B.K., Fry, S.T. and Kolodner, K. (1998). Ethical conflicts experienced by certified pediatric nurse practitioners in ambulatory settings. *Journal of Pediatric Health Care, 12*(4): 183–190. Available at http://dx.doi.org/10.1016/S0891-5245(98)90044-X

Camosy, C.C. (2011). Ethics for the pediatrician: Just distribution of health-care resources and the neonatal ICU. *Pediatrics in Review, 32*(5): 204–207. doi: 10.1542/pir.32-5-204

Centers for Disease Control. (2012). Child Maltreatment Prevention. Retrieved August 3, 2012. Available at http://www.cdc.gov/violenceprevention/childmaltreatment/

Chambers, M. (November 13, 1983), Initiator of 'Baby Doe' case unshaken. *New York Times,* Retrieved from http://www.nytimes.com/1983/11/13/nyregion/initiator-of-baby-doe-case-unshaken.html

Committee on AIDS. (1999). Disclosure of illness status to children and adolescents with HIV infection. *Pediatrics, 103*: 104–106. Available at http://pediatrics.aappublications.org/content/103/1/164.full.pdf

Committee on Bioethics. (1995). Informed consent, parental permission, and assent in pediatric practice. *Pediatrics, 95*: 314–317. Available at http://aappolicy.aappublications.org/cgi/content/abstract/pediatrics%3b95/2/314. Reaffirmed 2006.

Committee on Bioethics. (1997). Religious objections to medical care. *Pediatrics, 99*(2): 279–281. doi: 10.1542/peds.99.2.279 Reaffirmed October 2006.

Committee on Bioethics. (1999). Sterilization of minors with developmental disabilities. *Pediatrics, 104*(2): 337–340.

Committee on Bioethics and Committee on Hospital Care. (2000). Palliative care for children. *Pediatrics, 106*(2): 351–357.

Cummings, C.L. and Mercurio, M.R. (2010). Ethics for the pediatrician: autonomy, beneficence, and rights. *Pediatrics in Review,* 31(6): 252–255. doi: 10.1542/pir.31-6-252

Davies, B., Sehring, S.A., Partridge, J.C., Cooper, B.A., Hughes, A., Philp, J.C. and Kramer, R.F. (2008). Barriers to palliative care for children: Perceptions of pediatric health care providers. *Pediatrics, 121*(2): 282–288. doi: 10.1542/peds.2006-3153

Diekema, D.S. and the Committee on Bioethics. (2005). Responding to parental refusals of immunization of children. *Pediatrics, 115*: 1428–1431. doi: 10.1542/peds.2005-0316

Duff, R.S. and Campbell, A.G.M. (1973). Moral and ethical dilemmas in the special care nursery. *New England Journal of Medicine, 289*: 890–894. doi: doi:10.1056/NEJM197310252891705

Eckler, P., Worsowicz, G.M. and Dowley, K. (2009). Improving physician-patient communication. In: *Health Communication in the New Media Landscape* (pp. 283–302). J.C. Parker and E. Thorson (Eds.). New York, NY: Springer Publishing Company.

English, A. (2007). Sexual and reproductive health care for adolescents: legal right and policy challenges. *Adolescent Medicine State of the Art Reviews, 18*(3): 571–581.

Feierman, J., Lieberman, D., Schissel, A., Diller, R., Kim, J. and Chu, Y. (2002). Health Care & the Law: A Guide to the law on Minor's Rights in New York State. New York Civil Liberties Union Reproductive Rights Project. Available at http://www.nyclu.org/files/thl.pdf

Feikin, D.R., Lezotte, D.C., Hamman, R.F., Salmon, D.A., Chen, R.T. and Hoffman, R.E. (2000). Individual and community risks of measles and pertussis associated with personal exemptions to immunizations. *Journal of the American Medical Association, 284*: 3145–3150. doi: 10.1001/jama.284.24.3145

Feudtner, C., Kang, T.I., Hexem, K.R., Friedrichsdorf, S.J., Osenga, K., Siden, H. and Wolfe, J. (2011). *Pediatric palliative care patients: a prospective multicenter cohort study. Pediatrics, 127*(6): 1094–1101. doi: 10.1542/peds.2010-3225

Feudtner, C., & Marcuse, E. K. (2001). Ethics and immunization policy: promoting dialogue to sustain consensus. *Pediatrics, 107*, 1158–1164. doi: 10.1542/peds.107.5.1158

Fisher, M. A. (2011). Ethics for the pediatrician: caring for abused children. *Pediatrics in Review, 32*(7): e73-78. doi: 10.1542/pir.32-7-e73

Frey, D. R. (2004). Care of the dying adolescent: special considerations. *Pediatrics, 113*(2): 381–388. doi: 10.1542/peds.113.2.381

Friebert, S. and Huff, S. (2009). NHPCO's pediatric standards: A key step in advancing care for America's children. *NewsLine,* 9–13. Available at http://www.nhpco.org/files/public/chipps/Peds-Standards_article_NL-0209.pdf

Galowitz, P. (2012) Doctors: Limiting Medicaid prescriptions adds risk. *USA Today*. Available at http://www.usatoday.com/news/nation/story/2012-07-22/medicaid-prescription-limits/56464896/1

Gardner, M. and Steinberg, L. (2005). Peer influence on risk taking, risk preference, and risky decision making in adolescence and adulthood: An experimental study. *Developmental Psychology, 41*: 625–635. doi:10:1037/00012-1649.41.4.6625

Gilmour, J., Harrison, C., Asadi, L., Cohen, M.H. and Vohra, S. (2011). Childhood immunization: when physicians and parents disagree. *Pediatrics, 128* Suppl 4: S167–174. doi: 10.1542/peds.2010-2720E

Gladsjo, J.A., Breding, J., Sine, D., Wells, R., Kalemkiarian, S., Oak, J. and Friedlander, S.F. (2004). Termination of life support after severe child abuse: the role of a guardian ad litem. *Pediatrics, 113*(2): e141–145. doi: 10.1542/peds.113.2.e141

Goldman, E.B. and Quint, E.H. (2011). Arguments against sterilization of developmentally disabled minors. *Journal of Child Neurology, 26*(5): 654–656. doi: 10:1177/0883073811402077

Gonzales, J.L. (2011). Ethics for the pediatrician: genetic testing and newborn screening. *Pediatrics in Review, 32*(11): 490–493. doi: 10.1542/pir.32-11-490

Gust, D.A., Darling, N., Kennedy, A. and Schwartz, B. (2008). Parents with doubts about vaccines: which vaccines and reasons why. *Pediatrics, 122*: 718–725. doi: 10.1542/peds.2007-0538

Guttmacher Institute. (2012a). State Policies in Brief: Parental Involvement in Minors' Abortion. Available at http://www.guttmacher.org/statecenter/spibs/spib_PIMA.pdf

Guttmacher Institute. (2012b). State Policies in Brief: An Overview of Minors Consent law. Available at http://www.guttmacher.org/statecenter/spibs/spib_OMCL.pdf

Guttmacher Institute. (2012c). State Policies in Brief: Minors Access to Prenatal Care. Available at http://www.guttmacher.org/statecenter/spibs/spib_MAPC.pdf

Halperin, S.A. (2000). How to manage parents unsure about immunizations. *Canadian Journal of CME 2000, 12*: 62–75. Available at http://resources.cpha.ca/CCIAP/data/45e.pdf.

Hentschel, R., Lindner, K., Krueger, M. and Reiter-Theil, S. (2006). Restriction of ongoing intensive care in neonates: A prospective study. *Pediatrics, 118*: 563–569. doi: 10.1542/peds.2005-1615

Hussain, H., Omer, S.B., Manganello, J.A., Kromm, E.E., Carter, T.C., Kan, L. and Salmon, D.A. (2011). Immunization safety in US print media, 1995–2005. *Pediatrics, 127*: S100-S106. doi:10.1542/peds.2010-1722O

Hayeems, R.Z., Bytautas, J.P. and Miller, F.A. (2008). A systematic review of the effects of disclosing carrier results generated through newborn screening. *Journal of Genetic Counselor, 17*(6): 538–549. doi: 10.1007/s10897-008-9180-1

Hazen, E., Schlozman, S. and Beresin, E. (2008). Adolescent psychological development: A review. Pediatrics in Review, 29(5): 161–169. doi: 10.1542/pir.29-5-161

Howell, S. (2007). Pediatric palliative care. *Pediatrics, 120*(1) : 244–245. doi: 10.1542/peds.2007-0711

Janvier, A., Bauer, K.L., & Lantos, J.D. (2007). Are newborns morally different from older children? *Theoretical Medicine and Bioethics, 28*: 413–425. doi: 10.1007/s11017-00709052-y

Jent, J.G., Eaton, C.K., Merrick, M.T., Englebert, N., Dandes, S., Chaptman, A.V. and Hershorin, E.R. (2011). The decision to access patient information from a social media site: what would you do? *Journal of Adolescent Health, 49*(4): 414–420. http://dx.doi.org/10.1016/j.adohealth.2011.02.004

John, R. (2007). Beneficence, prescriptions, and the nurse practitioner. *Advance for Nurse Practitioner, 15*: 55–57.

Kaempf, J.W., Tomlinson, M.W., Campbell, B., Ferguson, L. and Stewart, V.T. (2009). Counseling pregnant women who may deliver extremely premature infants: medical care guidelines, family choices, and neonatal outcomes. *Pediatrics, 123*(6): 1509–1515. doi: 10.1542/peds.2008-2215

Kennedy, A., Basket, M. and Sheedy, K. (2011). Vaccine attitudes, concerns, and information sources reported by parents of young children: results from the 2009 HealthStyles survey. *Pediatrics, 127*: S92–S99. doi:10.1542/peds.2010-1722N

King, N.M. and Cross, A.W. (1989). Children as decision makers; guidelines for pediatricians. *Journal of Pediatrics, 115*: 10–16.

Kipnis, K. (2007). Harm and uncertainty in newborn intensive care. *Theoretical Medicine and Bioethics, 28*: 393–412. doi: 10.1007/s1107-007-9051-z

Kopelman, L. M. (2007). The Best Interest Standards for incompetent or incapacitated persons of all ages. *The Journal of Law, Medicine and Ethics, 35*(1): 187–196. doi: 10.1111/j.1748-720X.2007.00123.x

Kopelman, L.M., Irons, T.G. and Kopelman, A.E. (1988). Neonatologists judge the 'Baby doe' regulations. *The New England Journal of Medicine, 318*: 677–683. doi:10.1056/NEJM198803173181105

Kopelman, L. and Kopelman, A. (2007). Using a new analysis of the Best Interest Standard to address cultural disputes: whose data, which values? *Theoretical Medicine and Bioethics, 28*: 373–391. doi: 10.1007/s11017-9050-0

Kulkarni, R., Scott-Emuakpor, A.B., Brody, H., Weil, W.B., Ragni, M.V. and Gera, R. (2001). Nondisclosure of human immunodeficiency virus and hepatitis C virus coinfection in a patient with hemophilia: medical and ethical considerations. *Journal of Pediatric Hematology and Oncology, 23*(3): 153–158.

Ladd, R.E. and Forman, E.N. (2010). Ethics for the pediatrician: pediatrician/patient/parent relationships. *Pediatrics in Review, 31*(9): e65-67. doi: 10.1542/pir.31-9-e65

Lenhart, A. and Madden, M. (2007). Social networking site and teens, Pew Internet and American Life Projects. Available at http://www.pewinternet.org/Reports/2007/Social-Networking-Websites-and-Teens.aspx. Accessed July 20, 2012.

Lehavot, K., Barnett, J. E., & Powers, D. (2010). Psychotherapy, professional relationships, and ethical considerations in the myspace generation. *Professional Psychology: Research and Practice, 41*(2): 160–166. doi:10.1037/a0018709

Leikin, S. (1989). A proposal concerning decisions to forego life sustaining treatment for young people. *Journal of Pediatrics, 115*: 17–22.

Mercurio, M.R. (2010). Ethics for the pediatrician: imperiled newborns: limiting treatment. *Pediatrics in Review, 31*(2): 72–75. doi: 10.1542/pir.31-2-72

Mercurio, M.R., Adam, M.B., Forman, E.N., Ladd, R.E., Ross, L.F. and Silber, T.J. (2008). American Academy of Pediatrics policy statements on bioethics: summaries and commentaries: part 1. *Pediatrics in Review, 29*(1): e1-8. doi: 10.1542/pir.29-1-e1

Mercurio, M.R., Forman, E.N., Ladd, R.E., Maxwell, M.A., Ross, L.F. and Silber, T.J. (2008). American Academy of Pediatrics policy statements on bioethics: summaries and commentaries: part 3. *Pediatrics in Review, 29*(5): e28-34. doi: 10.1542/pir.29-5-e28

Mercurio, M.R., Maxwell, M.A., Mears, B.J., Ross, L.F. and Silber, T.J. (2008). American Academy of Pediatrics policy statements on bioethics: summaries and commentaries: part 2. *Pediatrics in Review, 29*(3): e15-22. doi: 10.1542/pir.29-3-e15

Moon, M., Taylor, H.A., McDonald, E.L., Hughes, M.T. and Carrese, J.A. (2009). Everyday ethics issues in the outpatient clinical practice of pediatric residents. *Archives of Pediatric and Adolescent Medicine, 163*(9): 838–843. doi:10.1001/archpediatrics.2009.139

Morahan-Martin, J.M. (2004). How Internet users find, evaluate, and use online health information: a cross-cultural review. *CyberPsychology & Behavior, 7*(5): 497–510. doi:10.1089/cpb.2004.7.497

National Conference of State Legislators. (2012). States with Religious and Philosophical Exemptions from School Immunization Requirements. Available at http://www.ncsl.org/issues-research/health/school-immunization-exemption-state-laws.aspx Retrieved on July 22, 2012.

National Newborn Screening and Genetic Resource Center. (2012). National Newborn Screening Status Report: Updated 7/1/2012. Available at: http://genes-r-us.uthscsa.edu/sites/genes-r-us/files/nbsdisorders.pdf. Retrieved July 22, 2012.

Okun, A. (2010). Ethics for the pediatrician: Children who have special health-care needs: ethical issues. *Pediatrics in Review, 31*(12): 514–517. doi: 10.1542/pir.31-12-514

Omer, S.B., Salmon, D.A., Orenstein, W.A., deHart, M.P. and Halsey, N. (2009). Vaccine refusal, mandatory immunization, and the risks of vaccine-preventable diseases. *New England Journal of Medicine, 360*(19): 1981–1988. doi: doi:10.1056/NEJMsa0806477

Orenstein, W.A. and Hinman, A.R. (1999). The immunization system in the United States—the role of school immunization law. *Vaccine, 17* (suppl 3): S19–24.

Paris, J.J. (2005). What standards apply to perinatology at the borderline of gestational age? *Journal of Perinatology, 25*: 683–684. doi:10.1038/sj.jp.7211401

Paris, J.J., Schreiber, M.D. and Moreland, M. (2007). Parental refusal of medical treatment for a newborn. *Theoretical Medicine and Bioethics, 28*: 427–442. Doi: 10.1007/s11017-007-9046-9

Paul, D. (2008). Patient advocacy in newborn screening: continuities and discontinuities. *American Journal of Medical Genetics Part C* (Seminars in Medical Genetics, 148C: 8–14. Doi 10.1002/ajmg.c.30166

Pineda, D. and Myers, M.G. (2011). Finding reliable information about vaccines. *Pediatrics, 127*: S134–S137. doi:10.1542/peds.2010-1722T

Pless, J. (1983). The story of baby doe. *The New England Journal of Medicine, 309*: 664.

Roberts, E. (1992). Refusal of treatment by 16–year-old. *The Lancet, 340*(8811): 108–109. doi: 10.1016/0140-6736(92)90417-2

Ross, L.F. (1998). *Children, Families and Health Care Decision Making.* Oxford, UK: Clarendon Press.

Ross, L.F. (2007). The moral status of the newborn and its implications. *Theoretical Medicine and Bioethics, 28*: 349–355. doi: 10.1007/s11017-007-9045x

Ross, L.F. (2008). Ethical and policy issues in pediatric genetics. *American Journal of Medical Genetics C Seminars in Medical Genetics, 148C*(1): 1–7. doi: 10.1002/ajmg.c.30162

Ross, L.F. (2009). Against the tide: arguments against respecting a minor's refusal of efficacious life-saving treatment. *Cambridge Quarterly of Healthcare Ethics, 18*(3): 302–315. doi: 10.1017/s0963180109090471

Ross, L.F. (2010). Forty years later: the scope of bioethics revisited. *Perspectives of Biological Medicine, 53*(3): 452–457. doi: 10.1353/pbm.0.0170

Ross, L.F. and Clayton, E.W. (2009). Clinical and ethical considerations in managing carrier detection. *American Journal of Public Health, 99*(8): 1348–1349. doi: 10.2105/ajph.2009.161554

Ross, L.F. and Frader, J. (2009). Hypoplastic Left Heart Syndrome: A Paradigm Case for examining conscientious objection in pediatric practice. *The Journal of Pediatrics, 155*(1): 12–15. doi:10.1016/j.jpeds.2009.03.008

Salmon, D.A., Haber, M., Gangarosa, E.J. Phillips, L., Smith, N.J., Chen R.T. (1999). Health consequences of religious and philosophical exemptions from immunization laws; individual and societal risk of measles. *Journal of the American Medical Association, 282*(1): 47–53. doi: 10.1001/jama.282.1.47

Shaw, A.J., Randolph, J. and Maynard, B. (1977). Ethical issues in pediatric surgery: a national survey of pediatricians and pediatric surgeons. *Pediatrics, 60*: 588–593.

Simpson, E. (2007, March). Kaine signs 'Abraham's law' bill on choice to refuse treatment. The Virginia Pilot. Available at http://hamptonroads.com/node/240161

Sklansky, M. (2001). Neonatal euthanasia: moral considerations and criminal liability. *Journal of Medical Ethics, 27*(1): 5–11. doi: 10.1136/jme.27.1.5

Solomon, M.Z., Sellers, D.E., Heller, K.S., Dokken, D.L., Levetown, M., Rushton, C. and Fleischman, A.R. (2005). New and lingering controversies in pediatric end-of-life care. *Pediatrics, 116*(4): 872–883. doi: 10.1542/peds.2004-0905

Spencer, G.E. (2000). Children's competency to consent: an ethical dilemma. *J Child Health Care, 4*(3): 117–122. doi: 0.1177/136749350000400305

Stokley, S., Stanwych, C., Avey, B. and Greby, S. (2011). Vaccination coverage among children in kindergarten—United States 2009–2010. *Morbidity and Mortality Weekly Review, 60*(21): 700–704.

Stotland, Nada L. (2007) Religion, conscience, and controversial clinical practices. *New England Journal of Medicine, 356*(18): 1889–1892. doi:10.1056/NEJMc070628

Swota, A.H. and Hester, D.M. (2011). Ethics for the pediatrician: providing culturally effective health care. *Pediatrics in Review, 32*(3): e39–43. doi: 10.1542/pir.32-3-e39

Talati, E.D., Lang, C.W. and Ross, L.F. (2010). Reactions of pediatricians to refusals of medical treatment for minors. *Journal of Adolescent Health, 47*(2): 126–132. doi: 10.1016/j.jadohealth.2010.03.004

Tarini, B.A., Burke, W., Scott, C.R. and Wilfond, B.S. (2008). Waiving informed consent in newborn screening research: Balancing social value and respect. *American Journal of Medical Genetics Part C: Seminars in Medical Genetics, 148C*: 23–30. doi 10.1002/ajmg.c.30164

Todres, I.D., Krane, D., Howell, M.C. and Shannon, D.C. (1977). Pediatricians' attitudes affecting decision-making in defective newborns. *Pediatrics, 60*: 197–202.

Townsend, S.F. (2012). Ethics for the pediatrician: obstetric conflict: when fetal and maternal interests are at odds. *Pediatrics in Review, 33*(1): 33–37. doi: 10.1542/pir.33-1–33

Turner, H.N. (2010). Parental preference or child well-being: an ethical dilemma. *J Pediatric Nursing, 25*(1): 58–63. doi: 10.1016/j.pedn.2009.04.007

Van der heide, A., van der Mass, P.J., van der Wal, G., de Graaff, C.L., Kester, J.G., Kollee, L.A. and Holl, R.A. (1997)Medical end-of-life decisions made for neonates and infants in the Netherlands. *Lancet, 250*: 251–255. doi:10.1016/S0140-6736(97)02315-5

Vannice, K.S., Salmon, D.A., Shui, I., Omer, S.B., Kissner, J., Edwards, K.M., and Gust, D.A. (2011). Attitudes and beliefs of parents concerned about vaccines: impact of timing of immunization information. *Pediatrics, 127*: S120–S126. doi:10.1542/peds.2010-1722R

Wells, K. and John, R. (2002). Culturally sensitive case study: A newborn with Down Syndrome. Newborn and Infant Nursing reviews, 2(4): 207–213. http://dx.doi.org/10.1053/nbin.2002.36081

CHAPTER 7

Ethics and Women's Health

CAROLINE M. HEWITT

Proponents of comprehensive women's reproductive health believe in a woman's decision to have a safe and satisfying sexual life including safe motherhood, access to diagnosis and treatment of sexually transmitted infections, management of reproductive tract malignancies, and protection against gender discrimination, gender inequity and inequality. Women—more specifically, their potential for reproduction—are often at the center of an ethical and political maelstrom. It is therefore important to understand the significance of the ongoing domestic and global debates surrounding women's reproductive rights (or lack thereof). This chapter will discuss two prevailing ethical approaches supporting women's right to reproductive health: Feminist Bioethics and Public Health Ethics. Also discussed will be the current United States legislative climate concerning women's reproductive rights and freedoms. Case studies will be presented at the end of the chapter applying both principles of feminist bioethics and public health ethics within our current health care environment.

7.1. FEMINIST BIOETHICS

Thomas Beauchamp and James Childress developed their influential approach to bioethics based upon the application of four general moral principles particular to ethical problems: autonomy, justice, nonmaleficence and beneficence (Beauchamp and Childress, 2009; Dodds, 2000). Despite Beauchamp and Childress's insistence that all four principles have a role to play in bioethics, some philosophers have argued that autonomy has become "the first among equals" (Beauchamp and Childress, 2009, p. 216). To quote from Beauchamp and Childress, regarding their definition of autonomy:

> *Autonomy is to be understood as 'personal rule of the self that is free from both controlling interferences by others and from personal limitations that prevent meaningful choice, such as inadequate understanding'. The principle of respect for autonomy requires respecting those choices made by individuals whose decisions are free from external interference or personal limitations (2009, p. 99).*

From a feminist perspective, the definition of autonomy provided by Beauchamp and Childress, with its emphasis on informed consent, is narrow and does not fully reflect women's experiences. For Dodds (2000), the notion of informed consent—within the paternalistic society in which we live and given the cultural association between "femininity" and "irrationality"—may actually limit women's autonomy. Feminist bioethics, therefore, is an attempt to reshape the 'conceptual terrain' on which women, and others subject to oppressive social conditions, are expected to make health care decisions; it is a discipline focused on identifying those features of healthcare that exacerbate, or ameliorate, oppression (Dodds, 2000). Feminist philosopher Susan Sherwin argues that feminist bioethics must be understood as an ethics of the oppressed:

> *"Feminists share a recognition that women are oppressed in our society and understanding that their oppression takes many different forms, compounded often by other forms of oppression based on features such as race, ethnicity, sexual orientation, and economic class. Because feminists believe that oppression is objectionable on both moral and political grounds, most are committed to transforming society in ways that will ensure the elimination of oppression in all its forms." (Sherwin, 1992, p. 48).*

7.1.1. Personhood

Control over a woman's reproductive life is an issue of concern in both feminist and public health bioethics. Whether about women's autonomy or welfare of a larger society, reproductive choices like abortion or the use of contraception continue to be debated nationally and internationally. Feminist bioethics is concerned with identifying and ameliorating features of health care which exacerbate oppression. The current United States abortion debate pits the rights of women against the rights of the fetus, also known as autonomy versus the moral rights of the fetus (Gibson, 2004). The essential conflict revolves around the disagreement over the moral status (personhood) of the fetus. According to Gibson (2004), there are three basic positions regarding the moral status of the fetus: conservative, moderate and liberal. The conservative view is that the fetus has a right to life from the moment of conception; the more moderate view is that the fetus comes into the possession of the right to life at some stage during pregnancy and the liberal view is that the fetus does not, at any stage of gestation, have a right to life. The abortion debate, therefore, is not so much over women's rights, but rather over the moral status of the fetus (Gibson, 2004).

Gibson (2004) goes on to suggest that the argument over fetal moral status rests on the concept of personhood, yet this very concept is essentially contested. As described by the three positions regarding the definition of fetal moral status, there is ongoing debate over the definition of personhood. When disagreement exists over the proper use of a concept or when no exemplar exists—and this concept is fundamental to the abortion debate—then, Gibson argues, this debate is irresolvable (2004).

7.1.2. Moral Absolutists

For those who approach the definition of the concept of personhood from a conservative position (commonly referred to as pro-life or anti-choice), fetal life begins at conception, and there is little ambiguity in the abortion debate. Taking a deontological approach to ethics—that is, an ethics consisting of duty and moral obligation—abortion is wrong. This conservative position is fundamentally deontological in its reliance on a single moral rule: do not kill. This is in opposition to teleological ethics which acknowledges more subtlety in the gradations between right and wrong. In other words, deontological ethics are concerned with determining the rightness or wrongness of actions, while teleological ethics are concerned with determining the goodness or badness of actions (Lake, 1985). In teleological ethics, actions themselves assume their distinctively moral character by virtue of their adherence to the rules. For these moral absolutists, circumstances have no bearing on the morality of abortion, including in cases of endangerment of a mother's life or rape. In all cases, abortion is intrinsically wrong by virtue of its violation of the moral rule against killing for a moral absolutist (Lake, 1985).

7.1.3. Relational Autonomy

The difference between non-feminist and feminist approaches to abortion lie in the relative attention each gives in its analysis of the interests and experiences of women. Feminist analysis regards the effects of unwanted pregnancies on the lives of women individually and collectively as a central element in the moral examination of abortion. Women must be regarded as full moral agents, responsible for making moral decisions about their own pregnancies (Sherwin, 1992). However, the moral status of the fetus needs to be considered as well. As described by Gibson (2004), this 'relational' conception of moral status views the mother and fetus not as two independent beings whose moral claims have to be balanced against one another, but rather focuses on the relationship between the fetus and mother. The moral status of the fetus is unique because a fetus exists only in relationship with a particular other on whom it is entirely dependent for existence. It is because of this relationship that the fetus is morally significant, as it is out of relationships that our moral obligations arise. However, fetuses do not have an absolute value because they have no existence independent of this relationship. Their value is that not of an individual human being, but of a human relationship. Personhood is understood in terms of social relations; for Sherwin, humans are fundamentally relational beings. The self is relational in that each of us develops as a person through our relationships with others. It is the variety of relationships and roles in which a human being participates in their membership of a community that gives them their value as persons (Sherwin, 1992). For feminists, therefore, personhood is understood in terms of social relationships; personhood is our capacity to participate in a variety of relationships. This feminist definition of autonomy is a re-working, rather than a rejection, of the Kantian ethics. Autonomy is viewed as something that resides in the individual self. But as the self is constituted and re-constituted within a network of relationships, so too is the capacity for autonomy (Gibson, 2004).

7.2. PUBLIC HEALTH ETHICS

Bioethics evolved around key principals of respect for persons—including the autonomy of persons capable of self-determination and protection of those who are incapable—the duty to do good (beneficence) and to do no harm (non-malfeasance) and justice. Public health ethics can be regarded as "macro" beneficence (Dickens and Cook, 2007). Whereas bioethics is concerned with protecting the rights of the individual through informed consent, in public health consent comes from legislated authority or from governmental mandates to protect populations from harm (Dickens and Cook, 2007). Utilitarianism is generally the moral theory most often applied to matters of public health. Utilitarianism is the moral theory concerned with the consequences of actions; the good consequence being that which most positively affects the greatest number of people. Utilitarians value well-being and accept only one principle of ethics: the principle of utility, the good to be maximized (Beauchamp and Childress, 2009). Hedonistic Utilitarians, such as Jeremy Bentham and John Stuart Mill, view utility entirely in terms of happiness or pleasure. More recent utilitarian philosophers argue that values other than happiness— knowledge, health, success, and enjoyment, for example—also contribute to well-being. This principle has been translated into the formula of doing the greatest good for the greatest number, and therefore has obvious applicability in public health policy and service (Beauchamp and Childress, 2009).

Utilitarians disagree whether the principle of utility pertains to particular acts in particular circumstances or to general rules that themselves determine which acts are right and wrong (Beauchamp and Childress, 2009). For 'Act' Utilitarians, the consequence of an act must first be considered. That action which results in the greatest good must be the action chosen. 'Rule' Utilitarians, on the other hand, first look to ethical rules which then direct the action to be taken.

7.2.1. Reproductive Health

Global unity concerning the urgency of improving women's reproductive health and rights is reflected in the historic 1994 International Conference on Population and Development (ICPD) held in Cairo, Egypt; confirmation about the fundamental rights of women and men was later made at the 1995 International Conference on Women in Beijing, China (Townsend, 2007). Both of these conferences recognized that reproductive health failures embodied in unsafe childbearing involve more than just clinical medicine and must also be addressed as public health concerns (Cook and Dickens, 2002).

Generally, reproductive health implies that people are able to have a satisfying and safe sex life, the capacity to reproduce, and the freedom to decide, if, and when, and how often to do so. This concept of reproductive health offers a comprehensive and integrated approach to health needs related to reproduction. It places women at the center of the process, and recognizes, respects and responds to the needs of all women, not only those of mothers. The 1988 World Health Organization (WHO) definition of reproductive health was adopted and expanded at the ICPD and International Conference on Women. It reads:

> *"Reproductive health is a state of complete physical, mental and social well-being and not merely the absence of disease or infirmity, in all mat-*

ters relating to the reproductive system and to its functions and processes. Reproductive health therefore implies that people are able to have a satisfying and safe sex life and that they have the capacity to reproduce and the freedom to decide if, when and how often to do so. Implicit in this last condition are the right of men and women to be informed and to have access to safe, effective, affordable and acceptable methods of family planning of their choice for regulation of fertility which are not against the law, and the right of access to appropriate health-care services that will enable women to go safely through pregnancy and childbirth and provide couples with the best chance of having a healthy infant." (UN, 1995)

Within this context, reproductive health care is defined as the constellation of methods, techniques and services that contribute to reproductive health and well-being by preventing and solving reproductive health problems. It also includes sexual health, the purpose of which is the enhancement of life and personal relations, and not merely counseling care related to reproduction and sexually transmitted diseases (Cook, Dickens and Fathalia, 2008).

7.2.2. Safe Motherhood

A major burden for females is related to their reproductive function and reproductive potential. Reproduction is not a disease (Cook, Dickens and Fathalia, 2008). A list of reproductive health indicators is as follows:

- Safe motherhood
- Fertility by choice (contraception, abortion)
- Sexually transmitted infections
- Female genital cutting (circumcision/mutilation)
- Infertility
- Cancers of the Reproductive Tract

The differential incidence of unsafe motherhood has been described as making the greatest discrepancy in any health statistic between developed and developing countries worldwide (Cook and Dickens, 2002). It is estimated that every year worldwide, about 515,000 women die of complications of pregnancy and childbirth. Furthermore, at least 7 million women suffer serious health problems after childbirth, and an additional estimated 50 million women suffer adverse health effects after childbirth (Cook and Dickens, 2002). To put these figures in context of developed and developing countries, the risk of pregnancy-related death for a Canadian woman is 1 in 8,700 compared to that of a woman in Rwanda which is 1 in 6 (Cook and Dickens, 2002). Safe motherhood depends on women's avoidance of untimely and otherwise inappropriate pregnancy.

Unsafe or otherwise unwanted pregnancies may result in unsafe abortions, either because abortion is not legally and safely available or, if legally available, there are no qualified practitioners to provide it; these situations raise obvious ethical concerns. The above-cited 1994 and 1995 watershed conferences both addressed the public health implications of unsafe abortion. The 1994 Cairo ICPD resolved "to strengthen their commitment to women's health to deal with the health impact of unsafe abortion as a major public health concern and to reduce the recourse to abortion through expanded and improved family planning services" (Cook and Dickens, 2002). The 1995 Beijing Conference developed a platform for action which resolved, "unsafe abortions threaten the lives of a large number of women, representing a grave public health problem as it is primarily the poorest and the youngest who take the highest risk" (Cook and Dickens, 2002).

7.3. CASE STUDIES

Two prevailing ethical approaches, feminist bioethics and public health ethics, recognize the centrality of women's experiences. There exist overlap in themes and interests between feminist bioethics and public health ethics, specifically that of the experience of the disenfranchised, which includes feelings of powerlessness and repression. Feminist and reproductive health advocates support and echo each other's concerns and approaches and similar ethical principles are argued from both perspectives. However, for purposes of academic purity, the following case studies will be presented from a feminist bioethical approach separately from public health (utilitarian) approaches.

7.3.1. Personhood and Partial Molar Pregnancy

Catherine, a 36 year old biochemist, and devout Roman Catholic, was thrilled to learn she was pregnant with her second child. She and her husband had been trying to get pregnant for the last six months. However, the couple was devastated to learn at the initial prenatal visit and sonogram, that this pregnancy was considered a "partial molar" and the viability of the fetus uncertain. Incidence of spontaneous abortion is high, and the likelihood of the birth of a viable fetus is very low. Partial molar pregnancies increase the risks of maternal preeclampsia, hypertension, hyperemesis and hyperthyroidism (Chiang and Berek, 2010). Catherine is faced with an ethical dilemma: who has a greater moral status, mother or fetus? Should Catherine proceed with an abortion or proceed with the pregnancy despite the risks to her own health and the very low likelihood of a viable infant? Catherine believes fully with the conservative view of personhood; that is, Catherine believes that life begins at the moment of conception. Even faced with the low likelihood that this fetus will be viable, for Catherine, conception has occurred and life exists; therefore, to do anything to interfere with this pregnancy is paramount to murder. Catherine views herself as a faithful Catholic who will do all in her power to follow the teachings of the Church. For Catherine, to follow the rules of the Church is more important than any circumstances which may interfere with this moral absolutism, even the potential for her own mortality.

Catherine's husband, Bob, however, does not share Catherine's moral absolutism. Bob is a feminist. Bob believes that personhood can only be understood in terms of social relationships. Since Catherine's fetus is only a fetus, and therefore unable to engage in any relationship other than the one with Catherine, and Catherine is an adult fully capable in engaging in many complex relationships, Catherine, therefore, holds a greater moral status than her fetus. Like Catherine, Bob understands the low likelihood that the pregnancy will ultimately progress to a viable infant, and he too understands the health risks for Catherine should she continue with the pregnancy. Bob reasons that Catherine holds a greater moral status than the fetus and therefore it is Catherine's right to exercise her own autonomy, and within a feminist bioethical framework, it is ethical for Catherine to choose to terminate her pregnancy. Bob further reasons that because Catherine is a full moral agent, responsible for making moral decisions about her own pregnancy, should she decide to continue with the pregnancy, based upon her own moral reasoning, then that is her own right.

What ethical principles are involved? How would you as a provider help them with a decision? What are your legal and ethical responsibilities to the patient? The fetus? The father?

7.3.2. Utility in Family Planning

Maria is a nurse practitioner working in a county health department's family planning clinic. She has just walked into an exam room to be greeted by a very nervous 16 year old female who wants contraception. The client reports being sexually active for six months with one partner and is using condoms inconsistently for contraception. Maria has an ethical dilemma: should she perform her "typical" new patient gynecologic exam (which includes a pelvic exam, pap smear and collection of cervical cultures for screening of sexually transmitted diseases) or follow the updated practice guidelines which negate the need to perform the above mentioned test in the traditional manner? Needing some context through which to think through this dilemma, Maria decides to apply the moral theory of Utilitarianism to help guide her practice.

Utilitarians themselves disagree whether the principal of utility pertains to particular acts in particular circumstances or to general rules that themselves determine which acts are right and wrong (Beauchamp and Childress, 2009). For Act Utilitarians, the consequence of an act must first be considered. That action which results in the greatest good must therefore be the action chosen. Rule utilitarians, on the other hand, first look to ethical rules which then direct the action to be taken. Maria needs to consider each type of utilitarianism within the context of her dilemma. Would following one or the other type of utilitarianism lead to a different outcome or a similar outcome?

7.3.3. Act Utilitarianism

"What would be the consequence of not performing the traditional exam", asks Maria, "which action would lead to the greatest happiness or well-being for the greatest number"? The most obvious and most directly experienced happiness would be enjoyed by the client. Maria imagines the client would be relieved she did not have to endure this uncomfortable, invasive and extremely embarrassing examination. Another positive outcome would be economic. From a bioethical utilitarian perspective, not performing the exam would more efficiently allocate limited healthcare resources: time and supplies. By not having to perform the exam, Maria would be spending less time with this client visit and thus have more time to attend to the 10 clients waiting to be seen. In terms of other resources, by not using the liquid-based pap now, it would be available for another client, for whom the pap test is indicated (according to national guidelines). The cost to the state laboratory would also be less. This is one less test to be run and interpreted both by the technician and pathologist. Lastly, supplies required to perform the pap would not be used; neither disposable speculum supplies nor the staff time and energy required to clean and sterilize the equipment would be required.

In addition to the two positive consequences of following the updated practice guidelines, Maria can also think of a negative consequence of this action. The remote possibility exists, reasons Maria, that this adolescent client could have an asymptomatic gynecologic neoplasm, which by virtue of not performing the full gynecologic exam, could be missed. This would be an undesirable consequence of not performing the traditional exam.

7.3.4. Rule Utilitarianism

Opposed to Act Utilitarianism, which is concerned with the consequence of actions, Rule Utilitarianism is concerned with rules as guidance for actions. The action of following the rule, opposed to the consequence of the action, is the motivation for Rule Utilitarianism. For Maria, the most obvious rule, in this context, is to do no harm. The principle of nonmaleficence is commonly used as the guiding principle in biomedical ethics (Beauchamp and Childress, 2009). Using the same process she used in examining her actions, Maria attempts to reason through which approach—to perform the exam or not to perform the exam—would cause the least harm. Maria is unsure if she should only consider potential harm for the client, or if she should consider potential harm to herself, as well. She reasoned that within the context of the rule of utility, if harm came to herself, the clinician, then she would be unavailable to care for other people in need, and thus would not be following rule utilitarianism.

In regards to what harm could be done to Maria if she were not to perform the exam, the harm would be financial. Most health insurance reimbursement rates to clinicians are based on time spent with the client as well as number of body systems examined. If no pelvic exam was performed, then Maria would bill the client's insurance company a lower fee. Less money would be coming into the clinic and less money paid to the clinician. "If do not perform the lengthier and more complex exam, I make less money and therefore will not be able to afford to continue to work in a public clinic and provide care to this underserved population," reasons Maria.

"Do no harm", thinks Maria, "what if I miss one of those asymptomatic gynecologic cancers? Although it is such a remote possibility, I still have to acknowledge the existence of that very small risk. It certainly would be harmful to the client if I were to miss a cancer."

Maria considered two potentially harmful outcomes for not performing the exam, and she now considers how not performing the exam would "do no harm" to the client. By not performing the exam, Maria would be avoiding inflicting discomfort (perhaps even pain), and embarrassment (perhaps trauma) on this individual. Before considering her arguments both through Act and Rule Utilitarianism, Maria wants to review the strength of the evidence which informed these "new national guidelines".

7.3.5. Implications for Practice

Maria has thought long and hard about how to best care for this client. Using utilitarianism as a guide, Maria has considered the consequence of her decision not to perform a pelvic exam. She has also considered what least harm will befall herself and the client if she were to follow the principal of nonmaleficence. Maria has also considered the current clinical evidence and national guidelines pertaining to adolescent reproductive health care.

In reviewing her arguments, Maria recalls how she thought of two positive consequences, in term of happiness for the greatest number, if she were to not perform the exam; the client would be happy and fewer health resources, including her own time, would be used. Maria does continue to worry about the very small risk that she may miss an asymptomatic gynecologic cancer. If she were to follow the principal of nonmaleficence, Maria imagines the greatest benefit to the client, in term of no harm, from not performing the exam. She does acknowledge the decrease in revenue by providing a shorter, less extensive visit, but she did not take a job in a public health clinic to get rich. Worrying about reimbursement when providing care at a clinic in which the majority of clients have no health insurance at all seems to be wrong, thinks Maria.

The risk of missing a gynecologic cancer would most certainly be doing harm. This thought haunts Maria. However, the risk of an adolescent presenting with an asymptomatic gynecologic cancer is extremely unlikely; studies looking at gynecologic cancers classify "young" as less than 50 (Grimes and Wallach, 1997). Also, considers Maria, the public health system is based upon allocation of limited resources to those at greatest risk. "I need to be more concerned about this client getting pregnant than I do having a rare vulvar cancer, and therefore I need to do everything in my power to provide evidence based, nonjudgmental care and education and ensure she will return to follow-up visits. Whether I follow Act or Rule Utilitarianism, both approaches seem to bring me to the same conclusion: I will follow the current evidenced-based practice and not perform the traditional pap."

Maria explains to the client that she did not need to perform a pelvic exam, but spends the time educating the client about contraception, STD prevention and safer sex practices. She collects a urine sample for screening of chlamydia and gonorrhea and a pregnancy test since the client reported inconsistent condom use. Maria prescribes oral contraceptive pills. The client is very pleased with the time and consideration she receives; she feels Maria really listened and feels secure she was prescribed the very best contraception for her.

7.3.6. Utility in Infertility

Issues relating to reproduction are often ethically fraught. Matters relating to assisted reproduction are medically complicated, financially expensive and present several ethical dilemmas. Customs, culture, religion and personal freedom may be at stake when the right to reproduce is threatened (or compelled), and when complex and expensive technologies are added to the mix, navigating one's way through this bioethical mine field is further challenging.

This third case study presents a reproductive choice scenario and discusses it from a Utility bioethical approach. Francis is a 43 year old single mother of a 14 year old daughter, and who is seeking fertility treatments to conceive a second child. She has saved enough money from her job as a manager at the local supermarket to pay for the donor sperm. The first two IVF cycles, covered by her health insurance, have been unsuccessful. Francis desires a third IVF cycle which her insurance will not cover. Francis's physician, a reproductive endocrinologist, supports her choice to seek another cycle.

Francis understands that the likelihood of a successful IVF conception is very low, and it has been explained to her both the maternal and fetal risks of pregnancy at her advanced maternal age: hypertension, preeclampsia, gestational diabetes, and preterm birth. Despite these medical risks, and the low likelihood of success, Francis is determined not to give up her dream "of having another child". Francis takes a second mortgage out on her house to raise the funds to pay for another IVF cycle.

From a mainstream autonomy perspective, it is Francis' decision alone to reproduce or not. However, from a Utilitarian approach (Act Utiliarianism), the possible consequences of her action (to proceed with another IVF cycle) must be considered. Is continuing with another IVF cycle a 'good action', one which most positively affects the greatest number of people? For Francis, the best consequence will be that she will have a healthy, term infant which will provide fulfillment of her desire to have another child. A 'bad' consequence may be as follows: a twin gestation causing numerous health problems for Francis and/or hypertension and gestational diabetes which might result in Francis' hospitalization for several weeks. If Francis were to develop uncontrollable preeclampsia and subsequently deliver 30 week infant twins, the infant twins would have to remain in the Neonatal Intensive Care Unit (NICU) for ten weeks (while Francis remained in the hospital with complications secondary to a pregnancy- related deep vein thrombosis).

The potential 'bad' consequences were not experienced by Francis and infants alone. Francis' 14 year old daughter would be required to stay with an elderly uncle while her mother was in the hospital, and might become increasingly despondent during her mother's absence. Francis' health insurance has an inpatient limit and most of her own hospital care and her infants' would not be covered and she would be responsible for majority of the costs. What costs Francis would not be able to pay would have to be covered by the hospital itself, which is a publicly funded hospital. Thus the ultimate burden would be paid by the taxpayers. Francis would default on her mortgage and lose her house.

As described in this case, the potential 'bad' consequences are numerous and affect many individuals and communities in addition to Francis. There is no one available to help Francis fully understand the potential consequences of her decision to proceed with another IVF cycle: Francis' physician has an ethically conflicting financial interest should she proceed with another IVF cycle. Francis cannot imagine the complexity of potential pregnancy-related health problems she may experience and Francis does not know that her health insurance plan has an inpatient limit.

Francis desires another child even though the potential consequences of her action to conceive another child through IVF are numerous and harmful. Francis does not fully understand these potential consequences and moves forward with another IVF cycle.

7.4. UNANALYZED CASES

1. Anastasia is a 23 year old Russian woman living in Moscow, who has been married for three years and desires contraception. She has had several prior abortions and she fears any further abortions will limit her ability to have a safe pregnancy when she is ready. Abortion in Russia is legal, safe and cheap. Contraception in Russia, conversely, is expensive and scarce. In fact, the state funded health insurance does not cover contraception, as the Russian population is below replacement level and the state is encouraging larger families. How would a Feminist and Utilitarian address this dilemma? Would their arguments differ or not? Why?

2. Ruby is a 21 year old woman who is very excited by her recent engagement and upcoming wedding. Ruby is an active member of a conservative evangelical Protestant community and she shares her community's values and cultural habits. However, Ruby did have unprotected intercourse with a former boyfriend. Ruby recently went to have her first annual well woman exam, and discovered that she has a high-risk strain of the Human Papilloma Virus (HPV). Her Pap test was normal. The HPV test was ordered in error, as typically it would not have been run if the Pap test was normal. Ruby now knows that she has a sexually transmitted infection (STI) that she could potentially pass to her future husband. It is unknown what, if any, ill effects HPV has on men. Should Ruby tell her fiancée that she has an STI, thus admitting she is not a virgin? What ethical issues are involved here?

7.5. REFERENCES

ACOG. (2009) Routine pelvic examination and cervical cytology screening (Committee Opinion Statement #431). *Obstetrics and Gynecology, 113*(5): 1190–1193. doi: 10.1097/AOG.0b013e3181a6d022

Beauchamps, T.L. and Childress, J.F. (2009). *Principals of Biomedical Ethics.* New York: Oxford.

Chiang, J.W. and Berek, J.S. (2010). Gestational trophoblastic disease: Epidemiology, clinical manifestations and diagnosis. *UpToDate.* Retrieved from http://www.uptodate.com/contents/gestational-trophoblastic-disease-epidemiology-clinical-manifestations-and-diagnosis?source=search_resultandsearch=hydatiform+moleandselectedTitle=2%7E38#H19.

Cook, R.J. and Dickens, B.M. (2002). The injustice of unsafe motherhood. *Developing World Bioethics, 2*: 64–81.

Cook, R., Dickens, B., and Fathalla, M. (2008). *Reproductive Health and Human Rights.* New York: Oxford.

Dodds, S. (2000). Choice and control in feminist bioethics. In: *Relational Autonomy* (pp. 213–235). C. Mackenzie and N. Stoljar (Eds.). New York: Oxford.

Dickens, B.M. and Cook, R.J. (2007). Reproductive health and public health ethics. *International Journal of Gynecology and Obstetrics, 99*: 75–79.

Feldman, S., Sirovich, B.E., and Goodman, A. (2012). Screening for cervical cancer: Rationale and recommendations. UpToDate. Retrieved from http://www.uptodate.com/contents/screening-for-cervical-cancer-rationale-and-recommendations?source=search_resultandsearch=pap+smearandselectedTitle=1%7E137.

Gibson, S. (2004). The problem of abortion: Essentially contested concepts and moral autonomy. *Bioethics, 18*: 221–233.

Grimes, D.A. and Wallach, M. (1997). *The Contraception Report.* New Jersey: Emron, Inc.

Lake, R. (1985). The metaethical framework of anti-abortion rhetoric. *Signs, 11*: 478–499.

Mosciki, A.B., Shiboski, S., Hills, N.K., et al. (2004). Regression of low-grade squamous intra-epithelial lesions in young women. *Lancet, 364*(9449): 1678–83.

Schlecht, N.F., Platt, R.W., Duarte-Franco, E., et al. (2003). Human papillomavirus infection and time to progression and regression of cervical intraepithelial neoplasia. *Journal of the National Cancer Institute, 95*(17): 1336–43.

Shafer, M.A. (1998). Annual pelvic examination in the sexually active adolescent female: what are we doing and why are we doing it? *Journal of Adolescent Health, 23*(2): 68–73.

Sherwin, S. (1992). *No longer patient: Feminist ethics and health care.* Philadelphia:Temple.

Szarewski, A. and Sasieni, P. (2004). Cervical screening in adolescents—at least do no harm. *Lancet, 364*(9446): 1642–4.

Townsend, J.W. (2007). Learning through conflict: Ethical debates in sexual and reproductive health. *Studies in Family Planning, 38*: 225–228.

UN, Department of Public Information. (1995). Platform for Action and Beijing Declaration, Fourth World Conference on Women, Beijing, China, 4–15 September 1995. New York: UN.

Workowski, K.A., and Berman, S.M. (2006). Sexually transmitted disease treatment guidelines. *MMWR Recommendation Report, 55*(RR-11): 1–94.

CHAPTER 8

Ethical Business Practices Overview

JENNIFER A. SMITH

8.1. INTRODUCTION

"In the evolutionary shift toward managed care, practitioners have been asked to embrace business values of efficiency and cost effectiveness, sometimes at the expense of their professional judgment and personal values. While some of these changes have been inevitable as our society sought to rein in out-of-control costs, it is not unreasonable for practitioners to call on payers, regulators and other parties to the health care delivery system to raise their ethical bar."
—Marcinko, D., The Business of Medical Practice, 2005

While not every nurse will set up his or her own practice, all will work within the context of a healthcare system that uses common business models and many will interact with insurance/managed care companies. Most health care professionals do not enter the field because they are intrigued by business or finance; in fact, to some it is considered 'anti-professional' to be concerned with the 'money end' of patient care. Nevertheless, it is important for providers to have a basic understanding of the financial under-pinning of the practices in which they work and the ethical and legal framework on which this is based. This chapter is meant to provide such an overview. While some examples described in this chapter may be physician-based, the principles apply to advanced practice nurses as well. Because of the diverseness of particular subject matter, individual topics are presented in alphabetical order for ease of reference.

8.2. ACCOUNTING

Financial information about a business is transmitted to the public via many mechanisms, foremost of which is accountancy, defined by the American Institute of Certified Public Accountants (AIPCA) as "the art of recording, classifying and summarizing in a significant manner and in terms of money, transactions and events which are, in part at least, of financial character, and interpreting the results thereof." The principles of accounting, the language of business, apply equally to healthcare institutions and practices, both for profit and non-profit.

The accounting profession is guided by its own code of ethics, and those that utilize the services of accounting firms should expect that these codes are enforced and followed. Just as in other fields, these codes are meant to provide users of these services with the confidence that the work provided is ethically sound. There are three major accounting associations, including the American Institute of Certified Public Accountants (AICPA), the Institute of Management Accountants (IMA), and the Institute of Internal Auditors (IIA); all have codes of ethics which apply to their members (Smith and Smith, Business and Accounting Ethics). These codes of professional conduct direct behavior and provide guidelines for ethical performance, often above and beyond required laws and regulations (Duska and Duska, 2003). Similar to medical/nursing codes of ethics, all three of these accounting associations' codes require that accounting professionals must maintain client/professional confidentiality, possess professional competence and act with integrity and objectivity.

Conflicts of interest may arise if an accountant has a vested interest in the company he/she is auditing or if the results of an audit may not be beneficial to the company, but are important for the shareholders to know, as it affects their investment.

Generally Accepted Accounting Principles (GAAP) are rules which currently frame financial accounting in the United States and are the basis for determining how accounting procedures are carried out. These are rules-based, as opposed to standards developed by the International Accounting Standards Board's International Financial Reporting Standards (IFRS), which are based on principles requiring professional judgment. Because of this, there is some question as to whether this is the proper basis for deciding accounting decisions; i.e., there is no context in which to inform decisions (Somerville, 2003). Work has been underway for several years by the Securities and Exchange Commission (SEC) to integrate IFRS and GAAP but as of January 2012, this has still not been accomplished.

Multiple large financial scandals in the 1980s and 90s (Enron, AIG, Arthur Anderson, etc.) (Alexander *et al.*, 2002) resulted not only in companies going out of business, but also the large accounting firms who were responsible for faulty/unethical accounting practices. In response, Congress passed the Sarbanes-Oxley Act of 2002 (also known as the Public Company Accounting Reform and Investor Protection Act of 2002). Sarbanes-Oxley is "to protect investors by improving the accuracy and reliability of corporate disclosures made pursuant to the securities laws . . ." and covers "public company accounting oversight board, auditor independence, corporate responsibility, enhanced financial disclosures, analyst conflicts of interest, commission resources and authority, studies and reports, corporate and criminal fraud accountability, white collar crime penalty enhancements, corporate tax returns, and corporate fraud and accountability." (SEC, 2002).

According to a 2007 survey of members of the International Federation of Accountants, some of the main factors which contribute to ethical failures for accountants are: "self-interest, failure to maintain objectivity and independence, inappropriate professional judgment, lack of ethical sensitivity, improper leadership and ill-culture, and failure to withstand advocacy threats." (Jackling *et al.*, 2007)

Business schools across the country also began to include business ethics in their accounting and other curricula as a result of these scandals. In 1988, Stephen Loeb proposed that ethics curricula should include seven goals:

- Relate accounting education to moral issues
- Recognize issues in accounting that have ethical implications
- Develop a sense of moral obligation or responsibility
- Develop the abilities needed to deal with ethical conflicts or dilemmas
- Learn to deal with the uncertainties of the accounting profession
- Set the stage for a change in ethical behavior
- Appreciate and understand the history and composition of all aspects of accounting ethics and their relationship to the general field of ethics (Loeb and Stephen, 1988; Dellaportas, 2006; Loeb, 1994).

Certified Public Accountants (CPAs) are regulated by individual states, which issue licenses to practice through the state board of accountancy. Because the state board may also include ethics language in its statutes, a breach of ethics may result in loss of license to practice. CPAs who audit financial statements of public corporations are also subject to regulation by the Securities and Exchange Commission (SEC). The SEC requires that all public firms' financial statements be audited by an independent CPA or accounting firm, thus promoting independence and avoiding potential conflicts of interest.

8.3. CONFLICTS OF INTEREST

In general usage, conflicts of interest develop when one is involved in two competing entities, usually of a financial nature, and which results in an unfair advantage for one and a disadvantage to the other.

In healthcare, conflicts of interest may arise when the best interests of a patient are put at risk because of a financial incentive or personal gain offered to their health care provider (perhaps by a pharmaceutical firm or medical device manufacturer) which goes against best evidence and standards of care. The American Medical Association offers a stated guideline:

> *"Under no circumstances may physicians place their own financial interests above the welfare of their patients. The primary objective of the medical profession is to render service to humanity; reward or financial gain is a subordinate consideration. For a physician to unnecessarily hospitalize a patient, prescribe a drug, or conduct diagnostic tests for the physician's financial benefit is unethical. If a conflict develops between the physician's financial interest and the physician's responsibilities to the patient, the conflict must be resolved to the patient's benefit" (AMA, 1994).*

How much money may be involved in such conflicts of interest for healthcare providers is reflected in the following example. In June 2011, the Senate Finance Committee began investigating the Medtronic Corporation about the $62 million they had given for over a decade to 15 surgeons. These surgeons, according to *Spine Journal*, failed to report serious complications observed in clinical trials in their research papers. The trials all involved a Medtronic bone-growth medication. Medtronic said it will "investigate questions surrounding researchers' potential conflicts of interest, refine our policies as warranted, and strive to lead the industry in ethical and transparent business practices" (Carreyrou, 2011).

Brennan *et al.*, (2006), in their article for *JAMA*, "Health Industry Practices that Create Conflicts of Interest—A Policy Proposal for Academic Medical Centers," state that academic medical centers must put more stringent policies in place "including the elimination or modification of common practices related to small gifts, pharmaceutical samples, continuing medical education, funds for physician travel, speaker's bureaus, ghostwriting, and consulting and research contracts."

The Institute of Medicine (IOM) Committee on Conflict of Interest in Medical Research, Education and Practice recommends that physicians should not:

- *accept items of material value from pharmaceutical, medical device, and biotechnology companies, except when a transaction involves payment at fair market value for a legitimate service;*
- *make educational presentations or publish scientific articles that are controlled by industry or that contain substantial portions written by someone who is not identified as an author;*
- *enter into consulting arrangements unless they are based on written contracts for expert services to be paid for at fair market value;*
- *meet with pharmaceutical and medical device sales representatives except by documented appointment and at the physician's express invitation; and*
- *accept drug samples, except in specified situations for patients who lack financial access to medications. (IOM, 2009)*

The IOM also recommends that:

> *"Pharmaceutical, medical device, and biotechnology companies and their company foundations should have policies and practices against providing physicians with gifts, meals, drug samples (except for use by patients who lack financial access to medications), or other similar items of material value, and recommends against asking physicians to be authors of ghostwritten materials. Consulting arrangements should be for necessary services, documented in written contracts, and paid for at fair market value. Companies should not involve physicians and patients in marketing projects that are presented as clinical research." (IOM, 2009)*

Many academic health centers and hospitals now require that all staff sign a yearly conflict of interest disclosure form that relates to research and patient care, if applicable, to prevent such issues. Columbia University's Conflict of Interest Policy states in part that:

> *"This Policy is designed to maintain the trust of the public, research volunteers, and the University research community and to help assure institutional compliance with applicable government regulations concerning outside financial relationships and research. The University recognizes the importance of relationships between faculty and commercial organizations, and seeks to encourage such relationships. These relationships can give rise to significant discoveries and to the translation of those discoveries into useful products. Productive relationships with commercial organizations also inspire new avenues of inquiry and provide opportunities to test academic research. However, the financial incentives that accompany such relationships may lead to financial conflicts of interest. Such conflicts of interest have the potential to create real or apparent bias in research. Conflicts of interest may affect research integrity and*

may place human research subjects at additional risk. Conflicts of interest, and even the appearance of conflict of interest, may reduce public confidence in the research enterprise." (Columbia University, 2011).

While much of the policy applies to the legal ramifications of noncompliance, the bases of the policy are the moral under-pinnings of honesty and the performance of duty for the common good.

Boston College posts a list of potential red flags that all managers and supervisors should be aware of, many of which relate to potential conflict of interests or fraud. They include: "marked personality changes in employees, financial pressures on employees, an employee living beyond his/her means, an employee having outside business interest, poor internal controls, rising department expenses, too much control in key employees, lax management and failure to pre-screen employees" (Boston College, 2011).

Conflicts may arise when a healthcare provider is asked to participate in fundraising or to solicit gifts from patients, which may not only affect the patient/provider relationship, but potentially the confidentiality and privacy of health information. The American Medical Association's Code of Ethics opinion regarding solicitation of gifts from patients states the following:

"Physicians should avoid directly soliciting their own patients, especially at the time of a clinical encounter. They should reinforce the trust that is the foundation of the patient-physician relationship by being clear that patients' welfare is the primary priority and that patients need not contribute in order to continue receiving the same quality of care. . . In particular, physicians should ensure that any patient information used for solicitation activities reveals only basic demographic data, not personal health information." (AMA, 2004)

Faculty members of Columbia School of Nursing, who have responsibilities for research, education, clinical service and administration, developed the school's own Conflict of Interest (COI) policy in 2010 (and revised in 2012).

"The purpose of this CUSON COI Policy is to reinforce some general principles set forth in University policies and to address in detail two areas particularly relevant to CUSON clinical care and nursing education. These critical CUSON activities must not be compromised by conflict of interest or even the appearance of conflict. Academic-industry collaborations are encouraged by the Bayh-Dole Act of 1980 and by long-standing policies of Columbia University. Relationships between CUSON faculty and commercial entities are present in clinical research

and educational activities. As a consequence of academic-industry relationships, potential questions may arise regarding the intellectual independence of faculty who are involved with commercial enterprises. Even perceived conflicts of interest can undermine the credibility of academic and clinical functions. Interactions with industry should be conducted to avoid or minimize conflicts of interest. When real or potential conflicts arise, they must be promptly and appropriately addressed.

To avoid, identify and, if necessary, address potential conflicts of interest, this Policy requires all full- and part-time CUSON Faculty, post-doctoral students and research scientists to adhere to the new policy described herein. This policy also requires that CUSON faculty, post-doctoral students and research scientists submit an annual Conflicts of Interest disclosure statement of significant commercial support (defined below) pertaining to education/training and clinical service, in addition to other University conflicts of interest disclosure requirements, such as those pertaining to research and administration.

This Policy adds to the existing University policies. To the extent there are other University policies or federal or state laws that govern COI issues, faculty must also abide by them. CUSON Faculty adherence to these policies for limiting potential or perceived conflicts will help avoid conflicts of interest. Annual disclosure in itself does not constitute avoidance or management of conflicts of interest. Failure to comply with mandatory policies will prompt formal review by the faculty COI Committee, with recommendations to the Dean, and may lead to sanctions up to and including non-renewal of appointment." (Columbia University, 2011)

There are additional sections in CUSON's COI policy including support for educational activities, gifts, consultation, continuing nursing education (CNE), non-CNE presentations and publications, travel, industry sponsored presentations, ghost authorship and ghost writing, inventions, drug and device representatives, and drug and device samples. Of course, not every contingency can be addressed, but these specifics do provide general guidance.

8.4. FRAUD

Fraud constitutes any unlawful activities undertaken to enrich the person committing the fraud and occurs in the healthcare arena just as in the rest of the business world. Fraud covers theft, embezzlement, incorrect financial reporting or expense reports, conflict of interest, software piracy, falsified insurance submissions, counterfeit prescriptions, deceptive advertising, DRG falsities, duplicate billing, split billing, and other deceitful practices. Every business enterprise must have safeguards in place to detect and prevent fraudulent behavior and systems to deal with any breaches in any such behavior. To state that such behavior is not only illegal, but unethical, is obvious.

Under the federal False Claims Act of 1863, an employee with knowledge of fraud against the government may file a lawsuit on behalf of the government. This law was created during the Civil War and was used against wartime defense contractors who billed the government for weapons that were not delivered as promised. It is now used by the Department of Justice in attacking healthcare fraud and abuse. Under its criminal statute, false claims are punishable by fine or imprisonment of up to five years, or both, for knowingly submitting a false statement for reimbursement. A key provision in the Act is entitled "qui tam", which allows an employee with knowledge of fraud against the government to file a lawsuit on behalf of the government (the employee is referred to as the *qui tam* plaintiff) and is entitled to a percentage of any recovery as well as protection from being "discharged, demoted, suspended, threatened, harassed or in any other manner discriminated against" (CMS False Claims Act). This provision is commonly known as the Whistleblower Act. Employees are the most common whistleblowers, as knowledge of 'inside' information is usually required to prove alleged fraud.

Innocent mistakes and mere negligence are not actionable under the False Claims Act, but acts such as bills for care not given, upcoding, providing substandard service but billing for standard care, or using someone else's Medicare/Medicaid number, are.

> *"You are exposed to civil penalty if you knowingly or recklessly present, or cause to be presented, to an officer or employee of the United States government . . . a false or fraudulent claim for payment or approval . . . or knowingly make, use, or cause to be made or used, a false record or statement to get a false or fraudulent claim paid or approved by the government" (CMS False Claims Act). "Reckless disregard as to the truth or falseness of a claim is sufficient to support a False Claims Act action" (CMS). In the case of United States v. Krizek, a psychiatrist's inadequate billing system and failure to supervise his billing agents was found to be reckless in the submission of duplicate claims, but the court found no fraud involved because there was no intent to defraud, only sloppy billing practices. Those who knowingly submit, "or cause another person or entity to submit, false claims for payment of government funds are liable for three times the government's damages plus civil penalties of $5,500 to $11,000 per false claim" (CMS False Claims Act).*

In 1997, a qui tam suit was brought by former employees of the pharmaceutical firm TAP, the maker of the drug Lupron. According to the whistleblowers, "TAP encouraged urologists to bill Medicare the average wholesale price of Lupron for samples that were provided free or at a steeply discounted price by the company. The company also engaged the urologists as consultants without specific deliverables, provided all-expense paid trips, and awarded unrestricted educational grants." (Birkhahn *et al.*, 2009, p.778). The government found that these actions constituted inducements to the physicians to prescribe Lupron (and bill to Medicare). The suit was settled when TAP agreed to pay the government $875 million and the whistleblowers received almost $100 million of the total (Birkhahn *et al.*, 2009).

Under the Deficit Reduction Act of 2005, Section 6032 requires that "any entity that receives or makes payments to the State Medicaid Program of at least $5 million annually, to provide Federal False Claims Act education to their employees." This was required because fraud costs the taxpayers huge amounts that could be otherwise spent on healthcare, as well as to alert all parties involved in the business side of health care to cut down on mistakes and negligence (CMS Deficit Reduction Act).

The Stark laws are part of the Social Security Act and overseen by the Centers for Medicare and Medicaid Services. It is also known as the Physician Self-Referral Law and is intended to prohibit physicians from profiting from their own referrals. They state that a physician cannot refer a patient covered by Medicare to a clinical laboratory where the physician or an immediate family member of the physician has a financial relationship. The Acts were initially enacted in 1989 to only cover clinical lab services, but in 1993 they were expanded to cover the rest of the designated health services (DHS). A physician many not refer a patient to certain DHS such as physical therapy, occupational therapy, radiation therapy, radiation services, durable medical equipment and supplies, parenteral and enteral nutrients, prosthetics, home health services, outpatient prescription drugs and other outpatient or inpatient services (CMS). In August of 2007, CMS issued additional regulations which prohibit physicians from referring patients for services and tests provided by businesses in which they or their family have a financial interest. The final revisions were in response to public comments and offered some flexibility when (for example) organizations recruit physicians to rural areas, or when hospitals wish to show appreciation to their staffs in annual events. CMS published the Medicare Self-Referral Disclosure Protocol (SRDP) in September 2010 as part of the Patient Protection and Affordable Care Act (PPAC). This protocol enables providers and suppliers to "self-disclose actual or potential violations of the physician self-referral statute" and allows leeway in reducing amounts due for violations (CMS Physician Self Referral).

CMS does allow some standard exceptions, including permitting the referral of a patient from one physician to another in the same group practice. In 2010, the in-office ancillary services exceptions were adopted that allow a physician within a group practice to refer a patient for MRI, CT or PET scans within the group practice, but at the time of referral must provide the patient with written notice that the patient may obtain these imaging services from a supplier other than the group practice and provide a list of alternatives. All this legislation is currently only applicable to physicians and does not yet pertain to advanced practice registered nurses (CMS Physician Self- Referral).

Additionally, CMS issued a new rule in 2008 which requires physicians to disclose to their patients, at the time of referral, if they have ownership or an investment in the hospital as well as for physician-owned hospitals to disclose to their patients the names of any physicians (and immediate family members) who have an ownership or investment in the hospital (CMS Changes to Disclosure of Physician Ownership in Hospitals and Physician Self-Referral Rules, 2008). Exceptions are allowed if proof can be established of qualifications as a sole rural provider or hospital. The Patient Protection and Affordable Care Act (ACA) of 2010 added other requirements for hospitals in order to qualify for the rural provider and hospital exceptions to the ownership or investment prohibition. Section 6001 of the ACA limits expansion to hospitals that have physician ownership or investment and mandates certain disclosure obligations for physician-owned hospitals and referring physicians that have an ownership or investment interest in a hospital.

The Anti-Kickback Statute deals with "Anyone who knowingly or willfully solicits or receives, either directly or indirectly, any remuneration (including any kickback, bribe, or rebate) in exchange for referring an individual for services under any federal healthcare program or in return for purchasing, leasing, or ordering any good, facility, service, or item paid for under a federal health care program shall be guilty of a felony" (CMS Anti-Kickback Rule). Each offense is subject to a fine of up to $25,000 or imprisonment for up to 5 years or both. Often kickbacks involve payments from one party to another (physician to physician or hospital to physician) with the intent to induce or reward referrals. "The 'one purpose' test is used by the federal government to determine if a hospital has unlawfully compensated a physician. If one purpose of the physician compensation is to induce referrals, then the statute (Anti-Kickback Rule) has been violated even though the compensation was for a professional service" (Mustard, 2009).

In addition to the False Claims Act and the Federal Anti-Kickback Statute, the Department of Health and Human Services also employs the Civil Monetary Penalties Law (CMPL) as means to regulate some aspects of the physician/provider-industry interaction. The Office of the Attorney General may use the CMPL to enforce the Anti-Kickback Statute and "provides for monetary penalties of up to $50,000 for each illegal act, assessments of up to three times the amount of the kickback, and the exclusion from participation in federal health care programs" (Birkhahn *et al.*, 2009).

Even when heavy fines are levied, collecting them is not always easy. Since 2005, the SEC and the Commodity Futures Trading Commission have imposed over $12.5 billion in fines (also including return of ill-gotten profits and repayment of restitution to investors for fraudulent activities). As of July 2011, only $8 billion has been recovered (WSJ, 2011).

Fraud involving HIPAA violations are now liable for criminal penalties enforced by the Department of Justice.

> *"An individual who knowingly obtains or discloses individually identifiable health information in violation of HIPAA faces a fine of $50,000 and up to one year imprisonment. The criminal penalties increase to $100,000 and up to five years imprisonment if the wrongful conduct involves false pretenses, and up to ten years imprisonment if the wrongful conduct involves the intent to sell, transfer, or use individually identifiable health information for commercial advantage, personal gain or malicious harm" (CMS Medicare HIPAA Eligibility).*

The Criminal Health Care Fraud Statute (18 U.S.C. Section 1347) specifically forbids the defrauding of any health care benefit program (i.e., Medicare or Medicaid) or to obtain "by means of false or fraudulent pretenses, representations, or promises any of the money or property owned by, or under the custody or control of, any health care benefit program in connection with the delivery of or payment for health care benefits, items, or services" (CMS Criminal Health Care Fraud). Penalties for violating the statute may include fines, imprisonment, or both.

The government utilizes multiple entities to coordinate and monitor fraud, including CMS, the Center for Program Integrity, the Office of the Inspector General, the Health Care Fraud Prevention and Enforcement Action Team and the General Services Administration.

8.5. GIFTS

Gifts given for the 'joy of giving' and with no expectation of return or reward are usually received with willingness and enthusiasm by the recipient. However, gifts given to healthcare professionals with a *quid pro quo* expectancy constitute major concerns of legality and ethics.

There is a long history of companies, particularly pharmaceutical and medical device manufacturers, marketing their products to physicians through:

> *"gifts, even of relatively small items, including meals; payment for attendance at lectures and conferences, including on-line activities; CME for which physicians pay no fee; payment for time while attending meetings; payment for travel to meetings or scholarships to attend meetings; payment for participation in speakers bureaus; the provision of ghostwriting services; provision of pharmaceutical samples; grants for research projects; and payment for consulting relationships" (Brennan et al., 2006).*

These gifts may compromise the professionalism and patient care given by physicians, and the guidelines suggested by such professional groups as the American Medical Association, the Accreditation Council for Continuing Medical Education and the American College of Physicians do not go far enough in protecting the welfare of patients or the integrity of research. Brennan *et al.* (2006) also dispute the commonly held belief that small gifts (pens, coffee mugs, etc.) do not influence physician behavior.

PhRMA, the Pharmaceutical Manufacturers Association, represents member companies and issued guidelines regarding gifts to physicians in 2002. Their voluntary guidelines suggest that gifts valued at less than $100 were allowed if the physician could prove a value to patients and that modest meals were acceptable if in the context of an educational setting. These PhRMA guidelines were endorsed by the Office of the Inspector General, which also issued its own guidelines in 2003. A revision by PhRMA in 2009 was stricter, disallowing all gifts (even pens and mugs for example) other than meals that "are modest as judged by local standards; are not part of an entertainment or recreational event; and are provided in a manner conducive to informational communication", sample medications and educational gifts (PHRMA Code, 2009). But self-regulation by the industry did not change either public perception or practice and in 2010, as part of the Affordable Care Act national health reform law, the Physicians Payments Sunshine Act was passed. This Act now requires all pharmaceutical companies to report all payments to physicians above $10 and pay penalties if they fail to do so ($150,000 for failure to report and $1 million for knowingly doing so). (Mizik, 2010). CMS is in the process of finalizing procedures for this reporting, which will likely begin sometime in 2012 (Yukhananvov, 2011).

The American Medical Association issued a number of guidelines to assist physicians (which have been endorsed by the American Academy of Pediatrics, the American College of Obstetricians and Gynecologists and the American College of Rheumatology):

- "Any gifts accepted by physicians individually should primarily entail a benefit to patients and should not be of substantial value. Accordingly, textbooks, modest meals and other gifts are appropriate if they serve a genuine education function. Cash payments should not be accepted. The use of drug samples for personal or family use is permissible as long as these practices do not interfere with patient access to drug samples. It would not be appropriate for non-retired physicians to request free pharmaceuticals for personal use or for use by family members.
- Individual gifts of minimal value are permissible as long as the gifts are related to the physician's work (e.g., pens and notepads).
- The Council on Ethical and Judicial Affairs defines a legitimate 'conference' or 'meeting' as any activity, held at an appropriate location where a) the gathering is primarily dedicated, in both time and effort, to promoting objective scientific and education activities and discourse (one or more educational presentations should be the highlight of the gathering), and b) the main incentive for bringing attendees together is to further their knowledge on the topic being presented. An appropriate disclosure of financial support or conflict of interest should be made.
- Subsidies to underwrite the costs of continuing medical education conferences or professional meetings can contribute to the improvement of patient care and therefore are permissible. Since the giving of a subsidy directly to a physician by a company's sales representative may create a relationship with the conference's sponsor who in turn can use the money to reduce the conference's registration fee. Payments to defray the costs of a conference should not be accepted directly from the company by the physicians attending the conference.
- Subsidies from industry should not be accepted directly or indirectly to pay for the costs of travel, lodging or other personal expenses of physicians attending conferences or meetings, nor should subsidies be accepted to compensate for the physician's time. Subsidies for hospitality should not be accepted outside of modest meals or social events held as a part of a conference or meeting.
- Scholarships of other special funds to permit medical students, residents, and fellows to attend carefully selected educational conferences may be permissible as long as the selections of students, residents, or fellows who will receive the funds are

made by the academic or training institution. Carefully selected educational conferences are generally defined as the major education, scientific, or policy-making meetings of national, regional, or specialty associations.

- No gifts should be accepted if there are strings attached. For example, physicians should not accept gifts if they are given in relation to the physician's prescribing practices. In addition, when companies underwrite medical conferences or lectures other than their own, responsibility for and control over the selection of content, faculty, educational methods, and materials should belong to the organizers of the conferences or lectures" AMA Medical Code of Ethics, Opinion 8.061).

The American College of Physicians statement on gifts says: "The acceptance by a physician of gifts, hospitality, trips, and subsidies of all types from the health care industry that might diminish, or appear to others to diminish, the objectivity of professional judgment is strongly discouraged. As documented by some studies, the acceptance of even small gifts can affect clinical judgment and heighten the perception and/or reality of a conflict of interest" (ACP, 2007).

Gifts from patients may present different challenges. According to the AMA Medical Code of Ethics opinion:

> *"Gifts that patients offer to physicians are often an expression of appreciation and gratitude or a reflection of cultural traditions, and can enhance the patient-physician relationship. . . . Physicians should make clear that gifts given to secure preferential treatment compromise their obligation to provide services in a fair manner. There are no definitive rules to determine when a physician should or should not accept a gift. No fixed value determines the appropriateness or inappropriateness of a gift from a patient; however, the gift's value relative to the patient's or the physician's means should not be disproportionately or inappropriately large" (AMA Code of Ethics—Gifts from Patients, 2003).*

At an academic healthcare center, faculty and student relationships might be influenced by inappropriate gift giving. Columbia University School of Nursing instituted a policy in 2009 to provide guidance for faculty should they be given a gift by a student. Generally, faculty may not receive gifts from students except small, non-personal, inexpensive tokens (not of greater than $50 in value). Faculty should be sensitive to students for whom giving of gifts is important and assure that students do not feel slighted, embarrassed or insulted (CUSON Accepting Gifts from Students Policy, 2009).

8.6. HUMAN RESOURCE MANAGEMENT

The workplace in healthcare consists of more than just patients and colleagues and requires specific and often complex knowledge of human resource issues, both legal and professional.

Human resource management (HRM) related issues in the workplace today can be overwhelming: recruitment, performance appraisals, training, compensation, benefits (pay equity), labor relations (unions, strikes), discrimination (ageism, gender, race, religion, disabilities, and sexual harassment), termination, occupational health and safety, and privacy (workplace surveillance, drug testing, and whistleblowing). In other words, any aspect of the work force concerned with employees and employers. While many of these issues are regulated by government agencies and legal compliance, many rely on the culture of the institution and how attuned it is to the welfare of its employees. Decisions made in business about any of these issues affect people's livelihoods and chances for future employment. The 'bottom line' is that employees and employers should be treated fairly and equitably and human resources management plays an important role in making sure that all parties know and understand the culture and values of the institution (Rose, 2007).

Winstanley and Woodall (1996) note ethical concerns arising from HRM practices including:

- *"Increased job insecurity arising from flexible work practices, short-term and temporary employment, fear of job loss due to outsourcing, increased stress and a widening imbalance of power between management and workforce;*
- *Increase in surveillance and control ranging from the use of psychometric tests to electronic surveillance to random drug screening/testing;*
- *Deregulation of the market place which may be seen as pushing HR into compromising 'good' practice for business needs—i.e., 'doing well vs. doing good';*
- *A decline in management integrity which contrasts an emphasis on managing organizational culture with a highly formulaic approach in employment contracts."*

Margolis, Grant and Molinsky propose three standards for ethical management of human resources which take into consideration the organization itself, the target of any harmful action and the HR managers. They provide a thoughtful, yet simple framework, to consider:

- *"Advance the organization's objective. Execute the task in question so that progress is made towards the objective that calls for it to be done in the first place—in other words, hiring and firing decisions, performance appraisals, etc., should serve a central organizational objective that has been decided in advance and is available to all staff and managers.*

- *Enhance the dignity of those who may be harmed by the action. When managers distribute opportunities and benefits, there may be some who do not receive those opportunities and benefits—or receive fewer than others. When companies go through cycles of destruction—restructuring, downsizing—individuals get harmed. In both instances, those who lose out are due treatment that respects their standing, fosters their resilience, and enables them to continue to function effectively.*
- *Sustain the moral sensibility of those executing morally ambiguous tasks. Someone must deliver the poor performance appraisal, announce the lay-off, or close the manufacturing facility or office. The difficulty and ambivalence which may occur when performing these tasks reflects an underlying uneasiness about fair treatment and fair outcomes, and managers ought to remain attuned to that uneasiness."*

Some companies/organizations publish their codes of ethics which become clear and visible statements of organizational culture and expectations. The HR department at Lehigh University states, in part:

> *"As human resources professionals, we are committed to: balancing organizational and individual employee needs and interests, showing respect for differences between individuals and groups and accommodating these differences whenever possible, managing our personal opinions and biases in the interest of objectivity and fairness to others, and using influence and authority appropriately" (Lehigh University, 2007).*

In the United States, the Sarbanes-Oxley Act of 2002, which covers all publicly traded companies, requires, among other things, that these companies have a code of ethics in place that includes detriments to financial wrong-doing and promotes integrity, specifically to senior financial officers and bans personal loans to executive officers or board of directors members. A company must affirm that they are committed to honest and ethical conduct and avoidance of conflicts of interest. Under the Act, companies must prove to the Securities and Exchange Commission that its financial statements are accurate, complete, timely and understandable. They must also comply with any applicable laws and regulations.

The Act also requires companies to develop a complaint system and non-retaliation policy that is clearly explained to employees. This protects whistleblowers and applies not just to the employees of a publicly traded company, but to anyone who works for such a company including contractors, agents, etc. Because of the anti-retribution and whistle-blower provisions in the Act:

> *"a company, officer, employee, contractor, subcontractor or agent is prohibited from discharging, demoting, suspending, threatening, harassing or otherwise discriminating in the terms and conditions of employment against an employee who...provides information or assists in an investigation regarding conduct that the employee reasonably believes is fraudulent or a violation of a rule or regulation of the SEC when such information or assistance is provided to or the investigation is conducted by (1) a federal regulatory agency or law enforcement, (2) a member of Congress or a committee, (3) a person with supervisory authority over the person or (4) a person who has authority to investigate, discover or terminate misconduct" (Sarbanes-Oxley Act of 2002).*

Being an ethically and socially responsible company can be an attraction for potential and current employees. Programs that encourage environmental responsibility, volunteerism and philanthropy, diversity, community and employee interactions, while ethically positive, are also good for business. Corporate social responsibility (CSR) is 'emerging as a business imperative' (Eide, P.). Non-publicly traded companies are also mirroring Sarbanes-Oxley requirements as the benefits of doing so are becoming more widely known. All impact HRM professionals. If employees know the rules, objectives and ethical expectations of the organization, and managers are expected to treat all employees fairly and are supported in their enforcement of rules and objectives, an ethical workplace will result.

8.7. INFORMATION TECHNOLOGY

It is almost impossible today not to have information technology (IT) play a role in business and personal lives. Employers are deciding whether or not to monitor emails and internet site visits and censorship, what security safeguards should be instituted to prevent hackers and spyware, should spam be utilized as a form of low cost marketing and what can and cannot be copyrighted when shared via IT (Reynolds, 2009).

The business side of health care is no different; from electronic health records (EHR) to computerized physician order entry (CPOE), to billing and claims systems to health information web sites to patient/practitioner emails, employers must develop policies and strategies for these and other contingencies. It is important that workplaces provide ethics instruction concerning IT issues to new employees and on a continuing basis in order to prevent unintentional violations and to provide information about consequences for unethical behaviors (Calluzzo and Cante, 2004).

Chief among the ethical issues involved with IT in healthcare is that of patient privacy/confidentiality. The Health Insurance Portability and Accountability Act of 1996 (HIPAA) was developed by the United States Department of Health and Human Services (HHS) in order to protect the privacy and security of certain health information. A Privacy Rule (the Standards of Privacy of Individually Identifiable Health Information, finalized in 2002) and a Security Rule (the Security Standards for the Protection of Electronic Protected Health Information, finalized in 2003) were established in order to implement HIPAA.

> *"The Privacy Rule standards address the use and disclosure of individuals' health information—called 'protected health information' by organizations subject to the Privacy Rule—called 'covered entities', as well as standards for individuals' privacy rights to understand and control how their health information is used. Within HHS, the Office for Civil Rights (OCR) has responsibility for implementing and enforcing the Privacy Rule with respect to voluntary compliance activities and civil money penalties. A major goal of the Privacy Rule is to assure that individuals' health information is properly protected while allowing the flow of health information needed to provide and promote high quality health care and to protect the public's health and well-being. The Rule balances necessary uses of information with protection of the privacy of people who seek health care. Because the health care marketplace has so many different participants, the Rule is designed to be flexible and comprehensive to cover the variety of uses and disclosures that must be addressed. HHS may impose penalties of $100 per failure to comply with a Privacy Rule requirement, not to exceed $25,000 per year for multiple violations. The Security Rule operationalizes the protections contained in the Privacy Rule by addressing the technical and non-technical safeguards that organizations called 'covered entities' must put in place to secure individuals' electronic protected health information (e-PHI)" (Health and Human Services Department, 2011).*

Both of these rules have revolutionized the way healthcare is delivered for providers, patients, payers and for a myriad of firms whose sole businesses are consulting, developing and selling solutions to these requirements.

The Health Information Technology for Economic and Clinical Health Act (the HITECH Act) of 2009 (as part of the American Recovery and Reinvestment Act of 2009) allocated $27 billion over ten years to support adoption of electronic medical records (EMR) and provides payments to doctors and hospitals when they adopt EMRs and demonstrate that their use of EMRs improves the quality, safety and effectiveness of patient care. Included in the program are provisions to improve security and privacy of the records (CMS, 2009).

The U.S. government now mandates that all health care providers use a unique identifier, the National Provider Identifier (NPI). This includes all covered entities such as health plans and health care clearinghouses and the number must be used for all administrative and financial transactions adopted under HIPAA (CMS, 2011). This is another system designed to protect both providers and patients from unauthorized sharing of confidential information.

Individual hospitals, healthcare systems, and practices also have developed safeguards and methods of communicating with their patients. For example, Kansas State University now has an employee code of ethics that all must agree to sign, with the understanding that violation of the agreement may result in disciplinary action which could include dismissal and legal action. Some salient points include: "I will take reasonable precautions to prevent unauthorized access to passwords, user identifications, or other information; I will limit access to information contained in the systems to only authorized people . . . I will not share, record, copy, transmit, delete or in any way alter information in these systems except when required to perform my duties . . ." (Kansas State Information Technology Employee Code of Ethics).

The American College of Healthcare Executives has adopted a policy position that "in addition to following all applicable state laws and HIPAA, healthcare executives have a moral and professional obligation to respect confidentiality and protect the security of patients' medical records. As patient advocates, executives must ensure their organization obtains proper patient authorization to release information or follow carefully defined policies and applicable laws in those cases for which the release of information without consent is indicated" (Board of Governors of the American College of Healthcare Executives, 2009).

The AMA's Code of Ethics clearly outlines systems that should be in place to protect the confidentiality of patient records and the use of computers and medical data stored in these computers and EMRs. (AMA Opinion 5.07 Confidentiality: Computers). It also has clearly defined standards for the use of email.

The AMA code also states that:

"Dedication to upholding trust in the patient-physician relationship, to

preventing harms to patients, and to respecting patients' privacy and autonomy create responsibilities for individual physicians, medical practices and health care institutions when patient information is inappropriately disclosed. When there is reason to believe that patients' confidentiality has been compromised by a breach of the electronic medical record, physicians should:

- *Ensure that patients are promptly informed about the breach and potential for harm, either by disclosing directly (when the physician has administrative responsibility for the EMR), participating in efforts by the practice or health care institution to disclose . . .*
- *Follow ethically appropriate procedures for disclosure . . . including describing what information was breached; how the breach happened; what the consequences may be; what corrective actions have been taken...and what steps patients themselves might take to minimize adverse consequences . . ." (AMA Opinion 5.10).*

The potential for breach of confidentiality, fraud and misuse of private information is growing exponentially along with the ease of use and acceptance of IT in everyday life. In 2011, UCLA Health System agreed to pay $865,500 as part of a settlement with federal regulators when hospital employees reviewed celebrity patient medical records without authorization. The US Department of Health and Human Services Office for Civil Rights found violations of HIPAA that included UCLA employees 'repeatedly and without a permissible reason' examined private electronic medical records of dozens of celebrities. Several employees were also fired and suspended (*L.A. Times,* 2011).

The use of IT is a world-wide phenomenon and Hongladarom and Ess (2007) believe that there are global implications for rules of intellectual property and that this perspective must be considered, especially in inter-cultural areas. Corporate IT ethics policies should be communicated clearly to all global partners.

8.8. LIMITED RESOURCES

Not having enough products or services to supply expectant customers can have a disastrous effect on a company's business. Demand exceeding supply may ruin current profits and curtail future growth. Similar issues arise in healthcare.

As healthcare costs continue to rise, government officials, politicians and most Americans have concerns about the system's ability to maintain support for funding programs already in existence, let alone future expansions. Limiting access and services may be fiscally responsible when attempting to balance budgets and woo voters, but presents equally compelling concerns such as rationing, quality of care and patients' right to care. If healthcare providers determine what tests, procedures, medications and treatments are necessary for the benefit of the patient, and all of these choices have attending costs associated with them; how then does this balance the conflicting rights of a provider to provide the best possible (and obviously most appropriate, evidence-based) care against the bottom-line only insurance authorization agent?

Most health care providers readily understand and agree with the concept of triage, meant to ensure that the sickest patients, who need immediate care, are taken care of first. This prioritizing of needs works well in the emergency room and on the battle field and helped to develop a national system to allocate organs for transplants. But as evidenced by the absence of agreement about every health care reform plan that has been proposed over the last several decades, the public may say it wants fairness and economic frugality for others in the system, but not when it applies to them as individuals. While there is no guaranteed 'right to health care' in the Constitution, allocation of limited and expensive health resources is now an integral part of health policy decisions. For example, in 1998, Oregon began a plan to rank Medicaid patients' medical procedures according to cost/benefit ratios—and reimburse accordingly. This was part of a cost savings strategy to enroll more Oregonians in the state health plan but was ultimately abandoned as too subjective (Jonsen, 1998; Fruits, 2010).

Some newer models evaluate allocation principles and suggest they be classified into four categories:

> *"treating people equally, favoring the worst-off, maximizing total benefits, and promoting and regarding social usefulness. No single principle is sufficient to incorporate all morally relevant considerations and therefore individual principles must be combined . . . recommend an alternative system which prioritizes younger people who have not yet lived a complete life, and also incorporates prognosis, saves the most lives, lottery and instrumental value principles" (Persad et al., 2009, p. 423).*

While intellectually satisfying, this model brings up many ethical concerns, including but not limited to fairness, justice and autonomy.

The American Medical Association's Code of Medical Ethics addresses financial barriers to health access in the following statements:

> *"Health care is a fundamental human good because it affects our opportunity to pursue life goals, reduces our pain and suffering, helps prevent premature loss of life, and provides information needed to plan for our lives. As professionals, physicians individually and collectively*

have an ethical responsibility to ensure that all persons have access to needed care regardless of their economic means. In view of this obligation:

- *Individual physicians should take steps to promote access to care for individual patients.*
- *Individual physicians should help patients obtain needed care through public or charitable programs when patients cannot do so themselves.*
- *Physicians, individually and collectively through their professional organizations and institutions, should participate in the political process as advocates for patients (or support those who do) so as to diminish financial obstacles to access health care.*
- *The medical profession must work to ensure that societal decisions about the distribution of health resources safeguard the interests of all patients and promote access to health records.*
- *All stakeholders in health care, including physicians, health facilities, health insurers, professional medical societies, and public policymakers must work together to ensure sufficient access to appropriate health care for all people" (AMA Medical Code of Ethics Opinion 9.0651).*

Critical care professionals were asked by survey in 1994 about their attitudes about rationing, as noted by Bloomfield, "The results of the study showed that quality of life of the patient, the probability of surviving, whether the acute illness could be reversed or not and the nature of a chronic disease all played a role in the provider's mind as to whether resources could be distributed fairly. Economic background of the patient did not play a role in this decision" (Bloomfield, 2009).

8.9. MANAGED CARE/THIRD PARTY PAYERS/BILLING AND COLLECTIONS

Payment is a requirement of services provided in all businesses, and the complicated relationship between patients, providers and third party payers/insurance companies is no exception.

If a health care professional's primary obligation is to his or her patients, then interactions with insurance companies and managed care organizations (MCO) may present ethical dilemmas related to issues such as denial of care, postponement of care, choice of medications/treatment and even provider choice. Terminology determined by business, which substitutes customer/client for patient and provider for health care professional, further blur the distinction between a financial transaction and appropriate patient care and stress competing interests.

Decisions regarding reimbursement may be made by non-healthcare professionals, widening the gap between those who deliver the care and those who say how it should be delivered (at least what will be paid for). Professional organizations may not help, "although physicians have an obligation to consider the needs of broader patient populations within the context of the patient-physician relationship, their first duty must be to the individual patient. This obligation must override considerations of the reimbursement mechanism or specific financial incentives applied to a physician's clinical practice." (AMA Code of Medical Ethics, Opinion 8.054, 2002). The American College of Physician's Ethics Manual goes so far as to state, "Whether financial incentives in the fee-for-service system prompt physicians to do more rather than less or capitation arrangements encourage them to do less rather than more, physicians must not allow such considerations to affect their clinical judgment or patient counseling on treatment options, including referrals" (ACP Ethics Manual, Sixth Edition).

The disruption of the patient-provider relationship may now be determined by reimbursement issues, rather than patient choice. Because managed care companies usually only pay for care provided by providers within their systems, patients may be forced to change providers if they wish their care to be covered by their insurance. Preferred provider groups will only reimburse fully to providers within their network, necessitating patients to 'pay extra' to continue to use an out-of network provider. Employers may change health plans offered to employees, employees may change jobs, and many MCOs require gatekeepers to specialists, all which can mean the loss of provider access.

Hospitals typically bill insured patients at a discounted or negotiated rate, but those who are uninsured or out of network are usually charged a much higher multiple of that rate (Hall and Schneider, 2008).

In Darragh and McCarrick's "Managed Health Care: New Ethical Issues for All" article (*Kennedy Institute of Ethics Journal,* 1996), they present a literature review compiled during the early years of the Clinton administration's attempt at health care reform and provide a basis for understanding why these concerns are still with us in the United States in 2011. "These cost-containment features now play an intimate role in clinical practice. When a managed care plan contracts with a physician, the doctor becomes a 'double agent' with contractual obligations to the plan to provide a preset amount of services and professional responsibilities to each patient to authorize necessary treatment" (Darragh and McCarrick, 1996).

The American Medical Association's statement concerning managed care states that:

"The expansion of managed care has brought a variety of changes to medicine including new and different reimbursement systems for physicians with complex referral restrictions and benefits packages for patients. Some of these changes have raised concerns that a physician's ability to practice ethical medicine will be adversely affected by the modifications in the system . . . the following points were developed . . .

- *"The duty of patient advocacy is a fundamental element of the patient-physician relationship that should not be altered by the system of health care delivery. Physicians must continue to place the interests of their patients first.*
- *When health care plans place restrictions on the care that physicians in the plan may provide to their patients . . . physicians must advocate for any care they believe will materially benefit their patients . . .*
- *When physicians are employed or reimbursed by health care plans that offer financial incentives to limit care, serious potential conflicts are created between the physicians' personal financial interests and the needs of their patients. Efforts to contain health care costs should not place patient welfare at risk . . .*
- *Physicians should encourage both that patients be aware of the benefits and limitations of their health care coverage and that they exercise their autonomy by public participation in the formulation of benefits packages and by prudent selection of health care coverage that best suits their needs" (AMA Medical Code of Ethics Opinion 8.13).*

For those who have no insurance, either by choice or not, the situation is often grim, yet affects even those who are covered. Rising insurance premiums, onerous labor contracts, and the exponentially rising costs associated with healthcare are some of the results of a system that must account for these millions of Americans. One example of the results of these escalating costs is described in a 2011 Wall Street Journal article (Anand, 2008) about Mennonites and Amish who believe that it is the religious duty of their community to provide care for each other when they are ill and consequently have never purchased any form of health insurance. However, as many of the children in these communities now suffer from genetic diseases (because of low rates of marriage to those outside these small communities), families are turning to the secular world's high-tech hospitals to provide care now available for hereditary diseases. While many healthcare systems offer some sort of charity care, which they must provide in order to receive tax subsidies from the government, the resulting bills can be astronomical and are a burden not only the patients, but the hospitals who must try to recover their costs. One of the hospitals in the article, Hershey Medical Center, said in a statement that "If a party chooses not to apply for medical assistance after we have counseled them and made the recommendation that they apply, they cannot be considered for charity care." (Anand, 2008).

The responsibility and understanding of what is covered/reimbursed (and what isn't) is not easily resolved, either for the patient or the providers who need to maximize their practices' profits. Authors Hall and Schneider suggest that physicians must decide between two different models of professionalism: "the transactional model which compares medical care to any other business transaction where payment is expected for services rendered, and the relational model which emphasizes the physician-patient relationship and discourages maximizing profit from this association" (Hall and Schneider, 2008).

Financial incentives for physicians are addressed by the AMA under their Code of Ethics. This opinion offers the following guidance:

- *"Although physicians have an obligation to consider the needs of broader patient populations within the context of the patient-physician relationship, their first duty must be to the individual patient. This obligation must override consideration of the reimbursement mechanism or specific financial incentives applied to a physician's clinical practice.*
- *Physicians, individually or through their representatives, should evaluate the financial incentives associated with participation in a health plan before contracting with that plan. The purpose of the evaluation is to ensure that the quality of patient care is not compromised by unrealistic expectations for utilization or by placing that physician's payments for care at excessive risk . . .*
- *Physicians also should advocate for incentives that promote efficient practice, but are not designed to realize cost savings beyond those attainable through efficiency . . .*
- *Patients must be informed of financial incentives that could impact the level or type of care they receive. Although this responsibility should be assumed by the health plan, physicians, individually or through their representatives, must be prepared to discuss with patients any financial arrangements that could impact patient care. Physicians should avoid reimbursement systems that, if disclosed to patients, could negatively affect the patient-physician relationship" (AMA Medical Code of Ethics Opinion 8.054).*

Similarly, the American College of Physicians' Center for Ethics and Professionalism, along with the Harvard Pilgrim Health Care Ethics Program and a sixteen member group of stakeholders, developed a statement of ethical principles; some of the points are:

- *Health plans, purchasers, clinicians and patients should be open and truthful in their dealings with each other;*

- *Health plans, purchasers, clinicians and patients should recognize and support the intimacy and importance of patient-clinician relationships and the ethical obligations of clinicians to patients;*
- *Resource allocation policy should be made through an open and participatory process;*
- *Clinicians have a responsibility to practice effective and efficient health care and to use health care resources responsibly;*
- *Health plans should engage purchasers in a discussion about what health care needs can reasonably be met, given a particular level of premium, and should explain the reasoning behind their coverage, exclusion, and cost determinations;*
- *Patients should have a basic understanding of the rules of their insurance;*
- *Health plans and health care organizations should not ask clinicians to participate in arrangements that jeopardize professional ethical standards. (Povar, 2004).*

8.10. MARKETING

Marketing is more than advertising—it is the entire spectrum of tools used to influence 'customers' to buy something, either a product or a service. Often considered pejoratively, it can be viewed as merely a basic communication tool necessary to provide essential information.

In the not so distant past, marketing of medical services was relegated to specialty journals rarely seen by the public. In *Goldfarb vs. Virginia State Bar*, the Supreme Court ruled that antitrust laws applied to professions and that restrictions on advertising by groups such as the American Medical Association were considered to unfairly restrict competition (Nisselson, 2008) Now, however, it is rare to not be bombarded by marketing campaigns known as direct-to-consumer advertising (DTCA) for hospitals, individual physicians, medications and insurance plans on television, billboards, Facebook and lay magazines.

There are a multitude of government agencies which are charged with protecting the public from unethical and/or false marketing claims. The Federal Trade Commission (FTC) and individual state agencies have responsibility for oversight of general marketing practices and for determining whether an advertisement is false, deceptive or misleading and for taking action against the advertiser. "Companies must support health advertising claims with solid proof. This is especially true for businesses that market food, over-the-counter drugs, dietary supplements, contact lenses, and other health-related products" (Federal Trade Commission, 2011).

The Food and Drug Administration (FDA) has responsibility for the safety of food and drug products and requires that "product claim ads give a fair balance of information about drug risks as compared with information about drug benefits" (FDA, 2011) Direct to consumer advertising began in the 1980s when drug companies began to provide consumers more information about their products instead of only to doctors and pharmacists. The FDA, under the Federal Food, Drug and Cosmetic Act, requires that advertisements for prescription drugs be accurate and not misleading. (FDA, 2011)

The Federal Communications Commission (FCC) regulates broadcast advertisements and "unless a broadcast advertisement is found to be in violation of a specific law or rule, the government cannot take action against it" (FCC, 2011). Consumers are advised, "depending on the nature of the advertisement, the appropriate agency should be contacted regarding advertisements that one believes may be false or misleading."

Misstating claims about the benefits of a product may not only be unethical, but may also be illegal. Weight loss products often overstate their success rates, or hide them in small print disclaimers or by using ambiguous language. Using sexual content and/or advertising products that could be seen as leading to promiscuous behavior such as condoms, birth control methods or sexual dysfunction medications, may be considered unethical to some consumers.

Because of the increasing scope of new unregulated media venues, many professional groups have developed their own ethical standards. The American Marketing Association's Statement of Ethics asks its members to be:

> *"honest (offer products that do what they claim they do in communications and honor all commitments), responsible (serve the needs of customers without using coercion), fair (refuse to engage in price fixing, predatory pricing or bait and switch tactics while keeping customer information private), respectful (avoid stereotyping while acknowledging the basic human dignity of customers), transparent (communicate openly and clearly and explain all risks) and be good citizens (fulfill economic, legal, and societal responsibilities)" (American Marketing Association Statement of Ethics, 1998).*

The American Medical Association's policy on advertising and publicity offers several key insights into healthcare marketing:

- *"A physician may publicize him or herself as a physician through any commercial publicity or other form of public communication...provided that the communication shall not be misleading because of the omission of necessary material information, shall not contain any false or misleading statement, or shall not otherwise operate to deceive.*

- *Because the public can sometimes be deceived by the use of medical terms or illustrations that are difficult to understand, physicians should design the form of communication to communicate . . . in a readily comprehensive manner. Aggressive, high-pressure advertising and publicity should be avoided if they create unjustified medical expectations or are accompanied by deceptive claims.*
- *. . . for example, testimonials of patients as to the physician's skill or the quality of the physician's professional services tend to be deceptive when they do not reflect the results that patients with conditions comparable to the testimoniant's condition generally receive.*
- *Because physicians have an ethical obligation to share medical advances, it is unlikely that a physician will have a truly exclusive or unique skill or remedy. Claims that imply such a skill or remedy therefore can be deceptive" (AMA Medical Code of Ethics Opinion 5.02—Advertising and Publicity).*

The American Psychological Association developed a code of ethics in 2002 which says that the advertisements of psychologists should not be false, deceptive or misleading about either their services or their fees (American Psychological Association, 2002).

The American Dental Association (ADA) Code Section 5.F, states that:

> *"Although any dentist may advertise, no dentist shall advertise or solicit patients in any form of communication in a manner that is false or misleading in any material respect . . . Advertising, solicitation of patients or business or other promotional activities by dentists or dental care delivery organizations shall not be considered unethical or improper, except for those promotional activities which are false or misleading in any material respect. . . . This shall be the sole standard for determining the ethical propriety of such professional activities" (American Dental Association, 2005).*

Patients with chronic pain are particularly affected by remedies offered by DCTA and may expect unrealistic results based on pharmaceutical and practitioner marketing strategies. Failure to note side-effects or the risk/benefit of treatments led the American Academy of Pain Medicine Ethics Council to develop standards which stress the need to "improve accountability for false or misleading advertising of pain treatments" (Taylor, 2011).

The American Society for Aesthetic Plastic Surgery (ASAPS) and the American Society of Plastic Surgeons (ASPS) developed a code of ethics partly in response to the increasing competition and numbers of physicians who perform elective cosmetic procedures and who rely on patient testimonials, patient (or model) images, and web/internet advertising in order to attract clients. The code specific to advertising stresses that members of the societies should not "deceive or mislead patients with their credentials, photographs, statements or testimonials." (Wong, 2010, p. 737). Practices prohibited by the ASAPS include: "promotional use of before and after photographs that use different lighting, poses or photographic techniques to misrepresent results, and exaggerated claims intended to create false or unjustified expectations of favorable surgical results" (ASAPS, 2000).

All of these marketing codes of ethics reflect the basic principles of respect for patient autonomy and nonmaleficence, as any attempts to recruit patients must not misrepresent the value of a service offered and must always consider how the average person/patient might interpret the information. Any offensive material, whether by using stereotypes or that is demeaning to a specific demographic or that targets vulnerable populations such as children, the elderly, and developing countries' consumers, is clearly in conflict with the ethical mores and should be avoided.

In the United States, one of the most controversial and continuing ethical issues is regarding marketing of the legally available known carcinogen—cigarettes. All cigarette and tobacco advertising was banned on television and radio in the early 1970s as a public health initiative by the FCC (The Public Health Cigarette Smoking Act). Warnings from the Surgeon General must be included now on any advertisements and on all packaging. The Family Smoking Prevention and Tobacco Control Act of 2010 prohibits cigarette companies from sponsoring any athletic or cultural events or using their logos on items of clothing. In 2011, new graphic images depicting the effects of smoking were required to be placed on all packaging (FCC, 2011).

8.11. RISK MANAGEMENT

Risk entails a potential loss as a result of an action and applies to all aspects of life. Managing that risk is important to the financial health of a business, just as it is important to the physical health of patients and their care providers.

Risk management in corporations may involve 'managing' ethics in the workplace through policies and procedures designed to educate, reinforce, and regulate acceptable and non-acceptable behaviors. "The very exercise of developing a code is in itself worthwhile; it forces a large number of people to think through, in a fresh way, their mission and the important obligations they, as a group and as individuals, have with respect to society as a whole." (DeGeorge, 1994). All risk management programs are undertaken because corporations wish to minimize any negative effects on their bottom line, either by purposeful or accidental losses of their products, reputation, market share or income. In the light of several well-known scandals such as Enron, Tyco, AIG and Arthur Anderson, the public (specifically customers and stakeholders) is now very much aware that corporations must integrate and enforce codes of ethics as they determine what levels of risk are acceptable.

The Caux Round Table (CRT), an international consortium of business leaders whose goal is to promote ethical business practices in global society, suggests that there are seven ethical risk principles relating to customers, employees, stakeholders, owners, suppliers, competitors and the public that should be considered in a risk management strategy, including: "civil law, criminal law, stakeholder specification, customer obligations, fairness, social values, and consequences" (Young, 2004, pp. 27–28). By answering questions and outlining possible scenarios in each of these categories, a framework for ethical corporate responsibility can be developed and used as a standard for all communities of interest.

Internal and external audits for financial reporting (Institute of Internal Auditors (IIA) Code of Ethics, 1988) are two of the main resources used in a risk management program, yet alone they do not address the underlying reasons such audits are necessary and legally required. A company must analyze all types of risks involving individual employees, management, board directors, investors, customers, and competitors—everything that concerns corporate legal compliance. The U.S. Sentencing Commission in 2005 amended its guidelines to require companies to expand their programs to include "compliance and ethics as a means to prevent and detect criminal conduct and foster an organizational culture that encourages ethical conduct and a commitment to legal compliance" (Federal Sentencing Guidelines Manual and Appendices, United States Sentencing Commission, effective 1 November 2005). This emphasis on organizational culture and corporate responsibility implies that compliance and ethics must be pervasive in a company, from top management on down.

"A typical ethics and compliance process may include an initial definition of ethics and compliance risk, the prevention of failures or lapses, the detection of noncompliance, the response to violations/allegations, and an evaluation and continuous improvement process" (LRN/Ethics and compliance risk management, 2007, p. 3).

Risks associated with compliance violations and ethics may include:

- *"accounting breakdowns including fraud, inaccurate record keeping, inappropriate record retention or destruction and noncompliance with the requirements of Sarbanes-Oxley;*
- *Business ethics failures, such as the exposure of confidential client information, conflicts of interest and giving and receiving inappropriate gifts;*
- *Employment related risks such as equal opportunity violations, workplace harassment and immigration offenses;*
- *Fair trading laws, which cover price fixing, abuse of dominance and collusion;*
- *Customer and workplace violations; for example, aiding and abetting illegal customer acts and creating unsafe workplace conditions and;*
- *Product issues such as product safety failures and intellectual property violations" (LRN/Ethics and compliance risk management, 2007, p.3).*

Public perception of a company's reputation is also a risk which may affect a company's performance and is now influenced by an ever growing world of twenty-four hour live communication channels. Public relations professionals who are specialists in handling the fall-out of bad publicity are now plentiful and are frequently employed by firms wishing to minimize the risk of financial damage resulting from a change in public opinion.

Risk management that is solely focused on legal compliance and requirements will not be effective unless there is an underlying culture that encourages ethical behavior through continuing education and support systems, while clearly and consistently enforcing code violations.

8.12. STAKEHOLDER ISSUES

In the broadest sense, a stakeholder is a constituent who can be affected by an organization's actions, while shareholders are those who own stock in a company. Healthcare stakeholders range from patients to the largest healthcare systems/hospitals and everything in between.

There are many different stakeholders and stakeholder groups in business and all are important, even those without a financial impact on the organization. Stakeholders differ from shareholders because, in theory, a corporation's responsibility to its shareholders is purely fiduciary, while the responsibility to stakeholders goes beyond financial responsibility. Stakeholders may include investors, employees, suppliers, customers, and also prospective employees and customers, trade associations, government bodies, competitors, the environment and the public. As explained by Grunig and Repper, the public differs from stakeholders because publics arise around issues and stakeholders are 'connected to the organization by consequences" (Grunig, 1992, pp. 171-57). As noted by Collins, ". . . the actions of individuals within the health care industry impact more than just the stockholders of the organization. In health care organizations, errors in management strategies and poor leadership decisions can impact all stakeholders and shareholders alike. This is mainly due to the fact that unlike most other industries, those in the health care industry understand that their actions could potentially create life-threatening consequences" (Collins, 2010, p. 343).

Research by Bowen demonstrates that many organizations showed "a preference for legalistic codes of ethics and governance documents seemed to pervade all but the most exemplary organizations in this sample." (Bowen, 2010). R. Edward Freeman (1984) suggests an idea of 'stakeholder theory' which states that a corporation/business firm should be managed in a way that achieves balance among the interests of everyone who bears a substantial relationship to the firm, i.e., its stakeholders. In one of his many lectures for the Darden School of Business's Business Roundtable Institute for Corporate Ethics, Freeman said, "Stakeholder theory says if you just focus on financiers, you miss what makes capitalism tick. What makes capitalism tick is that shareholders and financiers, customers, suppliers, employees, communities can together create something that no one of them can create alone" (Freeman, 2009).

Section 406 of the Sarbanes-Oxley Act of 2002 mandates that top officers in an organization have a code of ethics and defines a code of ethics as "standards as are reasonably necessary to promote honest and ethical conduct, including the ethical handling of actual or apparent conflict of interest between personal and professional relationships; full, fair, accurate, timely, and understandable disclosure in the periodic reports required to be filed by the issuer; and compliance with applicable governmental rules and regulations" (http://www.gpo.gov/fdsys/pkg/PLAW-107publ204/html/PLAW-107publ204.htm). Enactment of Sarbanes-Oxley has also motivated companies to put in place (and make public) policies and procedures that address ethical issues, not only for their employees, but for all stakeholders. Similarly, professional organizations are incorporating ethical behavior guidelines regarding stakeholders/shareholders into their codes of conduct (Association of Chartered Certified Accounts, 2007).

The 2010 Dodd-Frank act, put in place after the 2008 financial crisis, requires publicly held companies to give shareholders a 'say on pay' about executive compensation. In 2011, of 2,532 companies reporting, "shareholders at 39 of them rejected executive pay plans" (WSJ, July 8, 2011, B1), perhaps suggesting that excessive executive compensation may not meet the ethical standards of fair pay to company shareholders.

This emphasis on shareholder value being affected by ethics is not just occurring in the United States. Globalization and corporate social responsibility is now the norm in multi-national corporations. Archie Carroll has developed a pyramid framework for global institutions that states:

- *"Make a profit consistent expectations for international businesses (economic responsibility);*
- *Obey the law of host countries as well as international law (legal responsibility);*
- *Be ethical in its practices, taking host country and global standards into consideration (ethical responsibility); and*
- *Be a good corporate citizen, especially as defined by the host country's expectations (philanthropic responsibility)." (Carroll, 2004, p. 118)*

Corporate social responsibility may be initiated by stakeholders/shareholders rather than the 'conscience' of management, who may urge companies to 'do the right thing', but studies and surveys have shown that customers' purchasing decisions are increasingly influenced by the ethical conduct of the company and companies are listening (Kanovich, 2007).

8.13. TRANSPARENCY

Transparency in healthcare and business may take various forms, from publishing results of specific studies in the lay press, to detailing specific political background of supporters, to making financial reporting more readily accessible.

Beyond legal requirements, many companies now realize the benefits of providing the public clear statements of their ethical values and social responsibility (Bernard and Lacrosse, 2005; Jacobs, Cerfolio and Sade, 2009). Ernst and Young, the accounting firm, has a general section on their website about its corporate 'values' which says that it employs:

> *"People who demonstrate integrity, respect, and teaming. People with energy, enthusiasm, and the courage to lead. People who build relationships based on doing the right thing. Our values define who we are. They are the fundamental beliefs of our global organization. They guide our actions and behavior. They influence the way we work with each other—and the way we serve our clients and engage with our communities. Every day, each one of us makes choices and decisions that directly affect the way we experience each other and the way our clients and wider communities experience us. Our values give us confidence that we are using the same principles to help us make these decisions—throughout our global organization" (Ernst and Young Corporate Values, 2011).*

Merck pharmaceutical firm posts a more specific version of a code of conduct on its corporate website:

> *"Our chief compliance officer, who reports directly to the CEO, is responsible for ensuring high ethical standards and compliance across our business globally. This includes: making sure that the company complies with all applicable laws and regulations; through Merck's Office of Ethics, reinforcing the company's overall commitment to ethical business practices and behavior; and safeguarding individual privacy expectations through oversight of our global privacy program. Our Office of Ethics supports our commitment to the highest standards of ethics and integrity in all of our business practices. . . . We have taken significant steps recently to improve transparency, committing to public disclosure of our financial support for third-party groups and for healthcare providers who speak on behalf of Merck or our products . . ." (Merck Corporate Responsibility, 2011).*

The Commonwealth Foundation published a report in 2006 that said, "Transparency and better public information on cost and quality are essential for three reasons: (1) to help providers improve by benchmarking their performance against others; (2) to encourage private insurers and public programs to reward quality and efficiency; and (3) to help patients make informed choices about their care." The authors believe that to achieve transparency in our health system, the following steps should be taken:

- *"Medicare can assume a leadership role in making cost and quality information by provider and by patient condition publicly available...*
- *Create a National Quality Coordination Board within the U.S. Department of Health and Human Services, as the Institute of Medicine has recommended. The board will set priorities, oversee the development*

of appropriate quality and efficiency measures, ensure the collection of timely and accurate information on these measures at the individual provider level, and encourage their incorporation in pay-for-performance payment systems operated by Medicare, Medicaid, and private insurers.

- *Invest in health information technology . . .*
- *Make fundamental changes in current payment methods . . .*
- *Modify HSA legislation to reduce its potentially harmful effects on vulnerable populations . . ." (Commonwealth Fund, 2006).*

The federal government and individual states now publish specific hospital data on such measures as risk-adjusted mortality and morbidity, complication rates, specific rates for individual physicians, etc. In 2010, Health and Human Services in 2010 began an initiative, the Community Health Data Initiative (CHDI), which will provide free government health data directly to the public. Their mission is to "(1) raise awareness of community health performance, (2) increase pressure on decision makers to improve performance, and (3) help facilitate and inform action to improve performance." (HHS, 2010).

"This data set will consist of hundreds (ultimately, thousands) of measures of health care quality, cost, access and public health (e.g., obesity rates, smoking rates, etc.), including data produced for the Community Health Status Indicators, County Health Rankings, and State of the USA programs. It will include a major contribution of new national, state, regional, and potentially county-level Medicare prevalence of disease, quality, cost, and utilization data from the Centers for Medicare and Medicaid Services (CMS), never previously published, as well as data for measures tracked by Healthy People 2020. And it will include information on evidence-based programs and policies that have successfully improved community performance across many of these measures" (HHS, 2010).

This is all done in an effort to be more transparent to the public about publicly spent healthcare dollars.

Perhaps nothing could be more 'transparent' in the healthcare professions, than admitting to medical errors. Ethically sound, but fraught with concerns about malpractice, any admission of guilt has long been considered an unwise decision. However, in a study published in the Annals of Internal Medicine in 2010, a study was conducted of the University of Michigan Health System (UMHS), which began to fully disclose and offer compensation to patients for medical errors in 2001. The purpose of the study was to compare liability claims and costs before and after the new program—in other words, whether or not it cost more to 'do the right thing.' The results showed that rates of claims and lawsuits actually decreased, leading the authors to conclude that "the UMHS implemented a program of full disclosure of medical errors with offers of compensation without increasing its total claims and liability costs." (Kachalia, 2010).

8.14. CASE STUDIES

1. One of your patients with difficult to control hypertension has responded well to some drug samples for a new beta blocker that you gave him. You write him a prescription for the medication and are told by your office staff later that week, that the patient has called and told them that his insurance plan only covers the generic version of the drug. How should you handle the patient's request for the brand name drug? What if you believe there is no difference in efficacy? What if you believe there is reason to prescribe the brand name but it is far more expensive? What effects do requests such as these have on the health care system? Should you have used drug samples in the first place? Is it your responsibility, the managed care company's, the pharmaceutical firm's or the government's to determine what is in a patient's best interest, regardless of cost?
2. An undocumented, uninsured migrant worker is brought into the emergency room of a local community hospital with shortness of breath and chest pain. He was admitted to the hospital for evaluation and testing. Further exams showed congestive heart disease and severe atrial regurgitation. It is determined that the patient requires a valve replacement. Without being eligible for Medicaid because of his immigration status, and no way to pay for this expensive operation, what is your responsibility as a health care provider? What is the hospital's responsibility? How involved should the patient be in the decision making process? Do the principles of justice and beneficence hold here? Are there justifiable limits to the amount of care provided? What about allocation of scarce resources?
3. Mrs. X was at her annual gynecological exam with her nurse practitioner, Dr. Jones. Mrs. X is a healthy 45 year old who doesn't smoke, exercises regularly, and maintains her weight through good nutrition. All age appropriate and recommended screening tests have been negative in the past. Today she states that a new imaging center has opened up in her neighborhood and they are advertising a whole body CT scan. She asks Dr.

Jones to prescribe this for her, 'just in case' there's a problem that could only be seen by the scan. What is Dr. Jones responsibility to the patient? To the patient's insurance company? What ethical principles are at stake here or in any case when a patient requests a test or procedure that is not medically indicated? Is the imaging center utilizing ethical marketing practices by going directly to the consumer and implying there is a need for their product? Are patients entitled to expensive diagnostic procedures?

4. You have been invited by a pharmaceutical company to lead an informal discussion about high blood pressure, particularly in post-menopausal women. The discussion will be held in a restaurant and will be hosted by the company. There will be as many as twenty nurse practitioners attending, all with prescriptive privileges in your state. The pharmaceutical company sells a new and very expensive prescription product for reducing blood pressure. You are offered $500 to help recruit attendees and to lead the discussion. What ethical issues are involved? Are there any legal or professional concerns? Would you be more likely to prescribe this company's medication rather than another's or over lifestyle changes? If you sign a contract with a drug company to help recruit participants and lead an informal discussion, are you required to disclose this to your current employer's conflict of interest policy?

5. A patient of yours is experiencing premature ejaculation and has asked for your help. The anti-depressant medication sertraline (Zoloft) is commonly prescribed to treat this condition. The patient's insurance plan will pay for Zoloft only for treatment of depression. You wonder whether it is 'insurance fraud' to help the patient have the cost of his medication covered by his insurance company, by prescribing Zoloft for depression instead of for premature ejaculation treatment. What other issues might be involved? If you proceed with ordering the Zoloft, how would you chart/justify the reasons for doing so? Is this a legal issue? Would/should you involve the patient in the decision?

6. Your practice sees a mix of Medicare, Medicaid and privately insured patients. Over the past year, reimbursements from all these sources have been steadily declining and you are now forced with a choice: lay off two of your long-time front office/ billers who are the main source of income for their families or stop taking insurance altogether. You know that if you do stop taking insurance, you will lose many of your patients because

they will not be able to afford your new charges. What are the main ethical dilemmas presented by this case?

8.15. REFERENCES

Introduction

Marcinko, D. (Ed.) (2005) *The Business of Medical Practice: Advanced Profit Maximization Techniques for Savvy Doctors, 2nd Edition.* Springer Publishing Company.

Accounting

AICPA Code of Professional Conduct. (1988) Jersey City, NJ: American Institute of Certified Public Accountants.

AICPA Committee on Terminology. (1953) *Accounting Terminology Bulletin No. 1,* Review and Resume.

Alexander, D, Burns, G., Manor, R., McRoberts, F., and Torriero, E.A. (2002) The fall of Anderson. *Hartford Courant.* http://www.courant.com/news/nationworld/chi-0209010315sep01,0,2343149.story.

Dellaportas, S. (2006) Making a difference with a discrete course on accounting ethics. *Journal of Business Ethics, 65*: 391-404. DOI 10.1007/s10551-006-0020-7

Duska, R. and Duska, B. (2003) *Accounting Ethics.* Wiley-Blackwell, p. 28. ISBN 0-631-21651-0. http://books.google.com/?id=Y4LgynCsC&printsec=frontcover&dq=Understanding+Accounting+Ethics.

Institute of Internal Auditors. (1988) IIA Code of Ethics. Altamonte Springs, FL: Institute of Internal Auditors.

Institute of Management Accounts. (1997) Statements on Management Accounting: Objectives of Management Accounting, Statement No. 1B. New York, NY: Institute of Management Accounts.

Jackling, B., Cooper, B., Leung, P., and Dellaportas, S. (2007) Professional accounting bodies: perceptions of ethical issues, causes of ethical failure and ethics education. *Managerial Auditing Journal 22*(9): 928-944. Doi:10.1108/02686900710829426. http://proquest.umi.com.libproxy.sdsu.edu/pqdweb: did=1347117971&sid=1&Fmt=3&clientId-17862&RQT=309&VName+PQD.

Loeb, S. (1988) Teaching students accounting ethics: some crucial issues. *Issues in Accounting Education 3*:316–329. http://proquest.umi.com.libproxy.sdsu.edu/pqdweb?did=7569002&sid=1&2Fmt=7&clientId=17862&RQT=309&VName=PQD. Retrieved April 7, 2011.

Loeb, S. (1994) "Ethics and accounting doctoral education." *Journal of Business Ethics, 13*: 817–828.

Sarbanes-Oxley Act of 2002. www.sec.gov/about/laws/soa2002.pdf

Smith, K. and Smith, L. Business and Accounting Ethics, http://acct.tamu.edu/smith/ethics/ethics.htm. Retrieved April 7, 2011.

Somerville, L. (Feb. 28, 2003). Accounting changes boil down to principles vs. rules. *The Business Journal.* http://www.bizjournals.com/triad/stories/2003/03/03/focus2.html. Retrieved April 7, 2011.

Conflict of Interest

AMA Code of Medical Ethics – Opinion 8.03 – Conflicts of Interest: Guidelines http://

www.ama-assn.org/ama/pub/physician-resources/medical-ethics/code-medical-ethics/opinion803.page?

AMA Code of Medical Ethics—Opinion 10.018—Physician Participation in Soliciting Contributions from Patients. http://www.ama-assn.org/ama/pub/physician-resources/medical-ethics/code-medical-ethics/opinion10018.page?

Bernard, R. and Lacrosse, C. (2005) Corporate transparency: code of ethics disclosures. The CPA Journal.

Boston College Fraud Concepts and Business Ethics Red Flags http://www.bc.edu/offices/audit/fraud/redflags.html

Brennan, T.J., Rothman, D.J., *et al.* (2006) Health industry practices that create conflicts of interest: a policy proposal for academic medical centers. *JAMA 295*:429–33.

Campbell, E.G., Weissman J.S., *et.al.* (2007) Institutional academic industry relationahips. *JAMA 298*:1779–86.

Carreyrou, J. (2011) Senators look into Medtronic, doctors. *Wall Street Journal,* June 29, 2011, B1.

Columbia University Conflict of Interest Policy http://www.columbia.edu/cu/compliance/pdfs/COI_Policy.pdf)

Columbia University School of Nursing Conflict of Interest Policy, 2012. CUSON Faculty Handbook, CUSON Intranet.

Lo, B. and Field, M.J. (Eds.). (2009) Conflict of Interest and Medical Research, Education and Practice. Washington (DC): National Academies Press, 2009.

Jacobs, J., Cerfolio, R., and Sade, R. (2009) The ethics of transparency: publication of cardiothoracic surgical outcomes in the lay press. *The Annals of Thoracic Surgery. 87*:679–686.

Technology Transfer: Administration of the Bayh Dole Act by Research Universities. US General Accounting Office report to congressional committees. GAO/RCED-98–126, 1998. www.gao.gov/archive/1998/rc98126.pdf

Fraud

Birkhahn, R., *et al.* (2009) A review of federal guidelines that inform and influence relationships between physicians and industry. *Academic Emergency Medicine 2009: 16*:776–781.

Buppert, C. (2012) Nurse Practitioner's Business Practice and Legal Guide. Sudbury, MA: Jones and Barlett Learning, LLC.

CMS Anti-Kickback https://www.cms.gov/compliance/safe-harbor-regulations

CMS Changes to Disclosure of Physician Ownership in Hospitals and Physician Self-Referral Rules, Federal Register, October 3, 2008 https://www.cms.gov/acuteinpatientpps/ipps/itemdetail.asp?itemid=CMS1227598

CMS Deficit Reduction Act https://www.cms.gov/DeficitReductionAct/Downloads/Checklist1.pdf

CMS False Claims Act https://www.cms.gov/smdl/downloads/SMD032207Att2.pdf

CMS Health Care Fraud Statute https://www.cms.gov/MLNProducts/downloads/Fraud_and_Abuse.pdf

CMS Medicare HIPAA Eligibility https://www.cms.gov/Medicare HIPAA/Eligibility-TransactionSystemInquiriesRulesofBehavior.pdf

CMS Physician Self Referral https://www.cms.gov/PhysicianSelfReferral/01_overview.asp

Mustard, L. (2009) Questionable hospital financial relationships with physicians. *Medical Practice Management,* July/August 2009, pp. 41–43.

Patient Protection and Affordable Care Act, 2010, Public Law 111–148 http://www.gpo.gov/fdsys/pkg/PLAW-111publ148/content-detail.html

Gifts

AMA Medical Code of Ethics Opinion 8.061—Gifts to Physicians from Industry http://www.ama-assn.org/ama/put/physiican-resources/medical-ethics/code-medical-ethics/opinion8061.page?

AMA Medical Code of Ethics Opinion 10.017—Gift from Patients http://www.ama-assn.org/ama/put/physiican-resources/medical-ethics/code-medical-ethics/opinion10017.page?

Brennan, T.J., Rothman, D.J., *et al.* (2006) Health industry practices that create conflicts of interest: a policy proposal for academic medical centers. *JAMA 295*:429–33, 2006.

Columbia University School of Nursing. (2009) Accepting Gifts from Students Policy. CUSON Faculty Handbook, CUSON Intranet.

Mizik, N. (2010) The pharmaceutical industry interactions with physicians: the cost, the ethics, and the patient welfare. Columbia CaseWorks, Columbia Business School, pp. 1–7).

Pharmaceutical Research and Manufacturers of America. (2010) Code on Interactions with Healthcare Professionals. Washington, DC: Pharmaceutical Research and Manufacturers of America; c2010 [Revised 2008 Jun]. http://www/phrma.org/code_on_interactions_with_healthcare_professionals

Yukhananvov, A. (2011) Drugmakers get more time to record gifts to doctors. Reuters, Dec. 14, 2011. http://www.reuters.com/article/2011/12/15/us-cms-sunshine-idUSTRE7BE04N20111215

Human Resources

Eide, P. Introduction to the Human Resources Discipline of Ethics and Sustainability., http://www.shrm.org/hrdisciplines/ethics/Pages/EthicsIntro.aspx)

Lehigh University Code of Ethics. http://www.lehigh.edu/~inhro/code_of_ethics.html

Margolis, J., Grant, A., and Molinsky, A. (2007) Expanding ethical standards of hrm: necessary evils and the multiple dimensions of impact. In: Human Resource Management Ethics and Employment, pp. 237–251. A. Pinninton, R. Macklin and T. Campbell (Eds.). New York: Oxford University Press.

Rose, A. (2007) Ethics and Human Resource Management. McGraw Hill Publishers. http://highered.mcgrawhill.com/sites/dl/free/0077111028/536508/EHR_CO2.pdf))

Sarbanes-Oxley Act of 2002 www.sec.gov/about/laws/soa2002.pdf

Winstanley, D. and Woodall, J. (1996) Business ethics and human resource management. *Personnel Review, 25*(6): 5–12.

Information Technology

AMA Code of Medical Ethics—Opinion 5.07—Confidentiality: Computers http://www.ama-assn.org/ama/put/physician-resources/medical-ethics/code-medical-ethics/opinion507.page?

AMA Code of Medical Ethics—Opinion 5.10—A Physician's Role Following a Breach of Electronic Health Information Mail http://www.ama-assn.org/ama/put/physician-resources/medical-ethics/code-medical-ethics/opinion510.page?

American College of Healthcare Executives http://www.ache.org/policy/hiconf.cfm

Calluzzo, V. and Cante, C. (2004) Ethics in information technology and software use. Journal of Business Ethics, 51: 301–302.

CMS https://www.cms.gov/EHRIncentivePrograms/

HIPAA http://www.cms.gov/NationalProvidentStand/

Hongladarom, S. and Ess, C. (Eds.) (2007) Information Technology Ethics: Cultural Perspectives. Hershey, PA: Idea Group Reference, 2007. (ISBN 1-59904-310-6)

Kansas State University. Information Technology Employee Code of Ethics. https://www.ksu.edu/infotech/ethics/

LA Times. (2007) http://latimesblogs.latimes.com/lanow/2011/07/ucla-pays-865500-to-settle-celebrity-medical-record-snooping-case.html

Reynolds, G., 2009. Ethics in Information Technology. Cengage Learning, Boston, MA.

Limited Resources

AMA Medical Code of Ethics Opinion 9.051 http://www.ama-assn.org/ama/pub/physician-resources/medical-ethics/code-medical-ethics/opinion90651.page?

Bloomfield, E. (2009) The ethics of rationing of critical care services: Should technology assessment play a role? Anesthesiology Research and Practice, Article ID 915197, 8 pages.

Fruits, E. (2010) The Oregon Health Plan, A Bold Experiment that Failed. Portland, Oregon: Cascade Policy Institute.

Jonsen, A. (1998) Resource Allocation: Ethical Topic in Medicine. University of Washington School of Medicine. http://depts.washington.edu/bioethx/topics/resall.html

Persad, G., Wertheimer, A., and Emanuel, E. (2009) Principles for allocation of scarce medical interventions. *The Lancet January 31*, 2009; 373:423–31.

Managed Care/Third Party Payers/Billing and Collections

AMA Medical Code of Ethics Opinion 8.054—Financial Incentives and the Practice of Medicine, http://www.ama-assn.org/ama/pub/physician-resources/medical-ethics/code-medical-ethics/opinion8054.page?

AMA Medical Code of Ethics Opinion 8.13 – Managed Care, http://www.ama-assn.org/ama/pub/physician-resources/medical-ethics/code-medical-ethics/opinion813.page?

American College of Physicians. The Changing Practice Environment. In: ACOP Ethics Manual Sixth Edition,

http://www.acponline.org/running_practice/ethics/manual/manual6th.htm#finance

Anand, G. (2008) Opting out. Wall Street Journal June 28, 2008, A1.

Darragh, M. and McCarrick, P. (1996) Managed health care: new ethical issues for all. National Reference Center for Bioethics Literature, Scope Note 31, Kennedy Institute of Ethics Journal, 1996.

Hall, M.A. and Schneider, C.E. (2008) Patients as consumers; courts, contracts and the new medical marketplace. *Michigan Law Review 106*(4): 643–649.

Hall, M.A. and Schneider, C.E. The professional ethics of billing and collections. JAMA 300(15):1806–1808.

Povar, G. *et al.* (2004) Ethics in Practice: Managed Care and the Changing Health Care Environment, Medicine as a Profession Managed Care Ethics Working Group Statement. *Annals of Internal Medicine,* July 20, 2004, 141(2): 131–136.

University of Washington School of Medicine. Managed Care, Ethics in Medicine. http://depts.washington.edu/bioethx/topics/manag.html

Marketing

American Dental Association. Principles of Ethics and Code of Professional Conduct, With Official Advisory Opinions Revised to January 2005. Chicago: ADA.

American Marketing Association. Statement of Ethics. http://www.marketingpower.com/AboutAMA/Pages/Statement%20of%20Ethics.aspx.

American Medical Association. Medical Code of Ethics http://www.ama-assn.org/ama/put/physisicn-resources/medical-ethics/code-medical-ethics/opinion502.page?

American Psychological Association. (2002) Ethical principles of psychologists and code of conduct. American Psychologist, 57:1060–1073.

Ethical Moment—What ethical considerations are involved in offering introductory discounts to attract new patients?, *Journal of the American Dental Association, 139*(6): 769–771.

Ethics and Plastic Surgery: ASAPS position. July 20, 2000. http://www.surgery.org/media/news-releases/ethics-and-plastic-surgery-asaps-position

Federal Communications Commission. http://www.fcc.gov/cgb/consumerfacts/advertising.html

Federal Communications Commission. http://transition.fcc.gov/mb/audio/decdoc/public_and_broadcasting.html#_Toc202587565

Federal Communications Commission. http://transition.fcc.gov/mb/audio/decdoc/public_and_broadcasting.html#_Toc202587565

Federal Drug Administration. http://www.fda.gov/Drugs/ResourcesForYou/Consumers/PrescriptionDrugAdvertising/ucm072025.htm

Federal Trade Commission http://business.ftc.gov/advertising-and-marketing/health-claims

Taylor, M, (2011). The impact of the "business" of pain medicine on patient care. *Pain Medicine 12*:763–772.

Wong, W., Camp, M., Camp, J., and Gupta, S. (2010). The quality of internet advertising in aesthetic surgery: an in-depth analysis. *Aesthetic Surgery Journal, 30*(5): 735–743.

Risk Management

2005 Federal Sentencing Guidelines 8B2.1(a)(2). 2005 Federal Sentencing Guidelines Manual and Appendices, United States Sentencing Commission, effective 1 November 2005, http://www.ussc.gov/guidelin.htm

DeGeorge, R. (1994) In:, Military Ethics: Reflections on Principles – The Profession of Arms, Military Leadership, Ethical Practices, War and Morality, Education the Citizen-Soldier, p. 28. M. Wakin (Ed.). Diane Publishing.

Dienhart, J. (2010) Enterprise Risk Management: Why Ethics and Compliance Function Adds Value. Seattle, WA: The Ethics Resource and the ERC Fellows Risk Assessment Group, Seattle University.

Grunig, J.E. and Repper, F.C. (1992). Strategic management, publics and issues. In: Excellence in Public Relations and Communication Management, pp. 171–57. J.E. Grunig (Ed.). Hillsdale, NJ: Lawrence Erlbaum Associates.

Head, G. (2005) Why Link Risk Management and Ethics. International Risk Management Institute, February 2005. http://www.irmi.com/expert/articles/2005/head02.aspx

Institute of Internal Auditors (IIA) (1988) Code of Ethics. Altamonte Springs, FL: Institute of Internal Auditors.

LRN (2007) Ethics and compliance risk management, pp. 3,12.

Young, P. (2004) Ethics and risk management: building a framework. *Risk Management: An International Journal, 6*(3): 23–34.

Stakeholders

Association of Chartered Certified Accounts. (2007) Business Ethics Contribute Towards Shareholder Value. http://www.acca.co.uk/page/3011288

Bowen, S. (2010) An examination of applied ethics and stakeholder management on top corporate websites. *Public Relations Journal 4*(1).

Carroll, A. (2004) Managing ethically with global stakeholders: a present and future challenge. *Academy of Management Executives 18*(2): 114–119.

Collins, S. (2010).“Corporate social responsibility and the future health care manager. *The Health Care Manager 29*:4: 339–345.

Corporate Disclosures Act

http://www.gpo.gov/fdsys/pkg/PLAW-107publ204/html/PLAW-107publ204.htm

Freeman, R.E. (1984) Strategic Management: A Stakeholder Approach. Boston: Pitman.

Freeman, R. E. (2009) What is Stakeholder Theory? Business Roundtable Institute for Corporate Ethics, www.youtube.com/watch?v=bIRUalLcvPe8

Grunig, J. (1992) Strategic management, publics and issues. In: Excellence in public relations and communication management, pp. 171–57. J.E. Grunig (Ed.)

Kanovich, E. (2007) Stakeholder Theory, Ethics and the Return on Customer. http://www.slideshare.net/ekanovich/stakeholder-theory-ethics-and-the-return-on-customer

Transparency

Bernard, R. and Lacrosse, C. (2005) Corporate transparency: code of ethics disclosures. The CPA Journal.

Collins, S. and Davis, K. (2006) Transparency in Health Care: The Time Has Come. The Commonwealth Fund, March 15, 2006.

Ernst and Young. (2011) Corporate Values.www.ey.com/US/en?About-us/Our-values

Jacobs, J., Cerfolio, R., and Sade, R. (2009) The ethics of transparency: publication of cardiothoracic surgical outcomes in the lay press. The Annals of Thoracic Surgery 87:679-686

Kachalia, A., *et al.* Liability claims and costs before and after implementation of a medical error disclosure program. Annals of Internal Medicine 153(4): 213–221.

Merck Ethics Policy http://www.merck.com/responsibility/ethics-and-transparency/home.html

US Government Department of Health and Human Services. (2010) Community Health Data Initiative, 2010. http://www.hhs.gov/open/plan/opengovrnmentplan/initiatives/initiative.html

CHAPTER 9

Legal Issues for Advanced Practice Registered Nurses

ELIZABETH W. COCHRANE

This chapter is intended to provide APRNs with basic tools to allow them to understand and to stay abreast of the regulatory environment and requirements that will impact their own practices. As advanced practice registered nurses (APRN) continue to expand their scope of practice into areas that were previously reserved for physicians, APRNs will face increasing regulatory oversight and legal risk. Given the increasingly autonomous nature of APRN practice, APRNs have more responsibility and authority over their practice than do registered nurses. This results in a personal and professional mandate to stay current with legal and regulatory changes.

It is important to note that nothing in the following chapter is intended to be legal advice. APRNs have a responsibility to understand the legal framework in which they are operating, whether by their own research or by talking to legal and nursing professionals in their own jurisdiction. The Appendix to this Chapter provides a state-by-state analysis of the regulatory framework for nurse practitioners (as of the date of publication of this book). Given the rapidly evolving nature of advanced nursing practice and the oversight of advanced practice nurses, all APRNs should anticipate having to incorporate continued legal and regulatory education into their existing continuing education practices.

9.1. STATE REGULATION OF ADVANCED PRACTICE REGISTERED NURSES

The regulatory body that oversees APRN practice is generally a state's Board of Nursing. Illinois and Nebraska have created separate Advanced Practice Registered Nursing Boards to oversee APRNs. Other states have delegated APRN oversight to both the Board of Nursing and the Board of Medicine. These states include Alabama, Delaware,

Massachusetts, North Carolina, South Carolina, South Dakota, and Virginia.

States regulate APRNs through some combination of statute and regulation, each state with its own unique combination. A State's legislature may enact statutes to articulate the definition of licensure requirements, scope of practice and prescriptive authority of an APRN. These statutes are with one exception called Nurse Practice Acts. The exception to this is Michigan, which is the only state in the United States that does not have a Nurse Practice Act.

A state's legislature may delegate the authority to make rules and regulations governing the definition of licensure requirements, scope of practice and prescriptive authority of an ARPN to a state agency, such as the State's Board of Nursing. Statutes and regulations have equal weight from a legal perspective, but a regulation can never contradict a statute. This is why one may find more granularity in a state regulation versus a state statute.

9.2. ADVANCED PRACTICE NURSE PRACTITIONER SPECIALIZATION

As APRNs have expanded their roles into more specialized fields of care, there have been recent efforts by the APRN Consensus Work Group and the National Council of State Boards of Nursing's (NCSBN) APRN Advisory Committee to clarify titles and definitions of advanced practice through the Consensus Model for APRN Regulation. The Consensus Work Group's Licensure, Accreditation, Certification and Education Model (LACE) defines four APRN roles:

1. Certified registered nurse anesthetist (CRNA)
2. Certified nurse midwife (CNM)
3. Clinical nurse specialist (CNS)
4. Certified nurse practitioner (CNP)

The regulatory model proposed by the Consensus Work Group has a target implementation date of 2015. Many states have adopted these four APRN roles into their statutes and regulations, but others have yet to do so as of the date hereof (see Appendix).

As Boards of Nursing adopt this new regulatory language, nurses currently functioning as APRNs can expect that exemption of those already in the system (grandfathering) will occur. After the expected implementation of the LACE model, APRNs will be required to legally identify themselves as APRNs plus the specific role; for example, APRN CNP and, if appropriate, a specialty role preparation such as oncology.

9.3. DEFINITIONS

The American Academy of Nurse Practitioners (AANP) defines nurse practitioners (CNPs) as licensed independent practitioners who practice in ambulatory, acute and long term care as primary and/or specialty care providers. Standard definitions of the APRN roles of CNMs, CRNAs and CNSs are delineated below. Certified Nurse Midwives define their scope of practice as: "Midwifery as practiced by certified nurse-midwives (CNMs®) and certified midwives (CMs®) encompasses a full range of primary health care services for women from adolescence beyond menopause. These services include primary care, gynecologic and family planning services, preconception care, care during pregnancy, childbirth and the postpartum period, care of the normal newborn during the first 28 days of life, and treatment of male partners for sexually transmitted infections." (http://www.midwife.org/Our-Scope-of-Practice)

According to the American Association of Nurse Anesthetists, "Certified Registered Nurse Anesthetists (CRNAs) are registered nurses who have become anesthesia specialists by taking a graduate curriculum which focuses on the development of clinical judgment and critical thinking. They are qualified to make independent judgments concerning all aspects of anesthesia care based on their education, licensure, and certification. As anesthesia professionals, CRNAs provide anesthesia and anesthesia-related care upon request, assignment, or referral by the patient's physician or other healthcare provider authorized by law, most often to facilitate diagnostic, therapeutic, and surgical procedures. In other instances, the referral or request for consultation or assistance may be for management of pain associated with obstetrical labor and delivery, management of acute and chronic ventilation problems, or management of acute and chronic pain through the performance of selected diagnostic and therapeutic blocks or other forms of pain management." (http://www.aana.com/aboutus/Documents/scopeofpractice.pdf).

Finally, the National Association of Clinical Nurse Specialists offers the following definition: "Clinical Nurse Specialists (CNS) are licensed registered nurses who have graduate preparation (Master's or Doctorate) in nursing as a Clinical Nurse Specialist. Clinical Nurse Specialists are expert clinicians in a specialized area of nursing practice. The specialty may be identified in terms of population, setting, disease or medical specialty, type of care, or type of problem. Clinical Nurse Specialists practice in a wide variety of health care settings. In addition to providing direct patient care, Clinical Nurse Specialists influence care outcomes by providing expert consultation for nursing staffs and by implementing improvements in health care delivery systems. Clinical Nurse Specialist practice integrates nursing practice, which focuses on assisting patients in the prevention or resolution of illness, with medical diagnosis and treatment of disease, injury and disability." (http://www.nacns.org/html/cns-faqs1.php)

However, regardless of these standardized model definitions, there is no national standard definition of a nurse practitioner, as each state has its own definition and title for what it means to be a nurse practitioner. The variety of definitions between states is vast. Contrast the definition of an Advanced Practice Registered Nurse articulated by New York with that articulated by New Hampshire:

New York:

> *"The practice of registered nursing by a nurse practitioner, certifies under Section six thousand nine hundred ten of this article, may include the diagnosis of illness and physical conditions and the performance of therapeutic and corrective measures within a specialty area of practice in collaboration with a licensed physician qualified to collaborate in the specialty involved, provided such services are performed in accordance with a written practice agreement and written practice protocols" (N.Y. Educ. Law § 6902.3(a)).*

New Hampshire:

> *"Advanced Registered Nurse Practitioner" or 'A.R.N.P.' means a registered nurse currently licensed by the board under RSA 326-B:18" (N.H. Rev. Stat. Ann. §326-B:2.I.).*

Whereas New York uses the title "nurse practitioner", New Hampshire uses "Advanced Registered Nurse Practitioner". Whereas New York provides authority to diagnose and treat in collaboration with a physician in the definition of the nurse practitioner, New Hampshire is silent on the scope of practice in the definition of an ARNP. The distinctions between these two states alone highlight why a nurse practitioner must be familiar with how their own state defines and titles advanced practice nurses. The website for each state's nursing oversight authority is found at the end of the chapter.

9.4. WHAT ARE THE CERTIFYING/LICENSURE REQUIREMENTS FOR ADVANCED PRACTICE?

All states have an interest in who is licensed and/or certified to provide health care. To be an advanced practice nurse, all states require current licensure as a registered nurse. Almost all states require national certification as well as minimum of a master's degree. However, there are no nationally applicable standards. The National Council of State Boards of Nursing is (NCSBN) trying to reduce the variability between states and is moving to have all states adopt the APRN Consensus Model regulatory requirements. If adopted, all states would require:

1. Graduate level preparation at either the masters or doctoral level
2. National Certification and recertification to demonstrate continued competence
3. Acquisition of advanced clinical knowledge with significant educational emphasis on the direct care of individuals in an acute care or primary care setting
4. A practice built upon the competency of the RN
5. Educationally prepared to assume responsibility and accountability of care
6. Clinical experience of sufficient depth and breadth

However, until such a time as the APRN Consensus Model Regulatory requirements are universally adopted throughout the United States, APRNS should consult with their own state's Board of Nursing to become familiar with applicable certification standards in their state.

9.5. WHAT IS AN APRN'S SCOPE OF PRACTICE?

The NCSBN in their model Nurse Practice Act defines the scope of nursing practice as:

> *"Practice of Nursing. Nursing is a scientific process founded on a professional body of knowledge; it is a learned profession based on an understanding of the human condition across the lifespan and the relationship of a client with others and within the environment; and it is an art dedicated to caring for others. The practice of nursing means assisting clients to attain or maintain optimal health, implementing a strategy of care to accomplish defined goals within the context of a client*

centered health care plan and evaluating responses to nursing care and treatment. Nursing is a dynamic discipline that increasingly involves more sophisticated knowledge, technologies and client care activities." (NCSBN Model Nursing Practice Acts, page 3) (https://www.ncsbn.org/Model_Nursing_Practice_Act_March2011.pdf).

The NCSBN defines the scope of advanced nursing practice as:

"Practice of APRNs. Advanced practice registered nursing by certified nurse practitioners (CNP), certified registered nurse anesthetists (CRNA), certified nurse midwives (CNM) or clinical nurse specialists (CNS) is based on knowledge and skills acquired in basic nursing education; licensure as an RN; and graduation from or completion of a graduate level APRN program accredited by a national accrediting body and current certification by a national certifying body in the appropriate APRN role and at least one population focus.

Practice as an APRN means an expanded scope of nursing in a role and population focus approved by the BON, with or without compensation or personal profit, and includes the RN scope of practice. The scope of an APRN includes, but is not limited to, performing acts of advanced assessment, diagnosing, prescribing and ordering. APRNs may serve as primary care providers of record.

APRNs are expected to practice as licensed independent practitioners within standards established and/or recognized by the BON. Each APRN is accountable to patients, the nursing profession and the BON for complying with the requirements of this Act and the quality of advanced nursing care rendered; for recognizing limits of knowledge and experience; planning for the management of situations beyond the APRN's expertise; and for consulting with or referring patients to other health care providers as appropriate." (NCSBN Model Nursing Practice Acts, page 91) (https://www.ncsbn.org/Model_Nursing_Practice_Act_March2011.pdf)

These model definitions highlight that in general, the APRN scope of practice is an extension of nursing practice which allows for the diagnosing and treatment of disease. States vary as to scopes of APRN practice codified in their statutes and regulations. Again, statutes are created by state legislatures and rules and regulations are created by state agencies with authority granted to them by a state legislature. Again, it must be emphasized that statutes and regulations have the same force of law, but a regulation cannot contradict a statute.

The majority of states require nurse practitioners to have a collaborative relationship with a physician. Some states, such as California, only permit nurse practitioners to practice through standardized procedures developed in collaboration with physicians. Some states permit nurse practitioners to practice autonomously without the need for collaboration or oversight from a physician. These states include Alaska, Colorado, District of Columbia, Hawaii, Iowa, Idaho, Maine (after 24 months of oversight), Montana, New Hampshire, New Mexico, Oregon, Rhode Island, Utah (apart from prescriptive authority for Schedule II-III controlled substances which requires consultant/referral plan), Washington and Wyoming.

Some states require direct physician supervision. These states include Florida, North Carolina, Oklahoma, Tennessee and Virginia. Some states only permit nurse practitioners to practice pursuant to authority delegated to them by a physician. These states include Georgia, Michigan and South Carolina.

Beyond the variety of requirements for physician involvement, states also vary in the breadth of practice afforded to advanced practice registered nurses. Nevada permits nurse practitioners the authority to suture lacerations. Arizona, Oregon and Washington permit nurse practitioners to admit patients to the hospital. Most states explicitly permit nurse practitioners to diagnosis and treat medical conditions. Some states explicitly permit nurse practitioners to refer, teach and order tests.

All of the 50 States and the District of Columbia grant nurse practitioners some form of prescriptive authority; however, the scope, nature and conditions of that authority vary from state to state. Some states do not permit nurse practitioners to prescribe controlled substances. (Controlled substances are narcotics, depressants, stimulants and hallucinogenic drugs listed on DEA Schedules I-V.) Others permit nurse practitioners to prescribe controlled substances without restriction, while some states permit nurse practitioners to prescribe controlled substances under the supervision or in collaboration with a physician.

It is critical for APRNs to understand what is explicitly permitted under their state's scope of practice. They should not act in the absence of explicit authority (either by statute, regulation or physician collaboration/delegation/direction). There have been physician challenges to APRN scope of practice. For example, in *Sermchief v Gonzoles* (660 S.W2d 683. (Mo 1984)), nurse practitioners in collaborative practice with physicians were charged with violating their scope of practice for performing routine gynecological exams and tests, but the court found that the nurse practitioners were acting within legislative standard of their practice. Since the 1980s, these challenges have been fewer and far between. However, in the absence of clearly defined statutory or regulatory authority, a nurse practitioner is vulnerable to challenges that he or she is acting outside the scope of their practice and therefore practicing medicine without a license. Scope of practice is a major component in the analysis of medical malpractice claims against nurse practitioners, so it is vital that APRNs understand and function within the scope of practice in their individual state.

9.6. LEGAL ACTIONS AGAINST APRNs

In the litigious society of the United States, lawsuits are an unfortunate fact of life. The most common lawsuit brought against health care providers is a medical malpractice claim. A medical malpractice claim is (1) a tort that (2) alleges negligence. A tort is a civil wrong in which a person's actions or omissions have unfairly caused someone else to suffer loss or harm. A claim in tort may be brought by anyone who has suffered loss. Negligence is a legal theory that describes a failure to exercise the care that a reasonably prudent person would exercise in like circumstances.

To bring a medical malpractice claim against an APRN, a plaintiff has to prove:

1. *Duty:* The APRN owned the plaintiff a duty.
   a. An APRN has a duty to a person when there is a provider-patient relationship between the APRN and that person. While an office visit establishes an obvious provider-patient relationship, whenever an APRN provides professional advice or treatment in any setting (even over the phone), a provider-patient relationship may be established.
2. *Breach:* The APRN's conduct breached that duty (i.e., that the APRN's conduct fell below the standard of care)
   a. An APRN has a duty to act with a degree of care, skill and judgment that would be exercised by a reasonable nurse practitioner in the same or similar circumstances.
3. *Causation:* The APRN's conduct caused the plaintiff's injury.
4. *Harm:* The plaintiff was injured.

In order to succeed in court, the plaintiff must prove all of four elements of the claim (duty, breach, causation and harm). However, the plaintiff does not have to prove all four elements to file a lawsuit—they just have to be able to state that all four elements of the claim have occurred (i.e. that (1) the APRN owed a duty to a patient, (2) that the APRN's conduct breached that duty because the APRN did not act with the degree of care, skill and judgment that would be exercised by a reasonable nurse practitioner in the same or similar circumstances, (3) that the APRN's conduct was the cause of the patient's injury and that (4) the patient was injured). While filing a false claim is against the law, there are very few deterrents to prevent an injured person from filing a claim if they truly believe that an APRN has committed medical malpractice. Even the commencement of a suit can be costly and harmful to an APRN's practice.

The vast majority of lawsuits are settled. Very few lawsuits reach the courtroom and even fewer reach a verdict. Therefore, in order to understand the landscape of lawsuits filed, one must take claims settled into consideration. One malpractice insurer, CNA, has published a recent study, "Understanding Nurse Practitioner Liability," surveying claims it paid from 1998–2008 for nurse practitioners. CNA highlighted that "a threshold issue in such litigation often is the express regulatory authority of a nurse practitioner to render certain types of patient care." Of the claims surveyed, 39% were related to diagnosis, 28.3% were related to treatment and 17.7% were related to medication. While scope of practice claims accounted for only 1.1% of claims, those claims had the highest paid indemnity of an average of $450,000, whereas the average diagnosis indemnity was $186,168 (National Service Organization, 2011).

Malpractice insurers are also required by federal law to report damage awards paid on behalf of medical providers (including nurse practitioners) to the National Practitioner Data Bank. Of all claims reported to the National Practitioner Data Bank, diagnosis-related, treatment-related and medication-related incidents are the top malpractice allegations, accounting for approximately 44% of all malpractice claims against nurse practitioners (Miller, 2011).

9.7. FEDERAL LEGAL ISSUES FOR APRNs

While states and their respective boards of nursing are the entities charged with overseeing and regulating nurse practitioners, APRNs may also have to comply with the requirements of the federal government in certain areas. The following provides a brief overview of some of the federal legal issues APRNs may face in their practice.

9.7.1. DEA Registration

If a state's scope of practice permits APRNS to prescribe controlled substances, they must obtain a DEA number in order to do so.

9.7.2. Medicare & Medicaid

Medicare, which is a federal program funded out of Social Security to provide health care primarily for the elderly, and Medicaid, which is a joint federal-state program that provides healthcare and long-term care assistance to those who fall below a certain income level, both allow APRNs to bill Medicare and Medicaid directly for services provided. However, if an APRN bills Medicare or a state Medicaid program directly for their services, the APRN will receive only receive 85% of the physician fee schedule (CNMs receive even less). If an APRN's services are billed by a physician as "incident to" the services of the physician, the physician's practice will receive 100% of the physician fee schedule for the service. However, in order to qualify for "incident to" billing, the ". . . services must be performed under the direct personal supervision of the physician as an integral part of the physician's personal in-office service. Such direct personal supervision requires that the physician initiate the course of treatment for which the service being performed by the nurse practitioner is an incidental part and that the physician remain actively involved with the patient's care. The physician must also be physically present in the same office suite and be immediately available to render assistance if necessary. In addition, the nurse practitioner must be employed by the physician (or be a leased employee)." (American College of Nurse Practitioners - http://www.acnpweb.org/what-incident-billing, see also, https://www.cms.gov/Outreach-and-Education/Medicare-Learning-Network-MLN/MLNProducts/Downloads/Medicare_Information_for_APNs_and_PAs_Booklet_ICN901623.pdf and http://www.cms.gov/Outreach-and-Education/Medicare-Learning-Network-MLN/MLNMattersArticles/downloads/SE0441.pdf)

In order to stem the rising cost of health care in this country, federal and state governments are aggressively pursuing fraudulent billing practices. APRNs must be familiar with the requirements of Medicare and Medicaid billing and should expect to have their reimbursements audited. APRNs should also become familiar with the Medicaid eligibility and billing requirements for their own state.

9.7.3. HIPAA

Medical records have strict guidelines as to who can access records, for what reasons, how and how long they must be stored. With the Health Insurance Portability and Accountability Act of 1996 (HIPAA), most health care providers have to take steps to protect patient confidentiality in the use and disclosure of medical records. Generally, APRNs should ensure that access to medical records is limited to those individuals who have a need to see the information in order to do their jobs, should notify patients as to how their information will be used and disclosed and should only disclose confidential medical information with the written authorization of the patient. APRNs may disclose confidential medical information without the authorization of the patient to the Center for Medicare and Medicaid Services (CMS) and to state law officials if state law mandates that the provider report abuse, neglect or domestic violence.

Furthermore, all those covered by HIPAA must ensure that the patients receive a notice of privacy practices. Although patients are not required to sign that they have received this notification, most providers ask for a signed receipt. Also, the push to utilize electronic medical records (EMR) is being encouraged thru a series of incentives and penalties put forth in the American Recovery and Reinvestment Act of 2009. Substantial Medicare and Medicaid incentives are going to those who adopt the use of the EMR. In 2015, penalties will be imposed upon those who have not adopted such a system.

9.7.4. Stark Law

In order to curb abusive practices of referring patients to entities in which a physician has a financial interest, the Stark Law (42 U.S.C.S. § 1395nn) is a federal statute that prohibits physicians from making referrals to entities in which the physician or the physician's immediate family members have an interest unless an exception applies (e.g., physicians are permitted to make a referral if they are personally providing the service, or if the referral relates to the provision of clinical diagnostic lab testing, pathology exams, diagnostic radiology or radiation therapy). Stark is a strict liability statute, which means that if one acts in violation of the law, one is guilty of illegal conduct without regard to whether or not there was intent to act in a criminal manner (e.g., statutory rape).

APRN practice does not fall within the scope of the Stark Law, which applies only to physician services and physician financial arrangements. However, an APRN might still violate Stark. For example, if an APRN's referrals are directed, controlled or billed by a physician, an APRN's referrals may be imputed to the physician, even though the APRN is making the referral independently. Alternatively, if an APRN performs services pursuant to an illegal referral made by a physician in violation of Stark and the APRN bills or makes a claim for payment for the services performed, the APRN might be in violation of Stark and might also be in violation of Federal and/or State false claims acts.

9.7.5. The Federal Anti-Kickback Statute

The Federal Anti-Kickback Statute (AKS) (42 U.S.C.S. §1320-7b(b)) also makes it a crime to make payments for referrals of any service or item payable under a federal healthcare program. Specifically, the AKS makes it a crime to knowingly and willfully offer, pay, solicit or receive payment in cash or in kind, directly or indirectly, in return for (1) referring an individual to a person for the furnishing or arranging for any item or services, payable in whole or in part, under a federal health care program or (2) purchasing, leasing, ordering or arranging for any good, facility, service or item payable under a federal healthcare statute. The AKS requires proof of criminal intent and is punishable by up to 5 years in prison and fines of up to $25,000. Civil liability under the AKS can result in up to $50,000 in civil monetary penalties and damages of up to three times the amount of the illegal kickback. Unlike Stark, the AKS is applicable to APRNs, and therefore APRNs should be careful to avoid violation of this statute in any manner.

9.8. SPECIALIZED LEGAL ISSUES FOR APRNs

9.8.1. Genetic Testing

Since the 2003 mapping of the human genome, genetic testing has become more and more common. From the testing of newborns to that of adults, more and more of our genetic background is being discovered. We now can now determine the predilection to certain diseases as well as the actual presence of the genetic disease carrier. Companies such as 23andMe are opening the doors to non-prescribed genetic testing. Patients may come to appointments armed with their own genetic information. While much of the information is potentially helpful in treatment, there are serious privacy concerns associated with the knowledge that comes from genetic testing. As a result, APRNs should not obtain genetic materials for testing, nor share genetic findings, without consent.

In 2008, the Genetic Information Nondiscrimination Act was signed into law by President George W. Bush. This act prevents discrimination in insurance and the workplace based upon genetic information. Also, most states have developed safeguard legislation to protect individual rights in this area and to address the very serious consequences that can result from unprotected information sharing. There are five main areas of concern that also may be covered by state law. They are employment nondiscrimination, health insurance nondiscrimination, other insurance nondiscrimination, privacy issues and research issues.

Table 9.1 outlines the various levels of protection by state and represents information that should be shared with patients prior to any testing (http://www.genome.gov).

TABLE 9.1.

State	Employment Nondiscrimination	Health Insurance Nondiscrimination	Other Insurance Nondiscrimination	Privacy Protection	Research Protection
Alabama		yes	yes		
Alaska		yes	yes	yes	
Arizona	yes	yes	yes	yes	yes
Arkansas	yes	yes	yes	yes	yes
California	yes	yes	yes		
Colorado		yes	yes	yes	yes
Connecticut	yes	yes		yes	
Delaware	yes	yes		yes	yes
Florida	yes	yes	yes	yes	
Georgia		yes		yes	yes
Hawaii	yes	yes			
Idaho	yes	yes	yes		
Illinois	yes	yes	yes	yes	
Indiana		yes	yes		
Iowa	yes	yes		yes	yes
Kansas		yes	yes		
Kentucky		yes	yes	yes	
Louisiana	yes	yes		yes	yes
Maine	yes	yes	yes	yes	yes
Maryland		yes	yes		yes
Massachusetts	yes	yes	yes	yes	yes
Michigan	yes	yes		yes	
Minnesota	yes	yes	yes	yes	yes
Mississippi					
Missouri	yes	yes		yes	yes
Montana		yes	yes		yes
Nebraska	yes	yes		yes	yes
Nevada	yes	yes		yes	yes

(continued)

TABLE 9.1. (continued)

State	Employment Nondiscrimination	Health Insurance Nondiscrimination	Other Insurance Nondiscrimination	Privacy Protection	Research Protection
New Hampshire	yes	yes	yes	yes	
New Jersey	yes	yes	yes	yes	yes
New Mexico	yes	yes	yes	yes	yes
New York	yes	yes	yes	yes	yes
North Carolina	yes	yes	yes		
North Dakota		yes			
Oklahoma		yes			
Oregon	yes	yes	yes	yes	yes
Pennsylvania	yes	yes	yes	yes	yes
Rhode Island	yes	yes		yes	yes
South Carolina		yes		yes	yes
South Dakota	yes	yes		yes	
Tennessee		yes			
Texas	yes	yes		yes	yes
Utah	yes	yes			
Vermont	yes	yes	yes	yes	yes
Virginia	yes	yes			
Washington	yes			yes	yes
West Virginia		yes			
Wisconsin	yes	yes	yes		
Wyoming		yes			
District of Columbia	yes	yes			

Adapted from www.genome.com

9.8.2. Assisted Suicide

Assisted suicide is intentionally or knowingly aiding another person in taking his or her own life. In health care, knowledge of the assisted suicide laws is particularly important, as it is not uncommon for a patient to request medications from their providers in order to commit suicide. There are a variety of laws governing assisted suicide. Three states allow for the so-called 'death with dignity' provision whereby physicians may write medication prescriptions for those contemplating suicide. In other states, there are criminal repercussions for such acts. In all states, APRNs must adhere to prescription guidelines, document requests carefully and refer patients for evaluation if thoughts of suicide are suspected.

TABLE 9.2.

Description of Law	States
Common Law prohibition against Assisted Suicide	Alabama, District of Columbia, Massachusetts, West Virginia
Assisted Suicide is Manslaughter	Alaska, Arizona, Arkansas, Colorado, Connecticut, Florida, Hawaii, Missouri, Texas
Assisted Suicide is a Felony	California, Georgia, Indiana, Iowa, Kansas, Kentucky, Michigan, Mississippi, New Mexico, New York, North Dakota, Rhode Island, South Dakota, Tennessee, Wisconsin
Assisted Suicide is a Felony and/or Misdemeanor	New Hampshire, Pennsylvania
Prohibition against promoting suicide	Delaware, Illinois, Louisiana, Maine, Maryland, Minnesota, Nebraska, Ohio, Oklahoma, Virginia
Specific prohibitions against assisting with suicide for health care providers	Arkansas, Georgia, Ohio, Rhode Island, South Carolina, Virginia
Undetermined	Nevada, Utah
Death with dignity provisions for assisted suicide	Montana, Oregon, Washington

9.8.3. End of Life

End of life decisions have legal as well as ethical concerns based on autonomy and the loss of decision making capacity. To ensure that an individual's wishes are carried out, there are advanced directives which include living wills and health care proxies. The terms used vary by state. A living will may also be known as a health care directive, health care declarations or advanced directives. In general, advanced directives include the outline of care that an individual wishes to receive, medical power of attorney and do not resuscitate (DNR) orders. It often includes statements about nutrition, hydration, dialysis, and mechanical ventilation. Directives may also include information about organ donation. Health care proxies are appointed to ensure that the directives are adhered to, and/or to make decisions about items not covered in the advanced directives. All states have laws regarding advanced directives. In some states, the forms must be witnessed and notarized; in others, no action is needed. The National Hospice and Palliative Care Organization have the forms and directions for each state available on their website at http://www.caringinfo.org/i4a/pages/index.cfm?pageid=3289.

With the passage of the Patient Self-Determination Act of 1990, health care facilities must provide written information about advanced directives and patient rights for self-determination, including refusal of health care. Facilities also must ask about the presence of advanced directives, document their presence, educate their personnel about advanced directives and ensure there is no discrimination as a result of the patients' choices (http://www.americanbar.org/groups/public_education/resources/law_issues_for_consumers/patient_self_determination_act.html).

While many of the decisions seem clear-cut once a directive is signed, they are far from being so. It is not unusual for unwanted care to be rendered because the advanced directive was not readily available at the time a decision was made. Advanced directives from one state will not necessarily be honored in another and emergency medical technologists (EMTs) cannot honor advanced directives but must stabilize the patient and transport them to the nearest hospital. Also, the cost of end of life care that is perceived to be futile is coming under question in regards to a patient's wishes for ongoing expensive care.

The Agency for Healthcare Research and Quality, a division of the U.S. Department of Health & Human Services, publishes a website with up to date information on the research on advanced care planning (http://www.ahrq.gov). On the website, they note findings, such as up to 76% of all physicians with patients with advanced directives were unaware of the directives and only 12% of patients had input from their physicians in putting together their directives. The site also notes the many benefits to patients who have that discussion with the physician, including less fear and anxiety and more comfort from their physicians. The AHRQ website provides a five step process to be used for 'end of life' discussions.

9.8.4. Abuse

Nurses are required by law in most states to report child abuse as part of their professional duties. Only Oklahoma, New Jersey, North Carolina and Wyoming do not specifically mention a nurse's duty to report child abuse. West Virginia does not mention nurses but says medical professionals must report abuse, while Rhode Island specifically mandates that physician and certified nurse practitioners must do so. However, all states have mandatory reporting of child abuse by all people, which would cover nurses as citizens of the state.

The standard for making a report may vary, but in general requires a report whenever the nurse suspects, or has reason to believe, that a child has been abused or neglected or if there are conditions that could lead to harm. Also, in most instances, newborns who have drugs or alcohol in their systems at birth constitute a mandatory report situation. Unlike many other health care encounters, the statuary recognition of privileged communication is frequently suspended in these instances.

There are also provisions mandating the reporting of elder abuse in all 50 states. The age of the victim, what is covered under the law, what constitutes abuse, and how it is handled varies from state to state. The National Center on Elder Abuse of the Administration on Aging (http://www.ncea.aoa.gov) has a wide variety of resources, including state hotlines.

9.8.5. Declaration of Competence

Competence and capacity are important in the provision of health care, without which there can be no consent. Lack of informed consent can result in a charge of battery as well as malpractice. Capacity is defined as the clinical decision that an individual can use information to make a rational decision (Leo, 1999). Competency, on the other hand, is a legal determination that an individual can make a decision regarding a legal act, such as a health care decision. The two terms are not synonymous. However, an individual who has been found to lack the capacity to make health care decisions is usually also assumed to be de facto incompetent to do so.

Most adults are considered to have the capacity—and are competent—to make decisions about their own health care. There are exceptions. In an emergency when a decision must be made quickly, legal consent is assumed. In less serious situations, an effort is usually made to determine a surrogate decision maker. This generally is considered to be a spouse, adult child, parent, adult sibling or grandparent. However, if no surrogate is available and there is not imminent threat, caution should be taken. Any treatment should be well documented and be within the usual standard of care as the risk of battery and malpractice exists. In these cases, hospitals or providers will sometimes ask the court to appoint a guardian to protect patients' interests.

Capacity must be judiciously considered. When a clinical determination is made that a patient lacks capacity, it is wise to obtain a second determination before proceeding with treatment (Leo, 1999). To determine competence, it is necessary to seek expert consultation. Usually a psychiatrist will be asked to determine if the patient can understand and respond appropriately to treatment information, is rational in discussing treatment and understands the basics of the care decision and its consequences. With this information, a legal decision can be made by the courts as to the individual's competence. It should be noted that all adult individuals, even those with psychiatric disease or mental retardation, are considered competent unless they have been legally declared otherwise.

9.9. BUSINESS RISKS

In addition to the legal risks associated with practicing as an advanced practice nurse, APRNs should be cognizant of the legal risks associated with running a business. For example, if one enters into a partnership with another APRN or establishes a collaborative relationship with a physician, an APRN must ensure that these relationships are properly documented. The APRN must ensure that the legal duties and risks associated with any contract are fully understood before signing. Business risks are particular to each state and each type of business, and one should ideally consult with a licensed attorney prior to establishing a practice.

9.10. REFERENCES

American Academy of Nurse Practitioners. http://www.aanp.org/index.php. See in particular their survey of state practice environments. http://www.aanp.org/legislation-regulation/state-practice-environment

Buppert, C. (2012). *Nurse Practitioner's Business Practice and Legal Guide.* 4th Ed. Sudbury, MA: Jones & Bartlett .

Leo, R.J. (1999). Competency and the capacity to make treatment decisions: A primer for primary care physicians. *Journal of Clinical Psychiatry 1*(5): 131–141

Miller, K.P. (2011). Malpractice: Nurse practitioners and claimers reported to the National Practitioner Data Bank. *Journal for Nurse Practitioners 7*(9): 761–763.

National Council of State Boards of Nursing—APRN Consensus Campaign. https://www.ncsbn.org/428.htm

Nurses Service Organization. (2011) "Understanding Nurse Practitioner Liability: CNA HealthPro Nurse Practitioner Claims Analysis 1998-2008" available at: http://www.nso.com/nursing-resources/claim-studies.jsp?refID=nurseclaimreport2011The Hastings Center. http://www.thehastingscenter.org

9.11. APPENDIX—STATE-BY-STATE REGULATION OF NURSE PRACTITIONERS

The following sets forth basic information regarding the regulatory framework for nurse practitioners in each state. "Yes" means that the activity is explicitly stated in the state's APRN/Nurse Practice Act statute. "No" means that the activity is not contained in the statute.

Alabama

- **Recognized Nurse Practitioner Title(s)/Abbreviation(s):** Certified Registered Nurse Practitioner (CRNP); Certified Nurse Midwife (CNM), Certified Registered Nurse Anesthetist (CRNA), and Clinical Nurse Specialist (CNS)

- **Regulatory Authority:** Joint Committee of Board of Medical Examiners and Board of Nursing
- **Website:** http:\\www.abn.state.al.us
- **Required Physician Participation in Nurse Practitioner Practice:** Physician collaboration and physician-established protocols.
- **Nurse Practitioner Scope of Practice (as explicitly prescribed by statute or regulation):**

Diagnose	Yes ☑	No ☐
Treat	Yes ☑	No ☐
Prescribe	Yes ☑	No ☐
Admit to Hospital	Yes ☐	No ☑
Refer	Yes ☑	No ☐
Suture	Yes ☐	No ☑
Teach/Counsel	Yes ☑	No ☐
Order Tests	Yes ☑	No ☐

- **Statutory or Legislative Authority References:** Ala. Code. §34-21 et. seq.; Ala. Admin. Code r. 610-X-6 et. seq.

Alaska

- **Recognized Nurse Practitioner Title(s)/Abbreviation(s):** Advanced Nurse Practitioner (ANP), Registered Nurse Anesthetist (RNA)
- **Regulatory Authority:** Board of Nursing
- **Website:** http://www.dced.state.ak.us/occ/pnur.htm
- **Required Physician Participation in Nurse Practitioner Practice:** None
- **Nurse Practitioner Scope of Practice (as explicitly prescribed by statute or regulation):**

Diagnose	Yes ☑	No ☐
Treat	Yes ☑	No ☐
Prescribe	Yes ☑	No ☐
Admit to Hospital	Yes ☐	No ☑
Refer	Yes ☐	No ☑
Suture	Yes ☐	No ☑
Teach/Counsel	Yes ☑	No ☐
Order Tests	Yes ☑	No ☐

- **Statutory or Legislative Authority References:** A.S. 08.68 et. seq.; 12 ACC 44 et. seq.

Arizona

- **Recognized Nurse Practitioner Title(s)/Abbreviation(s):** Registered Nurse Practitioner (RNP) and Certified Registered Nurse Anesthetist (CRNA)

- **Regulatory Authority:** Board of Nursing
- **Website:** http://www.azbn.gov/
- **Required Physician Participation in Nurse Practitioner Practice:** None.
- **Nurse Practitioner Scope of Practice (as explicitly prescribed by statute or regulation):**

Diagnose	Yes ☑	No ☐
Treat	Yes ☑	No ☐
Prescribe	Yes ☑	No ☐
Admit to Hospital	Yes ☑	No ☐
Refer	Yes ☑	No ☐
Suture	Yes ☐	No ☑
Teach/Counsel	Yes ☐	No ☑
Order Tests	Yes ☑	No ☐

- **Statutory or Legislative Authority References:** A.R.S. §32.1601-1169 et. seq.; A.A.C. § R4-19 et. seq..

Arkansas

- **Recognized Nurse Practitioner Title(s)/Abbreviation(s):**
  —Registered Nurse Practitioner (NP or RNP)
  —Advanced Practice Nurse (APN) or any of:
    * Advanced Nurse Practitioner (ANP) or Advanced Registered Nurse Practitioner (ARNP);
    * Nurse Anesthetist, Certified Nurse Anesthetist or Certified Registered Nurse Anesthetist (CRNA);
    * Nurse Midwife, Certified Nurse Midwife, Licensed Nurse Midwife (CNM or LNM); or
    * Clinical Nurse Specialist (CNS).
- **Regulatory Authority:** Board of Nursing
- **Website:** http://www.arsbn.arkansas.gov/Pages/default.aspx
- **Required Physician Participation in Nurse Practitioner Practice:** Physician collaboration and physician-established protocols
- **Nurse Practitioner Scope of Practice:**

Diagnose	Yes ☑	No ☐
Treat	Yes ☑	No ☐
Prescribe	Yes ☑	No ☐
Admit to Hospital	Yes ☑	No ☐
Refer	Yes ☑	No ☐
Suture	Yes ☐	No ☑
Teach/Counsel	Yes ☐	No ☑
Order Tests	Yes ☑	No ☐

- **Statutory or Legislative Authority References:** A.C.A. § 17-87 et. seq.

California

- **Recognized Nurse Practitioner Title(s)/Abbreviation(s):** Nurse Practitioner, Nurse-midwife. No abbreviations specified by statute.
- **Regulatory Authority:** Board of Nursing
- **Website:** http://www.rn.ca.gov/
- **Required Physician Participation in Nurse Practitioner Practice:** General supervision/delegation from physician. Nurse Practitioners may only practice outside the scope of the practice beyond a Registered Nurse's scope of practice through standardized procedures developed by a physician in order to perform overlapping medical functions.
- **Nurse Practitioner Scope of Practice (as explicitly prescribed by statute or regulation):**

Diagnose	Yes ☐	No ☑
Treat	Yes ☐	No ☑
Prescribe	Yes ☐	No ☑
Admit to Hospital	Yes ☐	No ☑
Refer	Yes ☐	No ☑
Suture	Yes ☐	No ☑
Teach/Counsel	Yes ☐	No ☑
Order Tests	Yes ☐	No ☑

- **Statutory or Legislative Authority References:** Cal. Com. Code § Cal. Code Reg. tit. 16 §1485; Cal. BPC. Code §2834-2837 et. seq.

Colorado

- **Recognized Nurse Practitioner Title(s)/Abbreviation(s):** Advanced Practice Nurse (APN), Nurse Practitioner (NP), Certified Nurse Midwife (CNM), Certified Registered Nurse Anesthetist (CRNA), and Clinical Nurse Specialist (CNS)
- **Regulatory Authority:** Board of Nursing
- **Website:** http://www.dora.state.co.us/nursing/
- **Required Physician Participation in Nurse Practitioner Practice:** None.
- **Nurse Practitioner Scope of Practice (as explicitly prescribed by statute or regulation):**

Diagnose	Yes ☑	No ☐
Treat	Yes ☑	No ☐
Prescribe	Yes ☑	No ☐
Admit to Hospital	Yes ☑	No ☐
Refer	Yes ☑	No ☐
Suture	Yes ☐	No ☑
Teach/Counsel	Yes ☐	No ☑
Order Tests	Yes ☑	No ☐

- **Statutory or Legislative Authority References:** Colo. Rev. Stat. Ann. § 12-38 et. seq.

Connecticut

- **Recognized Nurse Practitioner Title(s)/Abbreviation(s):** Advanced Practice Registered Nurse (APRN)
- **Regulatory Authority:** Board of Nursing
- **BON Website:** None—see the Connecticut Department of Health Website for Board of Nursing information - http://www.ct.gov/dph/site/default.asp
- **Required Physician Participation in Nurse Practitioner Practice:** Physician collaboration and physician-established protocols
- **Nurse Practitioner Scope of Practice (as explicitly prescribed by statute or regulation):**

Diagnose	Yes ☑	No ☐
Treat	Yes ☑	No ☐
Prescribe	Yes ☑	No ☐
Admit to Hospital	Yes ☐	No ☑
Refer	Yes ☐	No ☑
Suture	Yes ☐	No ☑
Teach/Counsel	Yes ☐	No ☑
Order Tests	Yes ☐	No ☑

- **Statutory or Legislative Authority References:** Conn. Gen. Stat. Ann. §378-20-87a to §378-20-102a et. seq.

Delaware

- **Recognized Nurse Practitioner Title(s)/Abbreviation(s):** Advanced Practice Nurse (APN), Certified Nurse Midwife (CNM), Certified Registered Nurse Anesthetist (CRNA), and Clinical Nurse Specialist (CNS)
- **Regulatory Authority:** Board of Nursing and Board of Medical Practice
- **BON Website:** http://dpr.delaware.gov/boards/nursing/index.shtml
- **Required Physician Participation in Nurse Practitioner Practice:** None.
- **Nurse Practitioner Scope of Practice (as explicitly prescribed by statute or regulation):**

Diagnose	Yes ☐	No ☑
Treat	Yes ☑	No ☐
Prescribe	Yes ☑	No ☐
Admit to Hospital	Yes ☐	No ☑
Refer	Yes ☑	No ☐
Suture	Yes ☐	No ☑
Teach/Counsel	Yes ☑	No ☐
Order Tests	Yes ☑	No ☐

- **Statutory or Legislative Authority References:** Del. Cod. Ann. Tit. 24 § 1900 et. seq.

District of Columbia

- **Recognized Nurse Practitioner Title(s)/Abbreviation(s):** Advanced Practice Registered Nurse (APRN), Nurse Practitioner (NP), Certified Nurse Midwife (CNM), Certified Registered Nurse Anesthetist (CRNA), and Clinical Nurse Specialist (CNS)
- **Regulatory Authority:** Board of Nursing
- **BON Website:** http://hpla.doh.dc.gov/hpla/cwp/view,a,1195,q,488526,hplanav,|30661|,.asp
- **Required Physician Participation in Nurse Practitioner Practice:** None
- **Nurse Practitioner Scope of Practice (as explicitly prescribed by statute or regulation):**

Diagnose	Yes ☑	No ☐
Treat	Yes ☑	No ☐
Prescribe	Yes ☑	No ☐
Admit to Hospital	Yes ☐	No ☑
Refer	Yes ☑	No ☐
Suture	Yes ☐	No ☑
Teach/Counsel	Yes ☑	No ☐
Order Tests	Yes ☐	No ☑

- **Statutory or Legislative Authority References:** D.C. Code § 3-12 et. seq.

Florida

- **Recognized Nurse Practitioner Title(s)/Abbreviation(s):** Advanced Registered Nurse Practitioner (ARNP)
- **Regulatory Authority:** Board of Nursing
- **BON Website:** http://www.doh.state.fl.us/mqa/nursing/
- **Required Physician Participation in Nurse Practitioner Practice:** General supervision/delegation from physician.
- **Nurse Practitioner Scope of Practice (as explicitly prescribed by statute or regulation):**

Diagnose	Yes ☑	No ☐
Treat	Yes ☑	No ☐
Prescribe	Yes ☑	No ☐
Admit to Hospital	Yes ☐	No ☑
Refer	Yes ☐	No ☑
Suture	Yes ☐	No ☑
Teach/Counsel	Yes ☐	No ☑
Order Tests	Yes ☑	No ☐

- **Statutory or Legislative Authority References:** Fla. Stat. Tit. XXXII Ch. 464 et. seq.

Georgia

- **Recognized Nurse Practitioner Title(s)/Abbreviation(s):** Advanced Practice Registered Nurse (APRN)
- **Regulatory Authority:** Board of Nursing
- **BON Website:** http://sos.georgia.gov/plb/rn/
- **Required Physician Participation in Nurse Practitioner Practice:** General supervision/delegation from physician.
- **Nurse Practitioner Scope of Practice (as explicitly prescribed by statute or regulation):**

Diagnose	Yes ☑	No ☐
Treat	Yes ☑	No ☐
Prescribe	Yes ☑	No ☐
Admit to Hospital	Yes ☐	No ☑
Refer	Yes ☐	No ☑
Suture	Yes ☐	No ☑
Teach/Counsel	Yes ☐	No ☑
Order Tests	Yes ☑	No ☐

- **Statutory or Legislative Authority References:** Ga. Code Ann. § 43-26 et. seq., GA Comp R. & Regs. r. 410-12 et. seq.

Hawaii

- **Recognized Nurse Practitioner Title(s)/Abbreviation(s):** Advanced Practice Registered Nurse (APRN)
- **Regulatory Authority:** Board of Nursing
- **BON Website:** http://hawaii.gov/dcca/pvl/boards/nursing/
- **Required Physician Participation in Nurse Practitioner Practice:** None.
- **Nurse Practitioner Scope of Practice (as explicitly prescribed by statute or regulation):**

Diagnose	Yes ☐	No ☑
Treat	Yes ☐	No ☑
Prescribe	Yes ☐	No ☑
Admit to Hospital	Yes ☐	No ☑
Refer	Yes ☐	No ☑
Suture	Yes ☐	No ☑
Teach/Counsel	Yes ☑	No ☐
Order Tests	Yes ☑	No ☐

- **Statutory or Legislative Authority References:** Haw. Rev. Stat. §457 et. seq., Haw. Admin. Rules § 16-89 et. seq.

Idaho

- **Recognized Nurse Practitioner Title(s)/Abbreviation(s):** Advanced Practice Professional Nurse (APPN), Nurse Practitioner (NP), Certified Nurse Midwife (CNM), Registered Nurse Anesthetist (RNA), and Clinical Nurse Specialist (CNS)
- **Regulatory Authority:** Board of Nursing
- **BON Website:** http://ibn.idaho.gov/IBNPortal/
- **Required Physician Participation in Nurse Practitioner Practice:** None
- **Nurse Practitioner Scope of Practice (as explicitly prescribed by statute or regulation):**

Diagnose	Yes ☑	No ☐
Treat	Yes ☑	No ☐
Prescribe	Yes ☑	No ☐
Admit to Hospital	Yes ☐	No ☑
Refer	Yes ☐	No ☑
Suture	Yes ☐	No ☑
Teach/Counsel	Yes ☐	No ☑
Order Tests	Yes ☑	No ☐

- **Statutory or Legislative Authority References:** Idaho Code Ann. § 54-14 et. seq., Idaho Admin. Code § 23.01.01:280.

Illinois

- **Recognized Nurse Practitioner Title(s)/Abbreviation(s):** Certified Nurse Practitioner (CNP), Advanced Practice Nurse (APN), Certified Nurse Midwife (CNM), Registered Nurse Anesthetist (RNA), and Clinical Nurse Specialist (CNS)
- **Regulatory Authority:** Advanced Practice Nursing Board
- **APNB Website:** http://www.idfpr.com/profs/info/Nursing.asp
- **Required Physician Participation in Nurse Practitioner Practice:** Physician collaboration
- **Nurse Practitioner Scope of Practice (as explicitly prescribed by statute or regulation):**

Diagnose	Yes ☑	No ☐
Treat	Yes ☑	No ☐
Prescribe	Yes ☑	No ☐
Admit to Hospital	Yes ☐	No ☑
Refer	Yes ☐	No ☑
Suture	Yes ☐	No ☑
Teach/Counsel	Yes ☐	No ☑
Order Tests	Yes ☑	No ☐

- **Statutory or Legislative Authority References:** 225 Ill. Comp. Stat. § 65/15-5 et. seq., Ill. Admin. Code tit. 68, pt. 1300, sub-pt. D et. seq.

Indiana

- **Recognized Nurse Practitioner Title(s)/Abbreviation(s):** Advanced Practice Nurse (APN), Nurse Practitioner (NP) or Clinical Nurse Specialist (CNS)
- **Regulatory Authority:** Board of Nursing
- **BON Website:** http://www.in.gov/pla/nursing.htm
- **Required Physician Participation in Nurse Practitioner Practice:** Physician collaboration
- **Nurse Practitioner Scope of Practice (as explicitly prescribed by statute or regulation):**

Diagnose	Yes ☑	No ☐
Treat	Yes ☑	No ☐
Prescribe	Yes ☑	No ☐
Admit to Hospital	Yes ☐	No ☑
Refer	Yes ☑	No ☐
Suture	Yes ☐	No ☑
Teach/Counsel	Yes ☑	No ☐
Order Tests	Yes ☐	No ☑

- **Statutory or Legislative Authority References:** Ind. Code §25-23 et. seq.; Ind. Admin Code. tit. 848., r. 4-5 et. seq.

Iowa

- **Recognized Nurse Practitioner Title(s)/Abbreviation(s):** Advanced Registered Nurse Practitioner (ARNP) (Certified Nurse Practitioners, Certified Nurse Midwives, Certified Registered Nurse Anesthetist and Clinical Nurse Specialists are recognized specialties)
- **Regulatory Authority:** Board of Nursing
- **BON Website:** http://nursing.iowa.gov/
- **Required Physician Participation in Nurse Practitioner Practice:** Physician collaboration
- **Nurse Practitioner Scope of Practice (as explicitly prescribed by statute or regulation):**

Diagnose	Yes ☐	No ☑
Treat	Yes ☐	No ☑
Prescribe	Yes ☑	No ☐
Admit to Hospital	Yes ☐	No ☑
Refer	Yes ☐	No ☑
Suture	Yes ☐	No ☑
Teach/Counsel	Yes ☐	No ☑
Order Tests	Yes ☐	No ☑

- **Statutory or Legislative Authority References:** Iowa Admin. Code r. 655.7 et. seq.

Kansas

- **Recognized Nurse Practitioner Title(s)/Abbreviation(s):** Advanced Registered Nurse Practitioner (ARNP), Registered Nurse Anesthetist (RNA)
- **Regulatory Authority:** Board of Nursing
- **BON Website:** http://www.ksbn.org/
- **Required Physician Participation in Nurse Practitioner Practice:** General supervision/delegation from physician.
- **Nurse Practitioner Scope of Practice (as explicitly prescribed by statute or regulation):**

Diagnose	Yes ☑	No ☐
Treat	Yes ☑	No ☐
Prescribe	Yes ☑	No ☐
Admit to Hospital	Yes ☐	No ☑
Refer	Yes ☐	No ☑
Suture	Yes ☐	No ☑
Teach/Counsel	Yes ☑	No ☐
Order Tests	Yes ☐	No ☑

- **Statutory or Legislative Authority References:** Kan. Stat. Ann. § 65.1130-1134, Kan. Admin. Regs. § 60-11-101 - 60-11-121

Kentucky

- **Recognized Nurse Practitioner Title(s)/Abbreviation(s):** Advanced Registered Nurse Practitioner (ARNP)
- **Regulatory Authority:** Board of Nursing
- **BON Website:** http://www.kbn.ky.gov/
- **Required Physician Participation in Nurse Practitioner Practice:** General supervision/delegation from physician
- **Nurse Practitioner Scope of Practice (as explicitly prescribed by statute or regulation):**

Diagnose	Yes ☐	No ☑
Treat	Yes ☑	No ☐
Prescribe	Yes ☑	No ☐
Admit to Hospital	Yes ☐	No ☑
Refer	Yes ☐	No ☑
Suture	Yes ☐	No ☑
Teach/Counsel	Yes ☐	No ☑
Order Tests	Yes ☑	No ☐

- **Statutory or Legislative Authority References:** KY. Rev. Stat. Ann. § 314 et. seq.; 201 Ky. Admin. Regs. § 20:057 et. seq.

Louisiana

- **Recognized Nurse Practitioner Title(s)/Abbreviation(s):** Advanced Practice Registered Nurse (APRN), Nurse Practitioner (NP), Certified Nurse Midwife (CNM), Certified Registered Nurse Anesthetist (CRNA), Registered Nurse Anesthetist (RNA), and Clinical Nurse Specialist (CNS)
- **Regulatory Authority:** Board of Nursing
- **BON Website:** http://www.lsbn.state.la.us/
- **Required Physician Participation in Nurse Practitioner Practice:** Physician collaboration and physician-established protocols
- **Nurse Practitioner Scope of Practice (as explicitly prescribed by statute or regulation):**

Diagnose	Yes ☑	No ☐
Treat	Yes ☑	No ☐
Prescribe	Yes ☑	No ☐
Admit to Hospital	Yes ☐	No ☑
Refer	Yes ☑	No ☐
Suture	Yes ☐	No ☑
Teach/Counsel	Yes ☑	No ☐
Order Tests	Yes ☑	No ☐

- **Statutory or Legislative Authority References:** LA. Rev. Stat. 37:911 et. seq.; La. Admin. Code. Tit. 46, § XLVII et. seq.

Maine

- **Recognized Nurse Practitioner Title(s)/Abbreviation(s):** Advanced Practice Registered Nurse (APRN), Certified Nurse Practitioner (CNP), Certified Nurse Midwife (CNM), Certified Registered Nurse Anesthetist (CRNA), and Certified Clinical Nurse Specialist (CNS)
- **Regulatory Authority:** Board of Nursing
- **BON Website:** http://www.maine.gov/boardofnursing/
- **Required Physician Participation in Nurse Practitioner Practice:** Physician supervision for first 24 months of practice, thereafter none.
- **Nurse Practitioner Scope of Practice (as explicitly prescribed by statute or regulation):**

Diagnose	Yes ☑	No ☐
Treat	Yes ☑	No ☐
Prescribe	Yes ☑	No ☐
Admit to Hospital	Yes ☐	No ☑
Refer	Yes ☑	No ☐
Suture	Yes ☐	No ☑
Teach/Counsel	Yes ☑	No ☐
Order Tests	Yes ☑	No ☐

- **Statutory or Legislative Authority References:** ME. Rev. Stat Ann Tit. 32 § 2101 et. seq., Code Me. R. 8 02 380 §8 et. seq.

Maryland

- **Recognized Nurse Practitioner Title(s)/Abbreviation(s):** Nurse Practitioner (NP), Nurse Midwife (CNM), Nurse Anesthetist (CRNA), Nurse Psychotherapist (APRN/PMH)
- **Regulatory Authority:** Board of Nursing
- **BON Website:** http://www.mbon.org/main.php
- **Required Physician Participation in Nurse Practitioner Practice:** Physician collaboration
- **Nurse Practitioner Scope of Practice (as explicitly prescribed by statute or regulation):**

Diagnose	Yes ☑	No ☐
Treat	Yes ☑	No ☐
Prescribe	Yes ☑	No ☐
Admit to Hospital	Yes ☐	No ☑
Refer	Yes ☑	No ☐
Suture	Yes ☐	No ☑
Teach/Counsel	Yes ☐	No ☑
Order Tests	Yes ☑	No ☐

- **Statutory or Legislative Authority References:** COMAR 10.27 et. seq.

Massachusetts

- **Recognized Nurse Practitioner Title(s)/Abbreviation(s):** Nurse Practitioner Nurse Midwife, Psychiatric Nurse Mental Health Clinical Specialist, Nurse Anesthetist (No abbreviations specified by statute)
- **Regulatory Authority:** Board of Nursing and Board of Medicine
- **BON Website:** http://www.mass.gov/eohhs/provider/licensing/occupational/nursing/
- **Required Physician Participation in Nurse Practitioner Practice:** General supervision/delegation from physician.
- **Nurse Practitioner Scope of Practice (as explicitly prescribed by statute or regulation):**

Diagnose	Yes ☑	No ☐
Treat	Yes ☑	No ☐
Prescribe	Yes ☑	No ☐
Admit to Hospital	Yes ☐	No ☑
Refer	Yes ☐	No ☑
Suture	Yes ☐	No ☑
Teach/Counsel	Yes ☐	No ☑
Order Tests	Yes ☑	No ☐

- **Statutory or Legislative Authority References:** 244 Code Mass. Rules § 4.00 et. seq.

Michigan

- **Recognized Nurse Practitioner Title(s)/Abbreviation(s):** Michigan recognizes the nurse midwifery, nurse anesthetist and nurse practitioner specialties. No titles or abbreviations are specified by statute.
- **Regulatory Authority:** Board of Nursing
- **BON Website:** http://www.michigan.gov/lara/0,4601,7-154-35299_28150_27529_27542---,00.html
- **Required Physician Participation in Nurse Practitioner Practice:** No scope of practice in state law.
- **Nurse Practitioner Scope of Practice (as explicitly prescribed by statute or regulation):**

Diagnose	Yes ☐	No ☑
Treat	Yes ☐	No ☑
Prescribe	Yes ☐	No ☑
Admit to Hospital	Yes ☐	No ☑
Refer	Yes ☐	No ☑
Suture	Yes ☐	No ☑
Teach/Counsel	Yes ☐	No ☑
Order Tests	Yes ☐	No ☑

- **Statutory or Legislative Authority References:** There is no statutory or regulatory nurse practitioner scope of practice. There is no Nurse Practice Act. All rules promulgated by Board of Nursing or embedded in Public Health Code Act 368, Part 172 et. seq. Doctors may delegate authority to practice (including to prescribe) at their discretion. Mich. Comp. Laws. § 333.16215(1).

Minnesota

- **Recognized Nurse Practitioner Title(s)/Abbreviation(s):** Advanced Practice Registered Nurse Practitioner (APRNP). Minnesota recognizes the clinical nurse specialist, nurse anesthetist, nurse-midwife and nurse practitioner specialties.
- **Regulatory Authority:** Board of Nursing
- **BON Website:** http://mn.gov/health-licensing-boards/nursing/
- **Required Physician Participation in Nurse Practitioner Practice:** Physician collaboration.
- **Nurse Practitioner Scope of Practice (as explicitly prescribed by statute or regulation):**

Diagnose	Yes ☑	No ☐
Treat	Yes ☑	No ☐
Prescribe	Yes ☑	No ☐
Admit to Hospital	Yes ☐	No ☑
Refer	Yes ☐	No ☑
Suture	Yes ☐	No ☑
Teach/Counsel	Yes ☐	No ☑
Order Tests	Yes ☑	No ☐

- **Statutory or Legislative Authority References:** Minn. Stat. Ann. § 148.171 et. seq.

Mississippi

- **Recognized Nurse Practitioner Title(s)/Abbreviation(s):** Certified Nurse Practitioner (CNP), Certified Nurse Midwife (CNM), Certified Registered Nurse Anesthetist (CRNA), and Certified Clinical Nurse Specialist (CNS)
- **Regulatory Authority:** Board of Nursing
- **BON Website:** http://www.msbn.state.ms.us/
- **Required Physician Participation in Nurse Practitioner Practice:** Physician collaboration
- **Nurse Practitioner Scope of Practice (as explicitly prescribed by statute or regulation):**

Diagnose	Yes ☐	No ☑
Treat	Yes ☐	No ☑
Prescribe	Yes ☑	No ☐
Admit to Hospital	Yes ☐	No ☑
Refer	Yes ☐	No ☑
Suture	Yes ☐	No ☑
Teach/Counsel	Yes ☐	No ☑
Order Tests	Yes ☐	No ☑

- **Statutory or Legislative Authority References:** Miss. Code Ann. §73-15-17-20; Miss. Admin. Code. tit 30 §2840.

Missouri

- **Recognized Nurse Practitioner Title(s)/Abbreviation(s):** Advanced Practice Registered Nurse (APRN). Missouri recognizes the clinical nurse specialist, nurse anesthetist, nurse-midwife and nurse practitioner specialties.
- **Regulatory Authority:** Board of Nursing; prescription only under joint authority of the Board of Nursing and the Board of Medicine
- **BON Website:** http://pr.mo.gov/nursing.asp
- **Required Physician Participation in Nurse Practitioner Practice:** Physician collaboration.
- **Nurse Practitioner Scope of Practice (as explicitly prescribed by statute or regulation):**

Diagnose	Yes ☐	No ☑
Treat	Yes ☑	No ☐
Prescribe	Yes ☑	No ☐
Admit to Hospital	Yes ☐	No ☑
Refer	Yes ☐	No ☑
Suture	Yes ☐	No ☑
Teach/Counsel	Yes ☐	No ☑
Order Tests	Yes ☐	No ☑

- **Statutory or Legislative Authority References:** Mo. Ann. Stat. § 335 et. seq.; Mo. Code Regs. tit. 20 § 2200 et. seq.

Montana

- **Recognized Nurse Practitioner Title(s)/Abbreviation(s):** Nurse Practitioner (NP) or Advanced Practice Registered Nurse (APRN)
- **Regulatory Authority:** Board of Nursing
- **BON Website:** http://bsd.dli.mt.gov/license/bsd_boards/nur_board/board_page.asp
- **Required Physician Participation in Nurse Practitioner Practice:** None
- **Nurse Practitioner Scope of Practice (as explicitly prescribed by statute or regulation):**

Diagnose	Yes ☑	No ☐
Treat	Yes ☑	No ☐
Prescribe	Yes ☑	No ☐
Admit to Hospital	Yes ☐	No ☑
Refer	Yes ☑	No ☐
Suture	Yes ☐	No ☑
Teach/Counsel	Yes ☑	No ☐
Order Tests	Yes ☑	No ☐

- **Statutory or Legislative Authority References:** Mont. Code Ann. § 2-15-1734 et. seq.; Mont. Admin R. Mont. 24.159.1401 et. seq.

Nebraska

- **Recognized Nurse Practitioner Title(s)/Abbreviation(s):** Advanced Practice Registered Nurse (APRN), Nurse Practitioner (APRN - NP), Certified Nurse Midwife (APRN - CNM), Certified Registered Nurse Anesthetist (APRN - CRNA), and Certified Clinical Nurse Specialist (APRN - CNS)
- **Regulatory Authority:** Advanced Practice Registered Nurse Board
- **Website:** http://dhhs.ne.gov/publichealth/Pages/crl_nursing_nursingindex.aspx
- **Required Physician Participation in Nurse Practitioner Practice:** Physician collaboration
- **Nurse Practitioner Scope of Practice (as explicitly prescribed by statute or regulation):**

Diagnose	Yes ☑	No ☐
Treat	Yes ☑	No ☐
Prescribe	Yes ☑	No ☐
Admit to Hospital	Yes ☐	No ☑
Refer	Yes ☑	No ☐
Suture	Yes ☐	No ☑
Teach/Counsel	Yes ☐	No ☑
Order Tests	Yes ☑	No ☐

- **Statutory or Legislative Authority References:** Neb. Rev. Stat. §38-2301 et. seq.; 172 NAC 98 et. seq.; 172 NAC 100 et. seq.

Nevada

- **Recognized Nurse Practitioner Title(s)/Abbreviation(s):** Advanced Practitioner of Nursing (APN), Nurse Practitioner (NP), Nurse Midwife (CNM), Nurse Psychotherapist (APRN/PMH), Clinical Nurse Specialist (CNS)
- **Regulatory Authority:** Board of Nursing
- **BON Website:** http://nevadanursingboard.org/
- **Required Physician Participation in Nurse Practitioner Practice:** Physician collaboration and physician-established protocols
- **Nurse Practitioner Scope of Practice (as explicitly prescribed by statute or regulation):**

Diagnose	Yes ☑	No ☐
Treat	Yes ☑	No ☐
Prescribe	Yes ☑	No ☐
Admit to Hospital	Yes ☐	No ☑
Refer	Yes ☑	No ☐
Suture	Yes ☑	No ☐
Teach/Counsel	Yes ☑	No ☐
Order Tests	Yes ☑	No ☐

- **Statutory or Legislative Authority References:** Nev. Admin. Code § 632 et. seq.

New Hampshire

- **Recognized Nurse Practitioner Title(s)/Abbreviation(s):** Advanced Practice Registered Nurse (APRN)
- **Regulatory Authority:** Board of Nursing
- **BON Website:** https://www.nh.gov/nursing/
- **Required Physician Participation in Nurse Practitioner Practice:** None
- **Nurse Practitioner Scope of Practice (as explicitly prescribed by statute or regulation):**

Diagnose	Yes ☑	No ☐
Treat	Yes ☑	No ☐
Prescribe	Yes ☑	No ☐
Admit to Hospital	Yes ☐	No ☑
Refer	Yes ☑	No ☐
Suture	Yes ☐	No ☑
Teach/Counsel	Yes ☑	No ☐
Order Tests	Yes ☑	No ☐

- **Statutory or Legislative Authority References:** N.H. Rev. Stat. Ann. § 326-B:1 et seq.

New Jersey

- **Recognized Nurse Practitioner Title(s)/Abbreviation(s):** Advanced Practice Nurse (APN). New Jersey recognizes the nurse practitioner and clinical nurse specialist specialties.
- **Regulatory Authority:** Board of Nursing
- **BON Website:** http://www.state.nj.us/lps/ca/nursing/
- **Required Physician Participation in Nurse Practitioner Practice:** Physician collaboration and physician-established protocols
- **Nurse Practitioner Scope of Practice (as explicitly prescribed by statute or regulation):**

Diagnose	Yes ☑	No ☐
Treat	Yes ☑	No ☐
Prescribe	Yes ☑	No ☐
Admit to Hospital	Yes ☐	No ☑
Refer	Yes ☑	No ☐
Suture	Yes ☐	No ☑
Teach/Counsel	Yes ☑	No ☐
Order Tests	Yes ☑	No ☐

- **Statutory or Legislative Authority References:** N.J. S.A. § 45:1 et seq.; N.J.A.C. 13:37

New Mexico

- **Recognized Nurse Practitioner Title(s)/Abbreviation(s):** Certified Nurse Practitioner (CNP), Certified Registered Nurse Anesthetist (CRNA), Clinical Nurse Specialist (CNS).
- **Regulatory Authority:** Board of Nursing
- **BON Website:** http://nmbon.sks.com/
- **Required Physician Participation in Nurse Practitioner Practice:** None
- **Nurse Practitioner Scope of Practice (as explicitly prescribed by statute or regulation):**

Diagnose	Yes ☐	No ☑
Treat	Yes ☐	No ☑
Prescribe	Yes ☑	No ☐
Admit to Hospital	Yes ☐	No ☑
Refer	Yes ☐	No ☑
Suture	Yes ☐	No ☑
Teach/Counsel	Yes ☐	No ☑
Order Tests	Yes ☐	No ☑

- **Statutory or Legislative Authority References:** N.M. Stat. Ann. § 61-3 et. seq.

New York

- **Recognized Nurse Practitioner Title(s)/Abbreviation(s):** Nurse Practitioner (NP)
- **Regulatory Authority:** Board of Nursing
- **BON Website:** http://www.op.nysed.gov/prof/nurse/
- **Required Physician Participation in Nurse Practitioner Practice:** Physician collaboration
- **Nurse Practitioner Scope of Practice (as explicitly prescribed by statute or regulation):**

Diagnose	Yes ☑	No ☐
Treat	Yes ☑	No ☐
Prescribe	Yes ☑	No ☐
Admit to Hospital	Yes ☐	No ☑
Refer	Yes ☐	No ☑
Suture	Yes ☐	No ☑
Teach/Counsel	Yes ☐	No ☑
Order Tests	Yes ☐	No ☑

- **Statutory or Legislative Authority References:** N.Y. Educ. Law, Art. 139 § 6900 et. seq.

North Carolina

- **Recognized Nurse Practitioner Title(s)/Abbreviation(s):** Nurse Practitioner (NP) or Advanced Practice Registered Nurse (APRN)
- **Regulatory Authority:** Board of Nursing and Board of Medicine
- **BON Website:** http://www.ncbon.com/
- **Required Physician Participation in Nurse Practitioner Practice:** General supervision/delegation by a physician.
- **Nurse Practitioner Scope of Practice (as explicitly prescribed by statute or regulation):**

Diagnose	Yes ☑	No ☑
Treat	Yes ☑	No ☑
Prescribe	Yes ☑	No ☑
Admit to Hospital	Yes ☐	No ☑
Refer	Yes ☑	No ☐
Suture	Yes ☐	No ☑
Teach/Counsel	Yes ☑	No ☐
Order Tests	Yes ☑	No ☐

- **Statutory or Legislative Authority References:** 21 N.C.G.S. §90-171.19 et. seq.; N.C.A.C. 36.0101 et seq.

North Dakota

- **Recognized Nurse Practitioner Title(s)/Abbreviation(s):** Advanced Practice Registered Nurse (APRN)
- **Regulatory Authority:** Board of Nursing
- **BON Website:** https://www.ndbon.org/
- **Required Physician Participation in Nurse Practitioner Practice:** Physician collaboration
- **Nurse Practitioner Scope of Practice (as explicitly prescribed by statute or regulation):**

Diagnose	Yes ☑	No ☐
Treat	Yes ☑	No ☐
Prescribe	Yes ☑	No ☐
Admit to Hospital	Yes ☐	No ☑
Refer	Yes ☐	No ☑
Suture	Yes ☐	No ☑
Teach/Counsel	Yes ☑	No ☐
Order Tests	Yes ☐	No ☑

- **Statutory or Legislative Authority References:** N.D. Cent. Code § 43-12.1.01 et. seq.; N.D. Admin. Code § 54-05-03.1 et seq.

Ohio

- **Recognized Nurse Practitioner Title(s)/Abbreviation(s):** Certified Nurse Practitioner (CNP), Certified Nurse Midwife (CNM), Certified Registered Nurse Anesthetist (CRNA), Clinical Nurse Specialist (CNS).
- **Regulatory Authority:** Board of Nursing
- **BON Website:** http://www.nursing.ohio.gov/
- **Required Physician Participation in Nurse Practitioner Practice:** Physician collaboration
- **Nurse Practitioner Scope of Practice (as explicitly prescribed by statute or regulation):**

Diagnose	Yes ☐	No ☑
Treat	Yes ☐	No ☑
Prescribe	Yes ☑	No ☐
Admit to Hospital	Yes ☐	No ☑
Refer	Yes ☐	No ☑
Suture	Yes ☐	No ☑
Teach/Counsel	Yes ☐	No ☑
Order Tests	Yes ☐	No ☑

- **Statutory or Legislative Authority References:** Ohio Re. Code Ann. § 4723.01 et seq.

Oklahoma

- **Recognized Nurse Practitioner Title(s)/Abbreviation(s):** Advanced Registered Nurse Practitioner (ARNP), Certified Registered Nurse Anesthetist (CRNA), Certified Nurse-Midwife (CNM), Clinical Nurse Specialist (CNS).
- **Regulatory Authority:** Board of Nursing
- **BON Website:** http://www.ok.gov/nursing/
- **Required Physician Participation in Nurse Practitioner Practice:** General supervision/delegation by a physician.
- **Nurse Practitioner Scope of Practice (as explicitly prescribed by statute or regulation):**

Diagnose	Yes ☑	No ☐
Treat	Yes ☑	No ☐
Prescribe	Yes ☑	No ☐
Admit to Hospital	Yes ☐	No ☑
Refer	Yes ☑	No ☐
Suture	Yes ☐	No ☑
Teach/Counsel	Yes ☑	No ☐
Order Tests	Yes ☐	No ☑

- **Statutory or Legislative Authority References:** 59 O.S. § 567.1 et sq.; Okla. Admin. Code § 485:10-15-1 et. seq.

Oregon

- **Recognized Nurse Practitioner Title(s)/Abbreviation(s):** Nurse Practitioner (NP); Certified Registered Nurse Anesthetist (CRNA), Clinical Nurse Specialist (CNS)
- **Regulatory Authority:** Board of Nursing
- **BON Website:** http://cms.oregon.gov/osbn/Pages/index.aspx
- **Required Physician Participation in Nurse Practitioner Practice:** None
- **Nurse Practitioner Scope of Practice (as explicitly prescribed by statute or regulation):**

Diagnose	Yes ☑	No ☐
Treat	Yes ☑	No ☐
Prescribe	Yes ☑	No ☐
Admit to Hospital	Yes ☑	No ☐
Refer	Yes ☑	No ☐
Suture	Yes ☐	No ☑
Teach/Counsel	Yes ☑	No ☐
Order Tests	Yes ☐	No ☑

- **Statutory or Legislative Authority References:** O.R.S. § 678 et. seq., O.A.R. § 851-050-63 et seq.

Pennsylvania

- **Recognized Nurse Practitioner Title(s)/Abbreviation(s):** Certified Registered Nurse Practitioner (CRNP), Clinical Nurse Specialist (CNS)
- Regulatory Authority: Board of Nursing
- **BON Website:** http://www.portal.state.pa.us/portal/server.pt/community/state_board_of_nursing/12515
- **Required Physician Participation in Nurse Practitioner Practice:** Physician collaboration
- **Nurse Practitioner Scope of Practice (as explicitly prescribed by statute or regulation):**

Diagnose	Yes ☑	No ☐
Treat	Yes ☑	No ☐
Prescribe	Yes ☑	No ☐
Admit to Hospital	Yes ☐	No ☑
Refer	Yes ☑	No ☐
Suture	Yes ☐	No ☑
Teach/Counsel	Yes ☐	No ☑
Order Tests	Yes ☑	No ☐

- **Statutory or Legislative Authority References:** 49 PA Code § 21.251et. seq.; 49 PA Code § 21.801 et. seq.

Rhode Island

- **Recognized Nurse Practitioner Title(s)/Abbreviation(s):** Advanced Practice Nurse (APN), Certified Registered Nurse Practitioner (RNP), Certified Registered Nurse Anesthetist (CRNA).
- **Regulatory Authority:** Board of Nursing
- **BON Website:** http://www.health.ri.gov/for/nurses/index.php
- **Required Physician Participation in Nurse Practitioner Practice:** None
- **Nurse Practitioner Scope of Practice (as explicitly prescribed by statute or regulation):**

Diagnose	Yes ☐	No ☑
Treat	Yes ☐	No ☑
Prescribe	Yes ☑	No ☐
Admit to Hospital	Yes ☐	No ☑
Refer	Yes ☐	No ☑
Suture	Yes ☐	No ☑
Teach/Counsel	Yes ☐	No ☑
Order Tests	Yes ☐	No ☑

- **Statutory or Legislative Authority References:** R.I. Gen. Laws § 5-34, R.I. R. R5-34-Nur/Ed

South Carolina

- **Recognized Nurse Practitioner Title(s)/Abbreviation(s):** Advanced Practice Registered Nurse (APRN), Certified Registered Nurse Anesthetist (CRNA), Certified Nurse-Midwife (CNM), Clinical Nurse Specialist (CNS), Nurse Practitioner (NP).
- **Regulatory Authority:** Board of Nursing
- **BON Website:** http://www.llr.state.sc.us/pol/nursing/
- **Required Physician Participation in Nurse Practitioner Practice:** General supervision/delegation by a physician
- **Nurse Practitioner Scope of Practice (as explicitly prescribed by statute or regulation):**

Diagnose	Yes ☑	No ☐
Treat	Yes ☑	No ☐
Prescribe	Yes ☑	No ☐
Admit to Hospital	Yes ☐	No ☑
Refer	Yes ☐	No ☑
Suture	Yes ☐	No ☑
Teach/Counsel	Yes ☐	No ☑
Order Tests	Yes ☐	No ☑

- **Statutory or Legislative Authority References:** S.C. Code Ann. §40-33-5 et seq.

South Dakota

- **Recognized Nurse Practitioner Title(s)/Abbreviation(s):** Certified Nurse Practitioner (CNP); Certified Nurse Midwife (CNM).
- **Regulatory Authority:** Board of Nursing and Board of Medicine
- **BON Website:** http://doh.sd.gov/boards/nursing/
- **Required Physician Participation in Nurse Practitioner Practice:** Physician collaboration
- **Nurse Practitioner Scope of Practice (as explicitly prescribed by statute or regulation):**

Diagnose	Yes ☑	No ☐
Treat	Yes ☑	No ☐
Prescribe	Yes ☑	No ☐
Admit to Hospital	Yes ☐	No ☑
Refer	Yes ☑	No ☐
Suture	Yes ☐	No ☑
Teach/Counsel	Yes ☑	No ☐
Order Tests	Yes ☐	No ☑

- **Statutory or Legislative Authority References:** S.D. Codified Laws § 36-9A et seq.

Tennessee

- **Recognized Nurse Practitioner Title(s)/Abbreviation(s):** Advanced Practice Nurse (APN). Tennessee recognizes the nurse practitioners, nurse anesthetists, nurse midwives, and clinical nurse specialists as APNs.
- **Regulatory Authority:** Board of Nursing
- **BON Website:** http://health.state.tn.us/boards/nursing/
- **Required Physician Participation in Nurse Practitioner Practice:** General supervision/delegation by a physician for prescribing only. There is no other description of the scope of practice for nurse practitioners in Tennessee law.
- **Nurse Practitioner Scope of Practice (as explicitly prescribed by statute or regulation):**

Diagnose	Yes ☐	No ☑
Treat	Yes ☐	No ☑
Prescribe	Yes ☑	No ☐
Admit to Hospital	Yes ☐	No ☑
Refer	Yes ☐	No ☑
Suture	Yes ☐	No ☑
Teach/Counsel	Yes ☐	No ☑
Order Tests	Yes ☐	No ☑

- **Statutory or Legislative Authority References:** T.C.A. § 63-7 et seq.

Texas

- **Recognized Nurse Practitioner Title(s)/Abbreviation(s):** Advanced Practice Registered Nurse (APRN)
- **Regulatory Authority:** Board of Nursing
- **BON Website:** http://www.bon.texas.gov/
- **Required Physician Participation in Nurse Practitioner Practice:** General supervision/delegation by a physician.
- **Nurse Practitioner Scope of Practice (as explicitly prescribed by statute or regulation):**

Diagnose	Yes ☐	No ☑
Treat	Yes ☐	No ☑
Prescribe	Yes ☑	No ☐
Admit to Hospital	Yes ☐	No ☑
Refer	Yes ☐	No ☑
Suture	Yes ☐	No ☑
Teach/Counsel	Yes ☐	No ☑
Order Tests	Yes ☐	No ☑

- **Statutory or Legislative Authority References:** Texas Admin. Code § 221.1-17 et. seq.; TOC § 301 et. seq.

Utah

- **Recognized Nurse Practitioner Title(s)/Abbreviation(s):** Advanced Practice Registered Nurse (APRN), Certified Registered Nurse Anesthetist (APRN-CRNA-without prescriptive practice)
- **Regulatory Authority:** Board of Nursing
- **BON Website:** http://www.dopl.utah.gov/licensing/nursing.html
- **Required Physician Participation in Nurse Practitioner Practice:** None—however a consultation or referral plan is necessary for prescription of Schedule II-III controlled substances.
- **Nurse Practitioner Scope of Practice (as explicitly prescribed by statute or regulation):**

Diagnose	Yes ☑	No ☐
Treat	Yes ☑	No ☐
Prescribe	Yes ☑	No ☐
Admit to Hospital	Yes ☐	No ☑
Refer	Yes ☑	No ☐
Suture	Yes ☐	No ☑
Teach/Counsel	Yes ☑	No ☐
Order Tests	Yes ☐	No ☑

- **Statutory or Legislative Authority References:** Utah Code. Ann. § 58-31b-101 et. seq., Utah Admin. Code r. 156 et seq.

Vermont

- **Recognized Nurse Practitioner Title(s)/Abbreviation(s):** Advanced Practice Registered Nurse (APRN)
- **Regulatory Authority:** Board of Nursing
- **BON Website:** http://vtprofessionals.org/opr1/nurses/
- **Required Physician Participation in Nurse Practitioner Practice:** Physician collaboration
- **Nurse Practitioner Scope of Practice (as explicitly prescribed by statute or regulation):**

Diagnose	Yes ☑	No ☐
Treat	Yes ☑	No ☐
Prescribe	Yes ☑	No ☐
Admit to Hospital	Yes ☐	No ☑
Refer	Yes ☐	No ☑
Suture	Yes ☐	No ☑
Teach/Counsel	Yes ☐	No ☑
Order Tests	Yes ☐	No ☑

- **Statutory or Legislative Authority References:** Vt. Stat. Ann. Tit 26 § 1572(4); Vt. Code R. Ch. 4 Subchapter 8, III

Virginia

- **Recognized Nurse Practitioner Title(s)/Abbreviation(s):** Nurse Practitioner (NP)
- **Regulatory Authority:** Board of Nursing and Board of Medicine
- **BON Website:** http://www.dhp.virginia.gov/nursing/
- **Required Physician Participation in Nurse Practitioner Practice:** General supervision/delegation by a physician.
- **Nurse Practitioner Scope of Practice (as explicitly prescribed by statute or regulation):**

Diagnose	Yes ☐	No ☑
Treat	Yes ☐	No ☑
Prescribe	Yes ☑	No ☐
Admit to Hospital	Yes ☐	No ☑
Refer	Yes ☐	No ☑
Suture	Yes ☐	No ☑
Teach/Counsel	Yes ☐	No ☑
Order Tests	Yes ☐	No ☑

- **Statutory or Legislative Authority References:** Code of Virginia Ch. 29 § 54.1-2900 - § 54.1-2957.03.; 18 Va. Admin Code § 90-30-120A.

Washington

- **Recognized Nurse Practitioner Title(s)/Abbreviation(s):** Advanced Registered Nurse Practitioner (ARNP)
- **Regulatory Authority:** Board of Nursing
- **BON Website:** http://www.doh.wa.gov/LicensesPermitsandCertificates/NursingCommission.aspx
- **Required Physician Participation in Nurse Practitioner Practice:** None
- **Nurse Practitioner Scope of Practice (as explicitly prescribed by statute or regulation):**

Diagnose	Yes ☑	No ☐
Treat	Yes ☑	No ☐
Prescribe	Yes ☑	No ☐
Admit to Hospital	Yes ☐	No ☑
Refer	Yes ☑	No ☐
Suture	Yes ☐	No ☑
Teach/Counsel	Yes ☐	No ☑
Order Tests	Yes ☑	No ☐

- **Statutory or Legislative Authority References:** Wash. Rev. Code § 18.79.250, Wash Admin Code § 246.840-300.

West Virginia

- **Recognized Nurse Practitioner Title(s)/Abbreviation(s):** Advanced Nurse Practitioner (ANP)
- **Regulatory Authority:** Board of Nursing
- **BON Website:** http://www.wvrnboard.com/
- **Required Physician Participation in Nurse Practitioner Practice:** Collaboration with a physician for prescribing only.
- **Nurse Practitioner Scope of Practice (as explicitly prescribed by statute or regulation):**

Diagnose	Yes ☐	No ☑
Treat	Yes ☐	No ☑
Prescribe	Yes ☑	No ☐
Admit to Hospital	Yes ☐	No ☑
Refer	Yes ☐	No ☑
Suture	Yes ☐	No ☑
Teach/Counsel	Yes ☐	No ☑
Order Tests	Yes ☐	No ☑

- **Statutory or Legislative Authority References:** W.Va. Code §30-7-15 et. seq.

Wisconsin

- **Recognized Nurse Practitioner Title(s)/Abbreviation(s):** Advanced Practice Nurse (APN), Nurse Midwife (NMW)
- **Regulatory Authority:** Board of Nursing
- **BON Website:** http://drl.wi.gov/board_detail.asp?boardid=42&locid=0
- **Required Physician Participation in Nurse Practitioner Practice:** Collaboration with a physician.
- **Nurse Practitioner Scope of Practice (as explicitly prescribed by statute or regulation):**

Diagnose	Yes ☐	No ☑
Treat	Yes ☐	No ☑
Prescribe	Yes ☑	No ☐
Admit to Hospital	Yes ☐	No ☑
Refer	Yes ☐	No ☑
Suture	Yes ☐	No ☑
Teach/Counsel	Yes ☐	No ☑
Order Tests	Yes ☐	No ☑

- **Statutory or Legislative Authority References:** Wis. Admin Code § N8

Wyoming

- **Recognized Nurse Practitioner Title(s)/Abbreviation(s):** Advanced Practice Registered Nurse (APRN)
- **Regulatory Authority:** Board of Nursing
- **BON Website:** https://nursing-online.state.wy.us/
- **Required Physician Participation in Nurse Practitioner Practice:** None.
- **Nurse Practitioner Scope of Practice (as explicitly prescribed by statute or regulation):**

Diagnose	Yes ☐	No ☑
Treat	Yes ☑	No ☐
Prescribe	Yes ☑	No ☐
Admit to Hospital	Yes ☐	No ☑
Refer	Yes ☐	No ☑
Suture	Yes ☐	No ☑
Teach/Counsel	Yes ☐	No ☑
Order Tests	Yes ☐	No ☑

- **Statutory or Legislative Authority References:** Wyo. Stat. Ann. §33-21-120(a)(i).

Index